Sports Vision

Sports Vision

Edited by

Donald F.C. Loran
and
Caroline J. MacEwen

BUTTERWORTH
HEINEMANN

Butterworth-Heinemann
Linacre House, Jordan Hill, Oxford OX2 8DP
A division of Reed Educational and Professional Publishing Ltd

℞ A member of the Reed Elsevier plc group

OXFORD   BOSTON   JOHANNESBURG
MELBOURNE   NEW DELHI   SINGAPORE

First published 1995
Paperback edition 1997

© Reed Educational and Professional Publishing Ltd 1995

BO5887
617·75

British Library Cataloguing in Publication Data
A catalogue record for this book is available from the British Library.

Library of Congress Cataloguing in Publication Data
A catalogue record for this book is available from the Library of Congress.

ISBN 0 7506 3616 5

Composition by Genesis Typesetting, Laser Quay, Rochester, Kent
Printed and bound in Great Britain by The Bath Press, Avon

Contents

Preface

In our increasingly health and leisure conscious society, the majority of people are involved in sporting activities either as participants or spectators. Although participation in sports has undoubted benefits these have to be traded off against possible adverse effects, such as injury. Indeed sport is currently one of the principal causes of serious eye injury.

This book is intended for all those interested in sport and vision. These may include eye-care and sports medicine practitioners, optical and sports manufacturers in addition to sports scientists, participants, coaches (or trainers) and organizations. Because this book is addressed to a multi-disciplinary cross-section of potential readers, a glossary of technical terms is provided. The aim of this volume is to identify and introduce measures which optimize safe and efficient vision in sport.

The introduction of contact lenses, and more recently of refractive surgery, has helped to establish sports vision by offering new and expanded activities for ametropic sportspeople. Eye care practitioners gradually became aware of the role of vision in sporting performance and safety and vision testing is now an integral part of the screening of athletes at the Olympic Games and other sporting events. The information thus obtained is being used to establish a sports vision profile to facilitate future research.

Sports performance may be greatly assisted by the application of sports vision. Sportspeople will be more comfortable when glare is eliminated, more protected against injury by wearing suitable eye protectors and perform better when acuity is maximized and visual skills are improved. Additionally, coaching and sports vision enhancement training may help to develop superior anticipation and improve coordination and reaction times. While many sports require both physical fitness and a high visual performance, it is gratifying to note that opportunities also exist for the visually impaired and recognition of this is important. All of these areas combine to form sports vision and are explored in the following chapters.

As the importance of vision in sport was appreciated the need for more information became apparent. Sports vision education and qualifications were introduced and specialized publications and organizations became established, as outlined in the Bibliography and Appendix 1. It is intended that this book will fulfil educational requirements, stimulate an interest in sports vision and provide a reference source. New developments will progress rapidly and readers are strongly encouraged to keep up-to-date and help to establish sports vision as an accepted discipline by participation and research.

Each contributor is an acknowledged expert and the contents are aimed at an international market. Individual opinions may differ and contributors reside in different countries with different national sports and regulations. Additionally, as each section is independently written, some overlap is inevitable and even desirable. The editors have attempted to maintain a delicate balance by respecting authors' views, eliminating unnecessary duplication and catering for a multi-disciplinary audience.

This book would not have been possible without the work of our seventeen contributors drawn from five disciplines and we thank them for their valuable contributions. We are also grateful to Caroline Makepeace, Publisher of Butterworth-Heinemann for her continued assistance and encouragement throughout the preparation of the book.

Donald F. C. Loran
Caroline J. MacEwan

List of Contributors

Brian R. Ariel MSc FBCO FAAO
Optometrist and Sports Vision Practitioner, London

Alan Berman OD
Co-director, Institute for Sports Vision, Ridgefield, Connecticut

W. Neil Charman PhD DSc
Professor of Visual Optics, Department of Optometry and Vision Sciences, UMIST

Bradley Coffey OD FAAO
Associate Professor, College of Optometry, Pacific University, Forest Grove, Oregon

Michael Easterbrook MD FRCS(C) FACS
Associate Professor, University of Toronto

Nathan Efron BScOptom PhD FAAO FVCO MBCO
Professor of Clinical Optometry, Department of Optometry and Vision Science, UMIST

Ian Fell
Formerly Director, British Blind Sports, Elkington, Northants

John J. Gardner OD FAAO
The Eye Care Clinic, Hickory Hills, Illinois

Nicholas P. Jones BSc MB ChB DO FRCS FRCOphth
Honorary Consultant Ophthalmologist, Manchester Royal Eye Hospital

Donald F.C. Loran MSc FBCO AMCT DCLP
Director of Continuing Education, Department of Optometry and Vision Sciences, UMIST, Manchester; Visiting Senior Lecturer, Department of Vision Sciences, Aston University, Birmingham; Founder Chairman, The Sports Vision Association

Caroline J. MacEwen MB ChB MD FRCS FRCOphth
Consultant Ophthalmologist, Ninewells Hospital, Dundee, and Honorary Senior Lecturer, Department of Ophthalmology, University of Dundee

Henri Obstfeld MPhil FBOA:HD FBCO DCLP
Senior Lecturer, Department of Optometry and Visual Science, the City University, London

Roger Pope FBDO
Dispensing Optician, London

Alan W. Reichow OD FAAO
Associate Professor, College of Optometry, Pacific University, Forest Grove, Oregon

Emanuel S. Rosen BSc MD FRCS(E) FRCOphth FRPS
Consultant Ophthalmologist, Manchester Royal Eye Hospital

Arnold Sherman OD FAAO FCOVD
Merrick, New York

Steve P. Taylor PhD MSc FBCO FAAO
Vision Consultant, Bournemouth, and Visiting Research Fellow, Derby University

Foreword

Participation in sport has become increasingly popular and the media and marketing interest in sports events has developed in an unprecedented manner. Regular participation in sport is now widely accepted as beneficial to health and lifestyle in all age groups. Our school children are being encouraged to acquire the exercise habit and maintain it throughout their lives. However, in all activities, visual information and its processing fashion our body's responses. Any change in the quality of the visual stimulus due to poor lighting, soiled contact lenses, steamed-up spectacles or visual disability may alter that response and adversely affect performance.

Sport is also a major cause of serious eye injuries. These have become relatively more common as occupational and road-traffic-associated ocular injuries have declined. About a third of these are of a serious nature, requiring hospital admission for treatment. These injuries predominantly affect young men under 25 years including a large number of children, half of whom will suffer from permanent loss of visual acuity of field of vision.

Sports vision, therefore, is an important discipline in the field of sports medicine which, as part of its role, provides also for the protection of the sportsperson from illness, injury and disability.

Donald Loran and Carrie MacEwan have brought together contributions from both sides of the Atlantic to produce this outstanding text and I heartily congratulate them for this important contribution to sports medicine.

Greg McLatchie
Professor of Sports Medicine
University of Sunderland

Director of National Sports Medicine Institute
London

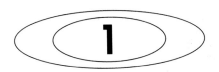

An overview of sport and vision

Donald F.C. Loran

Introduction

Play is an essential facet in the emotional and physical development of a child and encourages motor skills such as climbing, walking, jumping, throwing and catching and facilitates both eye–hand and eye–foot coordination. At about the age of four, when play begins to incorporate rules, it becomes a game (Sheridan, 1989). Thus play is an essential part of a child's development, leading to games with both individual and team participation, when it then becomes a sport.

Throughout history, competition and sport have been closely associated and different cultures have had different forms of participation. American Indians, somewhat macabrely, used the decapitated heads of enemies as a ball. Stones were used as early as 5200 BC for bowling and a ball game with the participants on horseback was described by the Persians in the Medan period (around 600 BC) when it was known as Chaugan (Jewell, 1977). Wrestling is traditionally recognized as the oldest and purest of combat sports and murals in the Egyptian tombs of Beni Hason dating back to 3000 BC illustrate wrestlers in combat.

In order to survive, animals, hominads and humans needed to develop highly coordinated sensory-motor responses such as running, tracking, swimming and fighting which involve sight, hearing and smell. Indeed when danger or arousal is imminent, a sophisticated and efficacious physiological response occurs in the sympathetic nervous system. The stimulus initiates a biochemical alarm which increases the flow of adrenaline, noradrenaline, endorphins and growth hormone and shunts the blood away from the gut to the muscles for rapid action (Hanson, 1988). The systemic blood pressure increases, as does the metabolic rate and circulating blood sugar. There is also a temporary inhibition of pain sensation. Thus, in a danger situation, 'Man the Hunter' initiates a capatoxic 'fight or flight' response and the body assumes a state of positive or beneficial stress which is essential for optimum performance. In contemporary society, 'Man the VDU Operator' may not be able to respond to alarm signals and frustration occurs, especially in response to a problem without an apparent solution. This may in turn lead to syntoxic, or negative, unproductive stress, which results in impaired performance and stress-related disorders such as neuroses, ulcers and vascular diseases (Figure 1.1). Therefore, in our health-conscious society physical activity has been seen as a panacea to reduce stress and to improve health and fitness.

The media are now promoting sport in an unprecedented manner and interest has increased enormously. Participation in sport is widely accepted as a beneficial, convenient

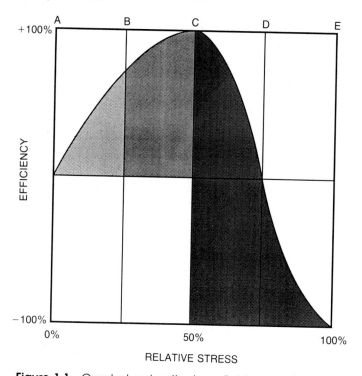

Figure 1.1   Graph showing the beneficial and adverse effects of stress on human performance, including sport. (After Hanson, 1988)

and popular means of exercise and improved fitness. This sports boom has been catalysed by the increase in school and community involvement, such as coaching schemes at local leisure centres, and by the increase in leisure time and healthy life expectancy, which means sports participation increasingly extends into and beyond middle age.

The General Household Survey (Office of Population Censuses and Surveys, 1987) showed that two out of five adults had participated in at least one sport in the four weeks before the interview, while in professional classes, this figure increased to four out of five. The type of sport also varied with social class. For example, the skilled manual group had the highest participation in darts and fishing whereas up to 95% of squash players were from managerial or professional groups (Loran, 1992).

While sports participation has undoubted advantages, such as improved physical fit-

ness, cardiovascular performance, strength, speed, response and reaction times, these have to be traded off against possible adverse effects. The latter may include penalties in terms of time, money and competitive stress which may result from performing poorly, but more seriously there is the risk of injury. (Indeed sports medicine, of which sports vision is a new and exciting discipline, has an important role in the protection of the sportsperson.) Hooliganism, professional fouls, assault, bribery, drug abuse, racism and political boycotts are also unwanted byproducts of sports today.

In the past, the rich and upper classes had more leisure time for sports participation, which was often developed at public schools, colleges and universities. County and Ivy League sports traditionally included rowing, rugby union, horse riding, golf and cricket. Conversely, the working class and immigrants typically had less time for leisure and generally became associated with the so-called 'working class' sports such as angling, darts, snooker, soccer and rugby league. Certain sports which enjoyed international success such as American, Canadian and Gaelic football and Australian rules football were probably derived from rugby football, while baseball was introduced into the United States by Abner Doubleday in 1839 and bears more than a superficial resemblance to the English game of rounders.

Instinct suggests that certain ethnic groups may specialize and excel in specific sports. This hypothesis is illustrated by the apparent dominance of Orientals in table tennis, swimming, gymnastics and ladies middle and long distance running, Asians in squash, hockey and cricket, while blacks seem to excel in speed events and boxing. Beashel and Taylor (1992), however, question the validity of ethnic athletic elitism solely associated with innate ability. They suggest that such apparent excellence is acquired and therefore more likely to be associated with the cultural and social background of the participants and believe that some ethnic minorities are attracted to certain sports such as boxing, athletics and soccer which require a minimum of equipment and organization. Furthermore, despite their disproportionate sporting predominance, only a minority of black sports people are appointed to officiating, administrative and managerial positions in the hierarchy of sport. It is heartening to note, however, that black participants have captained both the English soccer and British Olympic athletics teams in recent years.

The financial assistance offered by sponsorship to a sport, team or individual has gradually revolutionized contemporary sport thus enabling rich sportsmen to become richer; many have become millionaires many times over, especially in boxing, motor racing and golf (Temple, 1993). More importantly, however, sponsorship has enabled up-and-coming athletes to devote themselves full time to their sport and to avail themselves of top coaching and training facilities. However, sponsorship by tobacco and alcohol companies is still widespread in sport and considered by many to be contentious. Much of the success of American sport has developed from the excellent college and university sport scholarship system, while state support of young and developing elite athletes in the Republic of China and also former Soviet bloc countries has been reflected by their outstanding performances at international level. In today's sporting world the interest is enormous, the rewards at an all time high and the competition intense.

Sport is, by definition, competitive (Sinclair, 1991) and if there are two players or more, it follows there must be a winner and a loser or a draw, and that may, in turn, need to be settled by a penalty shoot-out or similar. Motivation is probably the strongest incentive and the concept of 'winning at all costs' is often initiated while at school or by parental pressure, and is to be deprecated. The incentive to win may vary from personal satisfaction, team spirit or national fervour to the high monetary awards accorded to professional sports persons. The most significant factor, however, in the winning formula is skill, which is partially innate and partially acquired (Cockerill and MacGillvary, 1981; Sheridan, 1989) and may therefore be optimized by coaching and training. Aptitude, in turn, is influenced by physique which may be classified as endomorphic or stocky, mesomorphic or muscular and the slim ectomorphs. Although the majority of competitors are not exclusive to a specific body type, physique does tend to influence and determine an athlete's best sport. In general, shorter athletes are more suited to events such as gymnastics, soccer and long distance running, tall individuals predominate in high jumping and basketball while the heavyweights are more likely to be attracted to combat sports, throwing and the defensive positions in rugby, Australian rules, Canadian, Gaelic and American football (Beashel and Taylor, 1992). A sports profile by somatyping is illustrated in Figure 1.2.

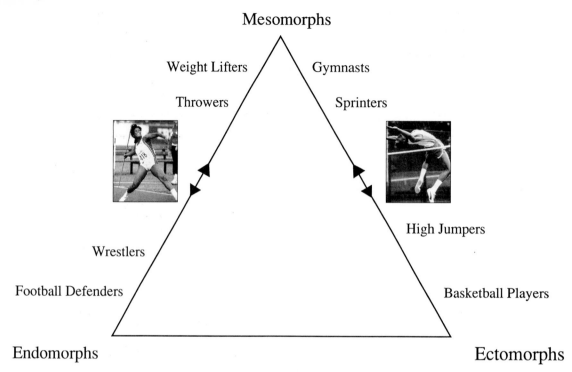

Figure 1.2   A sports profile by somatyping. (After Beashel and Taylor, 1992, by permission of Thomas Nelson Ltd. and also Mark Shearman)

It is probable that the majority of elite athletes have similar ability, physique, coaching and motivation and often the difference between winning and losing is marginal and recorded in millimetres or hundredths of a second. In order to improve their competitive edge, athletes may employ a variety of ancillary techniques such as **psychological variables** including the support or barracking of coaches, team mates or a partisan crowd, or the counselling effects of sports psychology, hypnotherapy, transcendental meditation and prayer. **Physiological factors** are many and varied and may include high-tech equipment and sportswear, diet, correct warming up procedures and fitness training. Sports science has endeavoured to predict athletic excellence by predetermining a profile of attributes necessary for success in specific sports (Beashel and Taylor, 1992) – a procedure which could also be adapted to vision in sports.

Vision in sporting activities

Optimum visual performance requires clear ocular media with the ability to focus objects sharply on to the retina from where the visual pathways conduct information to the primary cortex of the brain. This information is used in coordination with sensory, motor, perceptual and cognitive skills and Figure 1.3 illustrates the neuro-anatomical pathways involved in visual information processing.

In conventional sight testing, the examiner typically records visual acuity by instructing the patient to read high contrast letters at both 6 m and 40 cm. During testing the visual axes are normally parallel or converge symetrically on to an object of regard situated in the median plane. The advantages of such standardized test conditions are that they are simple and repeatable. Indeed, in our modern sedentary lifestyle, many activities such as

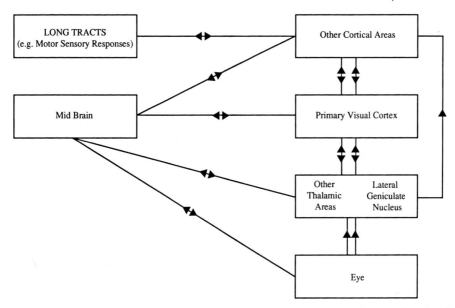

Figure 1.3 Diagrammatical illustration of the neuro-anatomical pathways involved in visual information processing. (After Trachtman and Kluka, 1993)

writing, reading, do-it-yourself (DIY) and watching television reflect, to some extent, the controlled laboratory type conditions of the refraction room. However, in order to consider visual function in a more realistic manner, it is necessary to apply the principles of task analysis to specific viewing conditions. This considers visual requirements while performing certain tasks and analysis should include factors such as the location and speed of both the object of regard and the observer, and take into account environmental factors such as lighting, contrast and glare. While task analysis is an integral part of the history, it is only recently that its significance to sports performance has been appreciated and applied as sports vision task analysis (see Glossary).

In many sporting activities the ball, puck or shuttlecock may approach at speeds of up to 140 mph. Alternatively, the observer may move at speeds which in sports such as Formula I or Indy Car racing may be in excess of 200 mph. Hubel and Weisel (1962) and Hubel (1988) have shown that the mammalian cerebral cortex is highly sensitive to contours

and movement as well as its precise retinal location. Any movement leads to processing information, and vision plays a vital role in spatial orientation, coincidal anticipation, reaction times, response times, eye–body coordination and static and dynamic balance. The efficacy of such activities needs to be considered, not only in a quiet laboratory, but more realistically by simulating the distractive background noise and stress of many competitive activities.

Traditionally, coaches instruct players to 'Keep your eye on the ball'. This advice may well be reasonable for a novice, for tracking a rapidly moving object in the far distance or for a slow-moving object close to the players, such as receiving a soccer throw-in. However, as players become more proficient, the projectile speed increases and it then becomes increasingly more difficult, if not impossible, to keep the eye on the ball. A vertically orientated hemisphere surrounding the body has been described in which a projectile would be moving too fast for the eyes to track; this has been termed the 'Zone of Fog' (Stein *et al.*, 1987). This zone is likely to affect all sports which require eye–body coordination but especially racquet sports in which the object is small and fast moving and the player is also moving at speed. The size and density of the zone varies with a number of factors, including dynamic visual acuity, illumination, contrast and fatigue (Stein et al., 1987). However, even if the so-called Zone of Fog did not exist, a neural time lag of about 1/5th of a second is believed to exist which is required to process visual information and to initiate the necessary corrective eye/hand movement (McCrone, 1993). This means there is an unbridgeable gap between the stimulus and the response so that it is additionally unlikely that the player can keep an eye on the ball.

Eye movements

Early experiments into eye movements suggested that most observers were unlikely to clearly track or follow moving objects travelling at velocities above 50 degrees per second or 25 mph (Ludvigh and Miller, 1958). Using cinematography, Hubbard and Seng (1954) determined that a pitched baseball cannot be followed during its final 8–15 ft of flight and, using a similar technique, Mowen (1976) determined that it was not possible to track a tennis ball for the 0.05–0.20 seconds prior to contact with the racquet. Hale (1992) also recorded the average visual reaction time of major league baseball players to be 0.24 seconds, during which a 90 mph pitched ball can travel 26 feet. In order to contact the ball, the striker must anticipate its position during its flight half way between the pitcher and the home plate.

According to McCrone (1993), top class cricket batsmen do not necessarily have quicker reaction times than the general population but have learned from experience how to anticipate the position of the ball in the final 200 milliseconds during which it cannot be seen. A spinning or swerving delivery often eludes the receiver by a last minute change of direction but top class batsmen will respond

by developing a repertoire of compensating strokes such as a hook or late cut.

A projectile, such as a tennis ball, needs to be followed when the player and the ball are both in motion, an exercise which inhibits clear vision (Ditchburn and Ginsborg, 1952; Ditchburn et al., 1959). Thus, the visual system is unable to follow and process a moving object clearly unless the gaze velocity or the combined conjugate speed of head and eye movements are able to stabilize the retinal image on the foveas. Motion therefore inhibits their vision but the ability to track a moving object, particularly when the player is also moving, is obviously a considerable advantage for participants in dynamic sports.

Many sports require players to follow targets and this may involve up to four types of eye movement: pursuit, saccadic, vestibulo-ocular and vergence eye movements (Bahill and La Ritz, 1984; R. V. Abadi, personal communication, 1994).

1. Pursuit eye movements are used to follow a slowly moving object travelling in a consistent direction, such as a high lobbed tennis ball, and might be used by a novice sports player. Pursuits attempt to match the eye movement with the speed of the target but these are relatively slow eye movements and if the target is moving rapidly this results in the inability to keep up, which needs to be corrected by a catch-up saccade.
2. Saccades are short, rapid and jerky eye movements used to catch up with a rapidly moving proximal object such as a tennis ball tossed prior to serving or to receive a tennis serve at speed (Stein et al., 1987). Vision during saccades is reduced due to a compensating mechanism known as saccadic suppression (Carpenter, 1988).
3. Vestibulo-ocular motor movements are utilized to maintain ocular fixation during head movements.
4. The vergence system is responsible for the observation of an approaching or receding object. The visual axes converge as an object approaches and diverge as it goes away. Visual tracking requires attention to be continual redirected from one object to another and if the target is either receding or approaching then the visual axes converge to form a triangle with the moving object located at the apex. This process,

termed triangulation by Sherman (1990), is one in which vergence and accommodation act as feedback to maintain a clear retinal image (Holland, 1993).

Each type of eye movement is normally tested clinically as a separate entity while the head is kept stationary. This approach is understandable as it facilitates analysis and repeatability. However, it fails to simulate the true situation in many sports where a combination of several types of eye and head movements is required either to follow or avoid a moving target. The peripheral retina is sensitive to movement and initiates corrective eye movements so that the object of interest becomes viewed by the central retina where the visual acuity is best. Two separate mechanisms, each with separate pathways to specific areas of the brain, are believed to control eye movements. The focal system is concerned with central vision and conscious object identification while the ambient system

is reflex, peripheral and controls fine movement (Trachtman and Kluka, 1993).

Successful players in visually demanding sports are believed to have fast smooth pursuits, suppression of the vestibulo-ocular reflex, and from time to time employ an anticipatory saccade (Bahill and La Ritz, 1984). In addition to keen dynamic visual acuity and quick, accurate depth perception, success in fast-moving sports requires a smooth and rapid vergence/accommodation facility. However, reaction times and visual performance may deteriorate under adverse conditions such as stress, fatigue or poor lighting (Wood, 1981; Leslie, 1993).

Vision in sport officials

Despite the advent of electronic scoring, line faults are still a source of dispute in tennis. Line judges and umpires would therefore require exceptional dynamic visual reactions

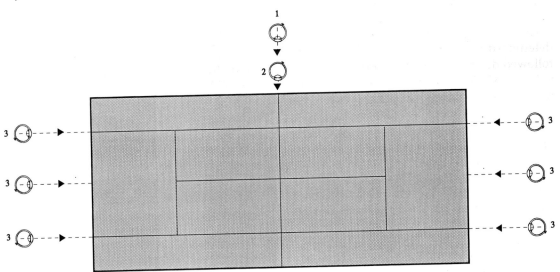

1 = Umpire
2 = Net Judge
3 = Line Judges or Linesmen

Figure 1.4 The strategic placing of tennis officials so that they are able to judge the relative position of a high velocity tennis ball with minimum eye movement in order to judge if a tennis ball, approaching at speeds up to 150 mph, is just in, or just out of play. The eye cannot follow the projectile at such high speed and the motion also inhibits vision. In tennis tournaments, seven stationary line judges are strategically placed as shown in Figure 1.4 so that they can directly align or sight an approaching ball without having to move their eyes. While neutral officials are sited in the optimum position to judge, they are obviously fallible, and borderline decisions frequently result in vociferous protest and tantrums from 'hyped up' players.

In sports such as American football and also cricket, officials now benefit from being able to watch video playback and slow-motion replays when making decisions, although some may find the ensuing interruption of play irksome. In contrast, replays are not generally available to soccer referees who are, however, assisted by two linesmen and often 'judged' both by partisan players and crowds. Soccer rules state 'that for a goal to be scored the whole of the ball must pass over the whole of the line' (International Football Association Board, 1991/92). This, in effect, often requires an instantaneous decision, the validity or otherwise of which may be re-enacted in 'trial by television' in front of millions of viewers.

Eye-body coordination

Sports action may be proactive, that is to say initiated by the player – for example baseball pitching or cricket bowling – or reactive, referring to the response by other players to that action – for example baseball or cricket batting (Acuvision, 1992). Such reactions are largely reflex and occur in milliseconds so that the eyes steer the body (Planter and Breedlove, 1993). The visual stimulus is the basis of the body's efficient reaction. Eye–hand coordination is utilized in racquet, bat and stick sports in addition to goal- and wicket-keeping, baseball, cricket and basketball. Association football (soccer) and sand soccer require

eye–foot, eye–head and eye–chest coordination whilst other forms of football such as American, Australian Rules, Canadian, Gaelic and rugby utilize both eye–foot and also eye–hand co-ordination.

Depth perception

Whilst depth perception clearly relates to many sports, an exact correlation between performance and depth perception is unclear and subject to debate (Olsen, 1956; Miller, 1960; Shick, 1971; ten Nepal 1993). Coffey and Reichow (1990) acknowledge that statistical correlations are not proven but nevertheless suggest, not unreasonably, that depth and distance judgements are visual task demands for most sports which involve target or competitive movement. In Table 2.1, Gardner and Sherman list a theoretical relationship between various sports and visual skills. This suggests that in two thirds of the sports considered perception is an important consideration for peak performance. In such situations, the athlete needs not only to judge the distance of objects but also to be able to do this quickly under dynamic and competitive stress.

Contrast

Contrast sensitivity testing gives a measure of the ability of the visual apparatus to filter and process information. This is, obviously, a significant sports vision skill and it is, therefore, most important that the contrast sensitivity function is measured and monitored in all athletes. This is especially the case where environmental variables are likely to reduce contrast. Sports affected by poor ambient illumination include skiing, cricket and baseball, motor rallying and motor cross. Additionally, soiled or deposited contact lenses, steamed up or dirty spectacle lenses or anomalies of the ocular media such as mild corneal oedema e.g. due to contact lenses, cataract or vitreous floaters might adversely affect contrast sensitivity and therefore sporting performance.

Information processing

Vision, in common with other sensory input systems, may be required to process complicated data selectively. For descriptive purposes this may be conveniently compared to a computer. The input receives information which is processed via neuronal networks and transferred to memory where it is interpreted and stored until it is required. Information processing systems are required to transmit items of information or 'bits' effectively at high speed. This is facilitated by a mechanism known as parallel processing in which data are simultaneously conducted through more than one pathway: each contains neurones with distinctive properties that process and filter the input in different ways and relay it to various parts of the brain. The real power of parallel processing is that many small processors work simultaneously, each using a small memory of its own. In actual brain networks, each neurone is effectively a small processor with its own small memory. In addition, groups of neurones may be condensed in nuclei or specialized areas which filter and process particular classes of input.

In man's visual system information from the retina is channelled along two major pathways, as shown in Figure 1.3.

1. The **retino midbrain** (Sadun, 1986; Kiernan, 1987), which relays information that controls pupil reactions and the visual accommodative response.
2. The **retino-geniculate** pathway projects from the retina via the lateral geniculate body (LGB) to the primary visual cortex (Hubel, 1988; Zeki, 1993). Within the geniculate body the input from the retina is separated into two subdivisions, the parvocellular (P) and the magnocellular (M). The output from the LGB to the cortex is, in turn, a combination of that from the two subdivisions. The P system relays information on high spatial and low temporal frequencies and is therefore concerned with the relay and analysis of visual

shape/pattern information. By contrast, the M system involves high temporal and low spatial frequencies which is more concerned with the detection and processing of information about visual movement (Kaplan *et al.*, 1989; Valberg and Lee, 1991; J.R. Cronly-Dillon, personal communication, 1994).

As previously noted, visual sensory input is related to a perceptual motor response which in many everyday activities may be suboptimal. However, under stress or tension a human subject may be able to quickly detect and process complex information because the information is processed in parallel. Apart from its relevance to sportspeople, other stressful and visually demanding occupations might include military jet fighter pilots, armed forces in combat or high speed drivers. Certain sports, as outlined in Chapter 3, however, do not require a high level of visual performance, or the sport may be adapted to allow participation of people who are visually handicapped. Sporting activities appropriate for the visually impaired include weight lifting, track and field events, tandem cycling, sky diving, rowing, canoeing or diving. Additionally other sports such as swimming, some ball games and skiing can, with some ingenuity, be suitably modified. A comprehensive overview of the visual skills required in a wide spectrum of sports is outlined in Chapter 2 by Gardner and Sherman (see Table 2.1) and Sherman (1990). Sports considered to be especially visually demanding include baseball, cricket, dynamic shooting (such as clay pigeon shooting), hockey and soccer goal-keeping, motor and motor cycle racing, most racquet sports, table tennis, volleyball and skiing.

Coaching and training

In a 90-minute game of soccer – which is arguably one of the most popular sports worldwide – the ball may only be in play for 60 minutes. If the game is relatively even, then each side should be in possession of the ball for roughly 30 minutes. During that time, however, it will also be in flight, so that in a

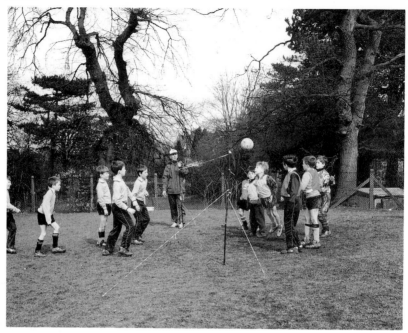

Figure 1.5 The author coaching primary school boys in soccer tennis. This training exercise, which has been developed from volleyball, enables junior players to develop and practise anticipation and those visual skills illustrated in Table 2.1 which are utilized in soccer

typical soccer game each player may only be in possession of the ball for as little as 2 minutes (Hughes, 1980). For the remainder of the game, players participate by encouraging, marking, covering, supporting and running off the ball (Widdows, 1989). More than 50% of soccer goals originate from set pieces (Hughes, 1980), and logically should improve with practice. Coaching aims to improve skills including anticipation and also possibly vision and perception by demonstration and repetitive learning, while training enhances strength, stamina, physical fitness, motivation and attention. Training and coaching sessions attempt to channel teaching into a concentrated period and during a typical 2-hour session football players and other athletes in training may practise skills which otherwise would take weeks, months or even a season to complete. Figure 1.5 shows junior soccer players practising soccer tennis, which employs many of the skills specific to soccer, including anticipation, dynamic visual acuity,

eye movements, binocular coordination, depth perception, proactive and reactive timing, accommodation/vergence facility, perceptual awareness and visualization in addition to eye–foot, eye–head and eye–body coordination.

While using a golf range, a player is able to practise repetitive golf swings from a supply of several hundred balls. Similarly tennis and cricket players may practise anticipatory skills in addition to strokes and shots from balls delivered at variable trajectories from a canon or delivery machine. Sports science attempts to establish the efficacy or otherwise of training and coaching and the same scientific rigour should be applied to sports vision enhancement techniques and their likely effect on performance, which is considered in Chapters 8 and 11.

In order to assess the validity or otherwise of training and coaching techniques, it is first necessary to establish baseline data. Sports scientists use physiological data to develop a profile of the successful athlete, which then forms a basis to monitor the effect of coaching and training. This is used to identify one sport with another, to compare sportspeople in a specific sport and to determine the effect of injury, illness and treatment on performance (Beashel and Taylor, 1992). A battery of standarized sports vision tests, known as the Pacific Sports Vision Performance Profiles (PSVPP), has been established and normal data published (Reichow et al., 1981; Coffey and Reichow, 1986; Coffey and Reichow, 1987; Coffey and Reichow, 1990). This information can now be used in a similar manner to the physiological and performance data in sports science to establish a vision profile of the elite athlete. Unlike sports science, however, sports vision is still in its infancy.

Vision screening

Vision screening of sportspeople, especially if undertaken on site, such as the changing rooms, sports field or Olympic village, is a valuable service which can be offered to the athletic community. Such activities were originally pioneered in the United States by the Sports Vision section of the American Optometric Association (Sherman, 1990) and have since been launched in the UK and elsewhere (Sports Vision Association, 1994). In 1992 and also 1994 detailed vision screening programmes were undertaken at the Olympic Games by an international team of sports optometrists and underwritten by one of the official sponsors (Bausch & Lomb). Seven hundred and twelve athletes, coaches and trainers were screened in 1992 by a battery of tests based on the PSVPP which included visual acuity, contrast sensitivity, depth perception, eye–hand coordination, reaction and response times.

The results from the 1992 Olympic vision screening (Table 1.1) indicate that one in two of the participants tested had never had their eyes tested before, although one in four experienced visual difficulties (Ivins, 1992; Edmunds, 1993). These results confirm pre-

Table 1.1 Screening demographics from the 1992 Olympic Games

	Winter Games	Summer Games
Total participants screened	282	430
Athletes	194	382
Coaches, trainers etc.	88	48
Countries represented	24	69
Events represented	13	>42
Visual performance history of atheletes		
Previous eye examination	54%	54%
Total contact lens wearers	15%	18%
Soft contact lens wearers	86%	86%
Rigid corneal lens wearers	14%	14%
Previous vision training	2%	4%
Utilizes visualization	54%	38%
Experiences visual difficulties	18%	33%

Source: Courtesy of Bausch & Lomb (1992)

vious work which shows that a significant proportion of elite athletes take part in their specific sports with uncorrected visual defects (Garner, 1977a, 1994; Sherman, 1990; Bausch & Lomb, 1992). It may well be that some of these athletes participate with a relatively low visual input, or that they compensate for their visual defects by developing other skills. Nevertheless, there is a clear message that sports vision practitioners have a vital role to play in screening and correcting visual defects in athletes with the realistic expectation of at least some improvement in performance.

An analysis of the results of screening the vision of athletes in the 1994 Winter Olympics is presented in Appendix 3.

Vision in sportspeople

For several years, there has been controversy regarding the relative standards of athletes' vision. Because a high visual input is a prerequisite for so many sports, it is tempting to speculate that elite sportspeople should manifest superior visual skills. This assumption has, however, been questioned, mainly by sports vision psychologists who argue that no visual skill predominates in successful athletes and that reported differences compared to non-athletes are not significant (Summers, 1974; Bietel, 1980; Mizusawa *et al.*, 1983; Starkes and Deakin, 1984). Conversely, there is now mounting evidence, mainly from sports optometry, to suggest that, compared to matched groups of recreational or non-athletes, top athletes do in fact display superior visual skills (Williams and Thier, 1975; Falkowitz and Mendel, 1977; Coffey and Reichow, 1990; Sherman, 1990; Vogel and Hale, 1992).

Visual skills tend to be sport-specific and athletes can, and do, compensate for vision defects. For example, long-standing monocular athletes are able to compete successfully in sports such as basketball, which requires critical depth perception. If, however, a binocular athlete suddenly loses vision in one eye, depth perception and hence sports performance are likely to be seriously impaired, with an increased risk of collisions (Stein *et al.*, 1987). There is, however, no sound evidence to suggest that improvements in visual performance arising from sports vision enhancement training actually result in a significant change in sporting performance (Stein *et al.*, 1987; Coffey and Reichow, 1990; ten Nepel, 1993). Abernethy (1986) believes that improving the reception of visual information by optical correction brings a parallel improvement in sporting performance. If, however, a similar improvement is to be achieved from sports vision enhancement training, then he suggests that attention should be directed towards the perceptual aspects of visual processing.

Compared to non-athletes, recall information from 'offensive' set pieces appears to be superior in top athletes (Allard, 1980/81), who are also likely to be able to retrieve perceptual information from memory accurately (Allard *et al.*, 1980). Additionally, the advanced athlete would appear to have excellent anticipatory skills (Abernethy, 1986) and also to be able to predict advance cues, for example the direction an opponent might flick a badminton shuttle, if a tennis serve is likely

to land on the forehand or the backhand, or whether a cricket batsman should play off the back or front foot. Abernethy concludes, 'Clearly what was done with the perceptory information was more important in determining sporting performance than the manner in which that information was acquired.'

It would appear, therefore, that top athletes are probably able to benefit from coaching to develop superior anticipation. This is explored and improved in some aspects of sports vision enhancement training. In addition, anomalies of vision should be detected and corrected as soon as possible in order to enhance optimal sporting performance.

Although acceptance of sports vision is slow, it is gratifying to note that athletes at all levels are becoming more aware that visual as well as physical fitness is important for successful sporting endeavour.

The history of sports vision

Television has introduced sport into our homes on an unprecedented scale and sporting activities and physical recreation have enjoyed increasing popularity for several decades. It has been estimated that 22 million people now participate in sports in Britain and of these up to 6.5 million are registered with clubs (Beaschel and Taylor, 1992). If these figures are truly representative, then almost half the population may engage in sporting activities, some of which are likely to be visually exacting or hazardous (see Table 1.2). Eye-care practitioners should therefore be mindful that one in two of their patients is likely to be involved in sport either as a participant or as a spectator.

The optimization of safe and efficient vision in sports, or 'sports vision', is of direct concern to all sportspeople and eye-care practitioners. Visual task analysis determines those skills and environmental variables necessary for a specific viewing situation, and a sports visual task analysis should be included in the history

Table 1.2 Sports participation in the UK, 1992

Sport	Men (millions)	Women (millions)	Total (millions)
Swimming	4.4	5.6	10.0
Rambling/hiking	2.6	1.8	4.3
Snooker	3.5	0.5	3.9
Keepfit/dance	N/A	3.9	3.9
Jogging/training	2.7	0.9	3.6
Badminton	1.8	1.6	3.4
Golf	2.9	0.5	3.4
Cycling	1.9	1.2	3.1
Darts	2.2	0.8	3.1
Weight training	2.1	0.7	2.8
Tennis	1.5	1.1	2.7
Football	2.2	0.1	2.4
Squash	1.5	0.6	2.1
Cricket	1.2	0.1	1.4
Table tennis	1.1	0.6	1.7
Bowls	0.9	0.4	1.4
Skiing	0.8	0.5	1.2
Climbing	0.5	0.2	0.7
Athletics	0.5	0.2	0.7
Rugby union	0.6		0.7
Windsurfing	0.3		0.3

n = 5.328. Data may not sum due to roundings.
Source: Mintel, 1993

of any comprehensive eye examination or any vision screening programme.

Vision is one of our most valued possessions, and nature has, in her wisdom, provided the eye with the following protective mechanisms against disease and injury.

1. The bony orbital cavities protect the eyes against glare and injury.
2. There is an adverse reaction to ocular irritation, whereby the protrusion of the eyebrows is increased, the vertical palpebral apertures reduce, the head turns away from danger while the hand may be used as a visor (Silver, 1986).
3. The iris and sclera absorb incident light which is further limited from entering the eyes when the pupils constrict to a bright stimulus.
4. The ocular media comprising the cornea, aqueous, lens and vitreous absorb non-ionizing radiation, especially in older eyes which have less transparent media.
5. Blinking clears and protects the eyes and may be initiated by a foreign body touching the lashes.
6. When threatened, Bell's Phenomenon occurs in which the eyes turn up and outward to protect the sensitive corneas from injury.
7. Reflex lacrimation increases the irrigating effect of sterile tears to flush debris, microbes and irritants from the conjunctival sacs.
8. Extreme sensitivity of the corneas and lid margins acts as feedback to initiate remedial action if the eyes are infected, irritated or damaged.

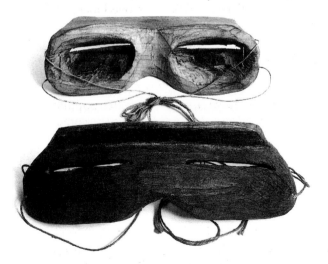

Figure 1.6 Early Eskimo spectacles incorporating two narrow horizontal slits to protect the eyes from glare arising from snow and ice. (© Wellcome Institute Library, London)

Headwear has traditionally been a prominent and important item of sportswear, serving the dual function of protecting the eyes from injury and also light reduction. Illustrations of early sporting events typically depict participants wearing a wide variety of headgear, for example visors in jousting. Today popular sports such as baseball, cricket and horse racing use protective headgear for the same reasons, although 'gentleman' cricketers should traditionally wear top hats (Jewell, 1977)!

Eskimos were arguably the first to produce sports spectacles – for hunting – by carving two horizontal stenopaeic slits into a mask of wood or bone thereby reducing glare from snow, ice and water (Daland, 1917) (Figure 1.6). It is possible, however, that the Chinese may have used coloured transparent pebbles gathered from river beds to serve the dual purpose of magnification and light protection (Duke-Elder, 1970). The earliest recorded use of 'sports sunglasses' was attributed to the Roman emperor, Nero. He reputedly viewed gladiators in combat through an emerald, presumably to absorb the intense solar radiation in the amphitheatre (MacGregor, 1992). The Chicago store of Sears, Roebuck and Co. offered both sunglasses and shooting spectacles in their 1886 catalogue (Gregg, 1987).

In 1909, the firm of Negretti and Zambra advertised in The Times of London that 'spectacles, close fitting and having extra large lenses are best for shooting and billiards'. The company also advertised thermoscopic lenses in the same issue to protect the eyes from glare (Obstfeld, 1993, personal communication). Sasini (1950) recommended that sports spectacles should be 'secure and designed with extra large eye sizes extended temporally to provide a wider field of vision'. He also described sports frames for billiards, shooting, fishing and swimming in addition to plastic and unsplinterable lenses to provide physical and photo protection in sporting activities. However, it was not until polycarbonate was introduced as an ophthalmic material that goggles and sports spectacles provided ade-

quate impact resistance for sports. At the time of writing, sports participation and assault constitute the major causes of serious eye injuries in the United Kingdom (MacEwen, 1989), despite the fact that sports-induced eye injuries are generally avoidable by the use of suitable eye protectors (Vinger, 1980).

Contact lenses were first suggested as a means of correcting vision in the early nineteenth century (Herschel, 1823). After the Second World War they generally became more widely available as an optical aid and effectively revolutionized sports participation by ametropic players. The early scleral or haptic lenses had a total diameter of about 25 mm or 1 inch and fitted snugly under the upper and lower eyelids. These lenses were relatively large, almost impossible to dislodge accidentally and were suitable for almost any sport where limited wear is acceptable. The minutes of the Contact Lens Society of Great Britain dated 26 January 1948 recorded an article which appeared in the Daily Mirror newspaper. This referred to well-known athletes such as soccer players who wore contact lenses, presumably of the larger scleral design, for their sport (N. Efron, personal communication, 1994). Indeed, sclerals are still today arguably the most suitable contact lenses for water and combat sports. The smaller corneal lenses which float on a thin layer of tears (Touhy, 1948; Graham, 1949; Touhy, 1963) are superior cosmetically and provide longer wearing times. However, they are considerably less secure and are not entirely suitable for activities requiring rapid eye movements, water sports or activities such as squash where there is a high risk of eye injury (Loran, 1992).

Soft contact lenses were introduced in Czechoslovakia in the 1960s (Wichterle and Lim, 1960) and proved to be an excellent sports lens. They are comfortable, cosmetically good, relatively easy to fit and secure when worn. Contact lenses generally opened vast new horizons for millions who were then able to participate in sports which were otherwise difficult, if not impossible to play in spectacles. Compared to glasses, contact lenses provided natural clear vision over a wider field of view, were virtually undetectable and secure in wear. For sporting activities, contact lenses, unlike glasses, are not obstructed by rain, snow, spray, condensation or perspiration. However, they still require over protectors for impact and water sports, and not everyone is suitable to wear contact lenses.

To see clearly without spectacles or contact lenses is the most attractive option and this apparent 'panacea' can now also be obtained by surgery. Radial keratotomy was one of the more successful types of refractive surgery and was discovered quite by accident in 1973 by Fyoderov, a Russian ophthalmologist. He was treating a short-sighted patient whose cornea was injured after his glasses were smashed in a cycling accident. When the bandages were removed, the patient could see clearly without glasses! A subsequent examination revealed that splinters of broken glass incised the cornea radially (like spokes on a wheel) which caused the corneal surface to flatten and thereby 'cure' the myopia (Rabkins, 1984). The various modalities available to correct vision in sports are discussed in more detail in Chapter 7.

There has been a traditional reluctance for sportspeople in general and professional players in particular to wear spectacles, which may appear to detract from their sporting image. Additionally, earlier spectacles were less than ideal for many sports. Fortunately, the phobia of wearing sports spectacles has now largely diminished, designs and materials have improved enormously and many elite sportspeople, such as top tennis players, have successfully won Grand Slam titles and other major tournaments while wearing spectacles. At the time of writing, however, there are no British, European or international standards for eye protection in sports and racquet players show a marked reluctance to wear eye protectors on the basis of informed consent (Loran, 1992).

In 1977, Garner estimated that in the United States alone almost 300 000 athletes required vision care, a figure which Gregg (1987) challenged as being too conservative. Gradually, sportspeople accepted the need for specialized vision care and eye-care practitioners today are appointed as team and athlete consultants. Typical services provided by sports vision practitioners include vision screening, evaluation of eye health care, refraction and the provision of eye protectors and optical appliances. Coaches are also instructed in simple eye care procedures, including first aid and the insertion, recentration and removal of contact lenses. Finally sports vision enhancement techniques are provided for sportspeople, and in baseball, for example, some cases of improved batting averages apparently resulted from vision training (Gregg, 1987). Baseball, basketball, ice hockey and to a lesser extent American football are all visually demanding sports, played extensively in North America. The exacting vision demands necessary for players to participate successfully in these and other sports no doubt acted as a catalyst for the development of sports vision.

Since 1979, optometrists have become involved in vision screening of athletes (Sherman, 1990). Manufacturers of contact lenses, sunglasses and ophthalmic lenses now sponsor major sporting events. Comprehensive facilities have been established to screen the vision of coaches, trainers and above all athletes in Olympic villages at both the summer and winter games (Edmunds, 1992; Ivins, 1992).

Sports vision has developed from a subspecialty of occupational vision to become a significant and important aspect of vision care in its own right. Indeed the subject now forms an integral part of the syllabus of many eye-care teaching institutions and professional bodies worldwide.

Sports medicine

Sports vision forms part of the larger discipline of sports medicine, which has now become well recognized as an established medical specialty. This area of medicine examines the effects of sporting activities on both health and disease. As such, it encompasses all exercise, training and sports and touches every medical and paramedical specialty.

Only part of this discipline deals with disease and injury associated with sport and the therapeutic aspects of management. In sports medicine the benefits of exercise and methods of maximizing physical potential are considered important. These areas of human performance currently form the basis of most of the research being carried out in this area. In addition, risk factors which contribute to the high injury rate in some sports are being recognized and isolated in order that the appropriate preventative strategies can be employed. Protective wear in many disciplines has been conceived and repeatedly improved and other preventative measures such as alteration in the rules to encourage safe play have also been employed. One of the overall strengths of this specialty, however, is its particular emphasis on education. This is employed to increase the knowledge of participants, observers and medical advisers alike. In so doing, it contributes towards improved health and fitness and a reduction in injury and illness associated with sporting activities. Sports medicine is active in encouraging a more thorough approach to all areas of health involved in sport (C.J. MacEwen, personal communication, 1994).

Sports vision worldwide

As eye-care practitioners began to appreciate the importance of vision in sports, the need to share information became apparent. Sports vision organizations, as illustrated in Appendix 1, were formed, specialized publications were made available and serious efforts made to establish sports vision as an accepted scientific discipline.

The subject was initially developed in the United States in the mid-1970s and some twenty years later is taught and examined worldwide in many vision training institutions. The sporting fraternity is gradually becoming aware of the need for safe and efficient vision in sporting activities and eye-care practitioners have an important role to play in publicizing this concept to sports participants and organizations.

The following overview is not necessarily comprehensive but illustrates the attempts which have been made in selected countries to establish sports vision. At the time of writing, detailed information of regional, national and international sports vision progress is not always readily available. The author therefore acknowledges with gratitude the personal communications from practitioners in Australia, Canada, Italy, the Low Countries, the United Kingdom and the United States. Apologies are also offered for inadvertent omissions.

Australia

The subcontinent offers an ideal environment for outdoor leisure activities and many popular Australian sports such as Australian rules football, cricket, rugby and tennis have a high visual profile (see Table 2.1). Additionally, outdoor pursuits, especially those on the beach and water, present potential light hazards to participants. Formal sports vision in Australia originated in 1987, with the formation of the Sports Vision section of the New South Wales, State Optometric Organization. In 1992, the Australian Optometric Association established a Sports Vision Section. This national organization was arguably the first to introduce a formal accreditation system by examination for practitioners wishing to practise sports vision. For some state and international teams in hockey and cricket, sports vision input is now an accepted factor in the coaching and training regime of players (Neil Murray, personal communication).

In 1992, the Standards Association of Australia became the first organization outside North America to agree and publish standards for eye protection in racquet sports (AS/NZ5 4066; Standards Association of Australia, 1992).

Canada

Skiing and ice-hockey (hockey) are popular Canadian sports which are both speed-orientated and potentially dangerous to players' eyes. Skiing requires photo-protection against glare and radiation whilst hockey players need physical eye protection to reduce the risk of injury from stick, puck or opponent.

In 1975, the Canadian Ophthalmological Association, shocked by the rising tide of head and eye injuries in hockey, undertook a prospective study into the problem. The results showed that, in a single season, forty hockey players, mostly in the 11–15 age group, suffered sight-threatening injuries (Pashby *et al.*, 1975; Pashby, 1977; Pashby, 1979; Rousseau *et al.*, 1982). Rule changes were subsequently introduced to prevent high sticking, the wearing of helmets was made mandatory in minor hockey and also in certain cities and provinces for all players. This impetus from ice-hockey then directed attention to preventing eye injury in racquet sports, and in 1982 Canada led the world by introducing standards for eye protection in racquet sports (Canadian Standards Association, 1982).

The Sports Vision Section of the Canadian Optometric Association was formed in 1987 and at its 1993 meeting there was a commitment to increase its membership from fifty (Granda, 1994).

Italy

On 15 April 1989, the city of Cervia in Italy sponsored a press conference to introduce journalists to the newly formed European Academy of Sports Vision (EASV). Some four years later, five Sports Vision Centres have been established and recognized by the Academy, which also publishes *Sports Vision Update*, a bi-annual journal.

EASV also collaborated with Ford Italiana in the selection and evaluation of aspiring young motor racing drivers. This programme emphasized the critical vision requirements for safe and efficient motor car driving. The Academy also organized sports vision screening and by 1993 had collated approximately 1000 specific sports vision diagnoses and recommended over 300 personalized vision training programmes (Roncagli, personal communication, 1994).

The Low Countries (Holland and Belgium)

From 1985 to 1988, a multinational optical manufacturer (Bausch & Lomb Inc.) sponsored and organized conferences in sports vision in the Low Countries, which in turn led to the formation of the Dutch Council in Sports Vision. Since its inception, members have been active in the vision screening of both national and international sports teams. In 1992, the council was renamed the Foundation of Sports Vision and membership comprised twelve optometrists and one ophthalmologist. This change in status widened the spectrum of sponsorship and members became active in fundamental research into sports vision enhancement, and sports vision programmes are being implemented in optometry practices. The Dutch Optometric Association was founded in 1993 and plans to establish a Sports Vision Section to supplement those in Contact Lenses and Low Vision. (R. Van't Pad Bosch, personal communication, 1994).

The United Kingdom

Industrial optometry concerns the eye at work and has for many years been an integral part of eye care in the UK. As leisure time increased, however, optometrists and other eye-care professionals began to appreciate the importance of vision in sports and recreation. Thus, since the early 1960s, sports vision in the UK was essentially taught and examined as a sub-specialty of occupational optometry.

In 1981, two psychologists at the University of Birmingham published what was arguably one of the first textbooks on vision and sport (Cockerill and MacGillivary, 1981). This was essentially based on visual space perception and addressed the psychological issues influencing how players learned and performed specific sports skills.

The Association of Optometrists (AOP) set up a sub-committee on sports vision in 1980 and was influential in contacting like-minded individuals to form the Sports Vision Association (SVA) in 1993.

Although eye protection standards for racquet sports were established in North America in the 1980s (Canadian Standards Association, 1982; American Society for Testing and Materials, 1988), at the time of writing there are no equivalent standards published in the UK. British Standards are available for eye protection for vehicle users (BS 4410), eye protection in industrial and non-industrial use (BS 2092) and also sun glare protectors for general use (BS 2724) (see British Standards Institution, 1979, 1987a, 1987b, respectively). While such standards undoubtedly enhance eye protection, they are neither designed for nor suitable for sports. A British Standards Institution Sub-Committee, PSM/2/9 was, however, established in 1993 specifically to consider eye protection for leisure activities. In 1994 the British Standards Institution published a Draft Standard for Eye Protectors for Squash and other Racquet Sports. It is intended to present the UK recommendation to the European Committee for Standardization (CEN) with a view ultimately to agreeing and publishing International Standards (ISO) for eye protection in sport.

The United States of America

Sports vision was essentially developed in the USA by optometrists and ophthalmologists as a result of the fitness boom of the 1960s. As a new discipline, it benefited from American innovation, an advanced national eye-care programme and generous financial backing from the optical industry.

In the 1920s, an Oklahoma optometrist, Alexander Skefft, developed behavioural optometry (Gregg, 1987) on the premise that visual skills are learned and could be further improved by training (Holland, 1993). Since 1979, the Sports Vision Section of the American Optometric Association (AOA) has undertaken vision screening of elite athletes in conjunction with the United States Olympic Committee (Sherman, 1990). In 1992, Bausch & Lomb became a worldwide sponsor of the Olympic Games and vision centres were subsequently established to screen the athletes' vision at Olympic villages (Albertville, France, 1992; Barcelona, Spain, 1992; Lillehammer, Norway, 1994).

Following the example of the Pacific University College of Optometry in 1980, other schools introduced sports vision into their curricula. Individual practitioners and universities, such as Pacific, set up sports vision clinics and also screened athletes' vision on site. Gradually optometrists and ophthalmologists were appointed as vision consultants to professional teams, especially in baseball (Gregg, 1987).

In 1984, the National Academy of Sports Vision (NASV) was formed by Dr A.I. Garner with the aim of maximizing visual performance and minimizing eye injuries in sport. To reflect the global aspects of sports vision, the organization changed its title to International and also assumed a multidisciplinary profile by organizing a joint conference with sports medicine. It also affiliated itself to more general sporting organizations such as the United States Sports Academy and the National Athletes Trainers Association. Both the Sports Vision Section of the AOA and the NASV promote a vigorous continuing education programme for their members through symposia and publications.

In the 1970s North American ophthalmologists jointly addressed the problem of sports-induced eye injuries. The result of their deliberations was the mandatory use of face masks in hockey (Rousseau *et al.*, 1982), standards were published to provide eye protection in racquet sports (CSA P400–M1, see Canadian Standards Association, 1982; and ASTM F803–88, see American Society for Testing and Materials, 1988) and the use of eye protectors was made compulsory in certain states (Jones, 1990) and tournaments (Chapter 11). Sports-induced eye injuries are preventable by players simply wearing suitable protectors and yet remain a significant cause of lost vision. It is nevertheless heartening to note (Prestage, 1990) that eye injuries arising in hockey and squash in North America have significantly reduced as a result of wearing eye protectors (A.F. Garner, 1993 and A. Reichow, 1994, personal communications).

Summary

Most people in the Western world are likely to be involved in sporting activities, either as participants or spectators. It is, therefore, perhaps surprising that most eye-care practitioners do not provide comprehensive and routine sports vision eye-care services. However, sports vision, a relatively new but exciting aspect of multidisciplinary eye care, is rapidly expanding to meet this need. Many optometrists, opticians and ophthalmologists, as well as sportspeople, organizations, trainers and coaches, are becoming aware of the advantages of safe and efficient vision in sport. How these criteria may be achieved is covered in the following chapters.

Acknowledgements

I wish to express my appreciation to those colleagues who offered advice, second opinions or unpublished data which is acknowledged under personal communication. Also my sincere thanks to Mrs Freda M. Taylor for typing the script.

References

Abernethy, B. (1986) Enhancing sports performance through clinical and experimental optometry. *Clinical and Experimental Optometry*, **69**, 189–196

Acuvision (1992) *CAS/Acuvision Training Manual*, Acuvision Systems Ltd, San Diego, Ca

Allard, F. (1980/81) Perception and sport skill. *Coaching Science Update*, **2**, 52–55

Allard, F. Graham, S. and Paarsalu, M.E. (1980) Perception in sport: basketball. *Journal of Sports Psychology*, **2**, 14–21

American Society for Testing and Materials (1988) F803–88 *Standard Specification for Eye Protectors for Use by Players of Racquet Sports*, ASTM, Philadelphia

Bahill, A.T. and La Ritz, T. (1984) Why can't batters keep their eyes on the ball? *American Scientist*, **72**, 249–253

Bausch & Lomb (1992) *Bausch & Lomb's Olympic Vision*, Monograph, Bausch & Lomb Inc., Rochester, NY

Beashel, P. and Taylor J. (1992) *Sport Examined*, 2nd edn, Thomas Nelson & Son, Walton on Thames

Beitel, P. (1980) Multivariate relationships among visual perception attributes and gross motor tasks with different environmental demands. *Journal of Motor Behaviour*, **12**, 20–40

British Standards Institution (1979) BS 4410 *Eye Protectors for Vehicle Users*, BSI, London

British Standards Institution (1987a) BS 2092 *Eye Protectors for Industrial and Non-Industrial Use*, BSI, London

British Standards Institution, (1987b) BS 2724 *Sun Glare Eye Protectors for General Use*, BSI, London

British Standards Institution Sub Committee (1993) Draft: PSM/219 *Specification for Eye Protectors for Squash and Other Racquet Sports*, BSI, London

Canadian Standards Association (1982) CSA P400–M1 *Racquet Sports Eye Protection*, CSA, Ontario

Carpenter, R.H.S. (1988) *Movements of the Eyes*, Pion, London, pp. 313–15

Cockerill, I.M. and MacGillivary, W. (1981) *Vision and Sport*, Stanley Thornes, Cheltenham

Coffey, B. and Reichow, A.W. (1986) Optometric evaluation of the elite athlete: optometric visual performance profiling–a report regarding the American Optometric Association, Sports Vision Section, National Sports Festival Vision Screening Programme. *American Optometric Association Sports Vision Section, News and Views*, **2**, 6

Coffey, B. and Reichow, A.W. (1987) Guidelines for screening and testing the athletes visual system, Part III: Optometric extension program foundation. *Curriculum II*, **59**, 355–368

Coffey, B. and Reichow, A.W. (1990) Optometric evaluation of the elite athlete: the Pacific Sports Visual Profile. *Problems in Optometry*, **1**, 32–58

Daland, J. (1917) Eskimo snow blindness and goggles. *Optometric Journal and Review of Optometry*, **39**, 1334–8

Ditchburn, R. and Ginsborg, B. (1952) Vision with

stabilized retinal image. *Nature*, **36**, 36–37

Ditchburn, R., Fenner, D. and Mayne, S. (1959) Vision with controlled movement of the retinal image. *Journal of Physiology*, **145**, 98–107

Duke-Elder, S. (1970) *System of Ophthalmology*, vol. 5, Henry Kimpton, London, p. 609

Edmunds, F.R. (1992) *Sports Vision Program*, Bausch & Lomb, International Professional Services, Rochester, NY

Edmunds, F.R. (1993) Olympic Vision Centre: preliminary results. *Contact Europe*, **1**, 11 (Bausch & Lomb, European Headquarters, Kingston upon Thames)

Falkowitz, C. and Mendol, H. (1977) The role of visual skills in batting averages. *Optometric Weekly*, **68**, 577–80

Garner, A.I. (1977a) An overlooked problem: athlete's visual needs. *Physician and Sports Medicine*, **5**, 74–82

Garner, A.I. (1977b) Visual aid prescribing for the athlete. *Californian Optometrist*, **3**, 18–19

Garner, A.I. (1994) Sports vision: then and now. *Sports Vision*, **10**, 42–44

Granda, J. (1994) *American Optometric Association Sports Vision Section, News and Views*, 15 April, p. 10A

Graham, R. (1949) The corneal lens. A progress report. *American Journal of Optometry and the Archives of the American Academy of Optometry*, **26**, 75–7

Gregg, J.R. (1987) *Vision and Sports: An Introduction*, Butterworths, Stoneham, Mass.

Hanson, P. (1988) *The Joy of Stress*, Pan Books, London

Hale, C.J. (1992) Vision in sports, *Sports Vision*, **8**, 26–9

Herschel, J.F.W. (1983) *Light Encyclopaedia Britannica*, 5th edn

Holland, K. (1993) Training the eye on sporting success. *The Optician*, **5412**, 16–18

Hubbard, A.W. and Seng, C.N. (1954) Visual movements of patterns. *Research Quarterly*, **25**, 42–57

Hubel, D.H. (1988) *Eye, Brain and Vision*, W.H. Freeman, London

Hubel, D.H. and Weisel, T.N. (1962) Receptive fields, binocular interaction and functional architecture in the cat's visual cortex. *Journal of Physiology*, **160**, 559–68

Hughes, C. (1980) *The Football Association Coaching Book of Soccer Tactics and Skills*, BBC Publishing, London

International Football Association Board (1991–92) *Referee's Chart and Player's Guide to the Laws of Football*, Pan Books, London

Ivins, P. (1992) Carrying the torch. *The Optician*, **5375**, 15–20

Jewell, B. (1977) *Heritage of the Past: Sports and Games*, John G. Eccles, Inverness

Jones, N.P. (1990) The incidence and severity of eye injuries in racquet sports. In *Eye Protection in Racquet Sports*, joint symposium organized by the Royal National Institute for the Blind and The City University, London

Kaplan, E., Lee, B.B. and Kulikowski, J.J. (1989) The role of P&M systems. In *Seeing and Colour* (eds J.J. Kulikowski,

C.M. Dickinson and I.I. Murray), Pergamon Press, Oxford, pp. 224–37

Kiernan, J.A. (1987) *Introduction to Human Neuro-Science*, J.B. Lippincott, Philadelphia

Leslie, S. (1993) Visual skills important for hockey. *Australian Optometry*, February, p. 16

Loran, D.F.C. (1992) Eye injuries in squash. *The Optician*, **5344**, 18–26

Ludvigh, E. and Miller, J.M. (1958) Study of visual acuity during ocular pursuit of moving test objects. I. Introduction. *Journal of the Optical Society of America*, **48**, 799–802

McCrone, J. (1993) Shots faster than the speed of thought. *The Independent on Sunday*, 27 June, p. 71

MacEwen, C.J. (1989) A prospective study of 5,671 cases. *British Journal of Ophthalmology*, **73**, 888–94

MacGregor, R.J.S. (1992) Collecting ophthalmic antiques. *Ophthalmic Antiques Collection Club*, Saltcoats, p. 32

Miller, D.M. (1960) The relation between some visual perception factors and the degree of success realized by sport performers. *Dissertation Abstracts International*, **21**, 1455–A

Mintel, (1993) Male and female participation in sport, 1992. *Recreation*, **52**, 8

Mizusawa, K., Sweeting, R.L. and Knouse, S.B. (1983) Comparative studies of color fields. Visual acuity fields and movement perception limits among varsity athletes and non-varsity groups. *Perceptual Motor Skills*, **56**, 887–92

Mowen, S. (1976) Eye tracking during the tennis forehand volley. Masters Thesis, Texas Women's University, Denton

Office of Population Censuses and Surveys, Social Security Division (1987) *The General Household Survey*, HMSO, London

Olsen, E.A. (1956) Relationship between psychological capacities and success in college athletes. *Research Quarterly of the American Association of Health and Physical Education*, **27**, 79–89

Pashby, T.J., Pashby, R.C., Chisholm, L.D.J. and Crawford, J.S. (1975) Eye injuries in Canadian hockey. *Canadian Medical Association Journal of Ophthalmology*, **113**, 663–6

Pashby, T.J. (1977) Eye injuries in Canadian hockey: Phase II. *Canadian Medical Association Journal*, **117**, 671–8

Pashby, T.J. (1979) Eye injuries in Canadian hockey: Phase III. *Canadian Medical Association Journal*, **121**, 643–4

Planter, P. and Breedlove, H. (1993) Youth sports and sports vision. *Sports Vision*, **9**, 22–8

Prestage, M. (1990) Eye protection in racquet sports: the need for a European Standard. In *Eye Protection in Racquet Sports*, joint symposium organized by the Royal National Institute for the Blind and The City University, London

Rabkins, S. (1984) Recent advances in sports vision: the pros and cons of radial keratotomy. Lecture delivered to Sports Vision, 84 West

Reichow, A.W., Coffey, B., Wacho, C.M. and Velnousky,

D.A. (1981) Visual evaluation of the elite athlete: optometric visual profiling. *American Journal of Optometry and Physiological Optics*, **63**, p. 80 (abstract)

Rousseau, A.P., Amyot, M. and Labelle, P.L. (1982) Winter sports: hockey and skiing. In *Sports Ophthalmology* (eds C.D. Pizzarello and B.G. Haig), Charles C. Thomas, Springfield, Ill., pp. 149–69

Sadun, A. (1986) Neuroanatomy of the human visual system Part I. Retinal projections to the LGN and pretectum as demonstrated with a new method. *Neuro-Ophthalmology*, **6**, 353–61

Sasini, L.S. (1950) *Spectacle Fitting and Optical Dispensing*. Hamond and Hamond, London

Sears, Roebuck & Co. (1896) *Catalogue*, Chicago, p. 463

Sheridan, M.D. (1989) *Spontaneous Play in Early Childhood*, Nfeb–Nelson Publishing Group, Windsor, pp. 9–19

Sherman, A. (1990) Sports vision testing and enhancement: implications for winter sports. In *Winter Sports Medicine* (eds M. Casey, C. Foster and E. Hixson), F.A. Davis, Philadelphia, pp. 74–84

Shick, J. (1971) Relationship between depth perception and hand–eye dominance and free throw shooting in college women. *Perceptual Motor Skills*, **33**, 539–42

Silver, J. (1986) Hazards of 'sunglasses'; towards simple standards for labelling and testing. In *Hazards of Light: Myths and Realities. Eye and Skin* (eds J. Cronly-Dillon, E. Rosen and J. Marshall), Proceedings of the First International Symposium of the Northern Eye Institute, University of Manchester, Pergamon Press, Oxford

Sinclair, J.M. (1991) *Collins English Dictionary*, 3rd edn, Harper Collins, Glasgow

Sports Vision Association (1994) Second International Conference. *Optometry Today*, **64**, 6

Standards Association of Australia (1992) AS/NZS 4066 *Eye Protection in Racquet Sports*, Standards Association of Australia, Sydney

Starkes, J.L. and Deakin, J. (1984) Perception in sport: A cognitive approach to skilled performance. In (eds W.F. Straub, and J.M. Williams), *Cognitive Sport Psychology* Lansing, NY, Sport Science Association, pp. 115–28

Stein, H., Slatt, B. and Stein, R. (1987) Visual approach to winning tennis. In *Sports Ophthalmology* (eds C.D. Pizzarello and B.G. Haig), Charles C. Thomas, Spring-field, Ill., pp. 81–104

Summers, E.F. (1974) Tennis ability and its relationship to Selon performance tasks. *Dissertation Abstracts International*, **34**, 5697

Temple, C. (1993) 'Lewis Christie shadowing could all be for nought', *The Sunday Times*, 16 May, Sport One, p. 8

ten Napel, J.A. (1993) Can visual training improve atheletic performance? In *Transactions of the First International Meeting of the Sports Vision Association*, The City University, London

Touhy, K.M. (1948) US Patent 2510438

Touhy, J.M. (1963) The birth of an idea. *Optometric World*, **50**, 14–20

Trachtman, J. (1991) Visual demands of minor league baseball players. *Sports Vision*, **7**, 8–11

Trachtman, J.N. and Kluka, D.A. (1993) Future trends in vision as they relate to sports performance. *International Journal of Sports Vision*, **1**, 1–7

Valberg, A. and Lee, B.B. (1991) *From Pigments to Perception*, Plenum Press, New York

Vinger, P.F. (1980) Sports-related eye injury. A preventable problem. In *Perspectives in Refraction* (ed. M.L. Rubin) (*Survey of Ophthalmology* 25); 47–51

Vogel, G. and Hale, R. (1992) Does participation in organized athletics increase a child's scoring ability on the Wayne Saccadic Fixater? *Journal of Behavioural Optometry*, **3**, 66–9

Wichterle, O. and Lim, D. (1960) Hydrophilic gels for biological uses. *Nature*, **185**, 117

Widdows, R. (1989) *The Hamlyn Book of Football Techniques and Tactics*, Treasure Press, London

Williams, J.M. and Thier, J. (1975) Horizontal and peripheral vision in male and female athletes and non athletes. *Research Quarterly of the American Association for Health and Physical Education*, **46**, 200–5

Wood, G.A. (1981) The effect of exercise-induced fatigue on visual reaction time. In *Vision and Sport* (eds I.M. Cockerill and W. MacGillivary), Stanley Thornes, Cheltenham, pp. 80–4

Zeki, S.M. (1993) *A Vision of the Brain*, Blackwell Scientific Publications, Oxford

2

Vision requirements in sport
John J. Gardner and Arnold Sherman

Introduction

The general heading of 'sport' covers a myriad of events which rely on varying degrees of skill, strength and endurance. The skill of the visual system is of paramount importance to many, if not most, athletic endeavours. This chapter provides descriptions of procedures used to test an athlete's visual input and motor responses related to the multiple anatomical, physiological and neurological aspects of vision that produce functional percepts. This is the information upon which the participant can act during the course of an athletic event.

Table 2.1 outlines a theoretical profile of the visual skills involved in a broad spectrum of sports. From this summary it can be seen that specific visual skills are often associated with certain sports but sporting activities generally require a wide and varied range of visual demands.

While it is generally agreed that vision is the primary sense modality used to obtain information from our environment, it is important to distinguish between sight and vision with regard to sport. Sight is the ability of the eye to resolve detail and to see clearly while vision is the interpretation of that which is seen. Sherman (1990) isolates the elements involved in the process of vision as the eyes, brain and body. Vision utilizes the eyes for input (sight); the brain integrates this information with other senses (inter-sensory matching) and stimulates the action systems of the body (neuromuscular) for output (response). Feedback is built into the visual system for correction, adjustment and refinement of vision and response. Sherman (1990) proffers that the entire process constitutes the visual system and therefore is not only limited to the external sense organs (eyes) (see Figure 2.1).

Vision, therefore, refers to the ability to gain meaning from the what the eyes see. Because of its integrative nature, vision depends on previous experience in order for the athlete to gather, analyse, process, store, retrieve and respond to the input quickly and efficiently in the context of an event. The speed with which this action is taken may distinguish winners from losers among athletes. For example, in baseball, it takes approximately 400 milliseconds (ms) from the time that the pitcher releases the ball until it reaches the home plate; and it takes approximately 200 ms to make the visual decision whether to swing or not to swing.

Visual assessment

In assessing sportspeople, one must first investigate the health and accuracy of the input system and the efficiency and accuracy

Table 2.1 Theoretical profile of the visual skills involved in a broad spectrum of sports

	Visual acuity	Dynamic visual acuity	Ocular-motor skills	Eye–hand coordination	Depth perception	Accommodation/vergence facility	Central–peripheral awareness	Visual reaction time	Visual adjustability	Visualization
Archery	4	1	3	5	2	3	5	1	5	2
Baseball hit and cricket	4	5	5	5	5	5	5	5	5	5
Baseball pitch	3	2	3	4	3	3	5	1	3	5
Basketball	3	3	4	5	5	3	5	5	5	5
Bowling/bowls	2	1	3	5	3	2	4	1	3	4
Boxing	2	2	5	5	3	3	5	5	5	4
Cricket wicket-keeper	4	5	5	5	5	5	5	5	5	3
Cricket bowler	3	2	3	4	3	5	5	1	3	5
Cricket fielding	4	5	4	4	4	4	3	3	3	2
Cycling (road racing)	5	5	5[a]	4	5	2	5	5	4	5
Darts	4	1	3	5	3	3	5	1	1	3
Diving (spring board and platform)	2	3	2	3	3	1	5	2	3	5
Football[d]	4	5	5	5	5	3	5	5	5	5
Golf	3	1	4	5	5	3	5	1	3	5
Gymnastics	1	3	3	5	5	3	5	5	5	5
Handball	4	5	5	5	5	3	5	5	5	3
High jump	3	3	4	3	5	3	5	4	3	5
Hockey (goalie)	4	5	5	5	5	5	5	5	5	3
Hurdles	4	4	4	4	4	3	4	3	4	5
Kayaking	4	4	4	5	5	3	5	5	3	5
Mountaineering	5[b]	3	2	5	5	3	5	5	3	5
Pool/snooker/billiards	2	1	4[a]	5	5	2	3	1	4	5
Race car driving	5	5	5	4	5	2	5	5	5	5
Racquetball/squash	4	5	5	4	5	4	5	5	5	5
Running	1	1	2	1	1	1	4	3	1	4
Shooters (clay pigeon, skeet, trap, hunting, long gun)	5	5	4	5	5	5	5	5	4	5

Table 2.1 Continued

	Visual acuity	Dynamic visual acuity	Ocular-motor skills	Eye-hand coordination	Depth perception	Accommodation/vergence facility	Central-peripheral awareness	Visual reaction time	Visual adjustability	Visualization
Shooters (range, fixed distance)	4	2	3	5	2	3	5	1	1	2
Skiing	5	5	5	5	5	3	5	5	5	5
Soccer[d]	3	4	5	5[c]	5	3	5	5	5	5
Soccer goal-keeping	4	5	5	5	5	5	5	5	5	3
Swimming	1	1	1	1	1	1	4	3	1	4
Tennis/table tennis	4	5	5	5	5	5	5	5	5	5
Track – high jump	1	3	3	4	4	3	3	4	4	4
Track – pole vault	1	3	3	5	5	3	4	4	4	5
Volleyball	4	5	5	5	5	3	5	4	4	5
Weightlifting	1	1	1	2	1	1	1	1	1	5
Wrestling	2	1	1	3	2	1	3	5	5	4

[a] A pattern ESO deviations or V pattern EXO deviations can significantly affect performance in these sports.
[b] Contrast sensitivity may be crucial (to the point of being life-saving) in this sport.
[c] Eye-body (foot–head–chest) coordination.
[d] Including American football, Australian rules football, Canadian rules football, Gaelic football, rugby league and rugby union.

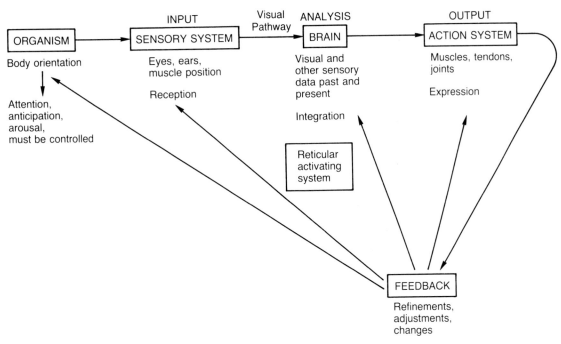

Figure 2.1 Elements involved in visual processing

of the output system. It is important, therefore, to consider:

1. General ocular health
2. Static visual acuity
3. Contrast sensitivity
4. Dynamic visual acuity
5. Binocular vision performance
6. Depth perception/stereopsis
7. Accommodation
8. Eye–hand coordination
9. Eye–body coordination
10. Central peripheral awareness

General ocular health

The good health of the eyes, ocular adnexa and visual pathway is mandatory for optimal sporting performance. Baseline examination of the eyes includes full anterior segment and fundus examination plus charting of the visual field. Any abnormality must be noted, photographed if possible and fully explained to the player. Since most of the equipment necessary to undertake the entire battery of the ocular health tests is too cumbersome to take to the site of a screening, it is recommended that a letter (and/or legal release) explaining this be given to each athlete at the time of the on-site screening and an appointment be made for a subsequent eye health examination.

Visual acuity

Three forms of visual acuity (see Glossary) are generally considered by vision professionals. They are:

1. Static visual acuity (VA)
2. Contrast sensitivity
3. Dynamic visual acuity (DVA)

1. Static visual acuity

Players must be tested with their full correction in place if worn for their sport. If the player does not wear a correction while performing their sport, they should be tested without this. In compensation for ametropia, the benefits of correction must be weighed against the detriment of the corrective device. In small refractive errors, spectacles or contact lenses may improve visual acuity on a letter chart, but may interfere with the sport (e.g. running) more than they help to accomplish the task.

Static visual acuity is the ability to see a non-moving target at a fixed distance. Conventional letter charts are used (Snellen letters and Landolt rings) at 20 feet (6 m) to test the static visual acuity. Binocular readings are taken first and the player is asked by the examiner to read the 'smallest line that you can see'. In this test of static visual acuity, neither the target nor the player is moving–a situation not encountered in many sports events.

Some examples of sports illustrated in Table 2.1 with high, medium and low demand of static visual acuity are as follows:

(a) High demand: target sports such as archery, static pistol, rifle shooting and darts are all examples of high demand, static acuity activities.

(b) Medium demand: basketball demands medium visual acuity. The player playing defence must watch the eyes of the opponent to see whether the opponent is going to look upwards towards the basket or look in one direction or another towards a team mate to whom they may pass. Often, this change of gaze must be seen from some distance to be able to determine the best defensive action.

(c) Low demand: an example of low demand of visual acuity is the lineman in American football. This player must concern himself with a relatively large, relatively slow-moving object, i.e. the opponent, usually no more than 3–10 feet away. Therefore, he does not necessarily have to see exceptionally small objects at great distances. A second example, although this one is debatable, is that of gymnasts on the rings or on the asymmetric bars who do not have to see very small images at great distances in order to perform their task accurately.

2. Contrast sensitivity

Tests of contrast sensitivity (see Glossary) can be conducted on commercially available units, some of which, because of size and portability, are appropriate for on-site testing (e.g. The Stereo-optical Co. Holladay Contrast Acuity Test) while others can be integrated into in-

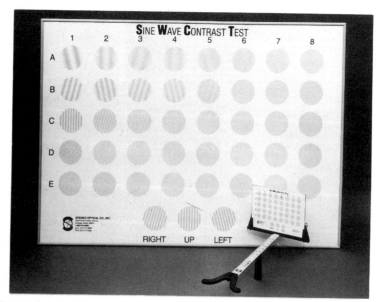

Figure 2.2 Distance and near contrast sensitivity tests designed for office/practice use. (Courtesy Stereo Optical Co. Inc.)

office sports vision testing (e.g. the Vistech and Stereo-optical Sine Wave Contrast Test), which is shown in Figure 2.2. The tests assess the player's ability to detect separation of areas of different contrast levels. They can be in the form of a projected chart or a fixed wall chart and near charts are also available. Coffey and Reichow (1990) observed that most sports involve visual discrimination of contrast that is much more subtle than the black on white high contrast of the Snellen letter chart. Further, the authors report that the athlete's performance on a Vistech unit exceeds the norms published by that company for a 'normal' population.

These contrast sensitivity tests cannot be memorized and the correct answers conveyed from one person to the next. This aspect of the contrast sensitivity target protects the integrity of the results.

3. Dynamic visual acuity

Dynamic visual acuity (DVA) is also known as kinetic visual acuity and is the visual acuity as determined when either the test target or the observer is in motion. It is the ability to detect the detail of an object in the field of vision when there is relative movement between the player and the object. This test is conventionally performed under binocular conditions and is closely related to the on-court visual demand.

Ludvigh and Miller (1958) introduced a test to assess would-be pilots, which Sherman (1990) has described as being useful for evaluating the DVA of athletes. In this test, a Landolt ring suddenly appears on a screen travelling at a constant angular velocity. The object is seen and the athlete being tested estimates the direction and angular velocity of the movement in degrees per second. The brain then sends a message to the extra-ocular muscles, causing innervation appropriate to place and to hold the image of the object in the vicinity of the fovea for a sufficiently long period of time to permit the resolution of the

critical detail. It is the total efficiency of this complex process that is measured by the DVA test.

DVA may also be tested with a Kirschner rotator, which is an oculorotor device utilizing a Snellen chart projected on to a rotating mirror with an arc diameter of 55 cm at 3 m (10 ft) testing distance. Sherman (1985) devised a sports vision disc (illustrated in Figure 2.3) which can be used to test and train dynamic visual acuity and ocular motor accuracy. The large letters are 10/30 and the small letters are 10/15. Using a simple children's gramophone or phonograph, DVA can be scored at 78, 45 and 33 rpm. The norm established utilizing more than 1000 athletes is 10/15 acuity at 45 rpm (Sherman, 1981). Coffey and Reichow (1990) described a similar method of measuring DVA with rotating targets. Targets sweeping across the field of vision have also been used by other researchers (Long and Penn, 1987, Long and Garvey, 1988; Rouse et al., 1988). It is likely that, with emerging advances in computer technology and virtual reality, it will soon be possible to measure a player's visual demand in three dimensions and also to train increased recognition skills.

Dynamic visual acuity is typically faster in goal- and wicket-keepers, baseball and cricket batsmen and tennis players. Conversely, it is less critical in athletes whose sports do not require them to follow fast-moving targets. Sanderson and Whiting (1978) indicated that DVA and baseball catching performance are related, whereas static visual acuity is unrelated to both DVA and baseball catching performance. It should be emphasized that the major factor in DVA is precise ocular-motor coordination.

The eye health-care professional can modify acuity by limiting exposure time of the target utilizing a slide projector with a short exposure attachment, known as a tachistoscope (LaFayette Engineering). This is commercially available as a 'tach unit' (Wayne Engineering). The target is presented for 0.01 seconds and the player is asked to write down the numbers

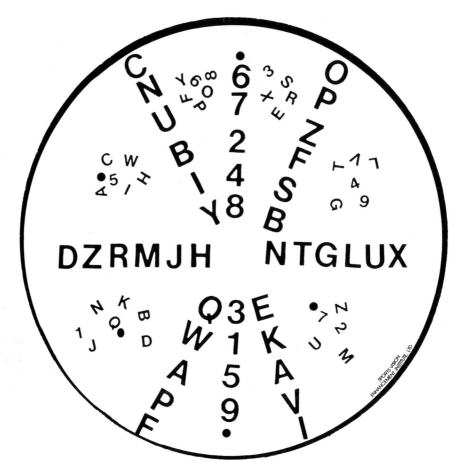

Figure 2.3   The Sherman Dynamic Acuity Disc

or patterns seen. Sherman (1990) uses tic-tac-toe (or noughts and crosses) patterns for testing and number, word or domino patterns for training. Such recognition accuracy appears to be critical to such high-speed sports as baseball, cricket, tennis, hockey and car racing. Training with tachistoscopic presentation improves the attention and concentration which is necessary for good athletic performance.

The following are some examples from Table 2.1 of sports with high, medium and low demand of dynamic visual acuity.

(a) High demand: the baseball or cricket batsman, who must see the ball moving towards him at high speed and must determine how to instruct the neuromuscular system to perform, i.e. to swing or not to swing at a given pitch has a high demand for dynamic visual acuity. Another example is the American footballer who is receiving the punt or the rugby player going for the 'up-and-under'. He must be able to judge the speed and the distance of the ball as well as the height of the ball relative to where he is going to catch it. At the same time, he must make judgement with quick glances towards the oncoming opponent who is going to tackle him after he catches the ball.

The tennis player, while hitting an overhead, must look up to determine the distance, speed and direction of the overhead shot and make some assessment of the position of his opponent to receive his shot. Further examples include the hockey goaltender who has to determine the relative movement between him-self and the hockey puck. Similar demands are required of soccer goal-keepers, cricket wicket-keepers and clay pigeon shooters.

(b) Medium demand: the basketball player who is trying to determine the speed at which the ball is moving as it is passed from one opponent to the next has a medium demand of dynamic visual acuity. At the same time, he is working to position himself to intercept the pass and attempting to determine how quickly his oppo-nent is moving to receive that pass. Another good example is soccer, where players must determine the speed of the ball and the angle at which it is moving and be able to position themselves accordingly to receive the pass, intercept or interrupt play.

(c) Low demand: there is a low demand of dynamic visual acuity in golf, where there is virtually no movement of either the ball or the player provided the player's head stays still. The position of the ball and the fixed position of the player's head negates any necessity to use dynamic visual acuity because there is no relative movement between the player and the object.

At this point in the evaluation, the eye health-care professional can state that the player has healthy eyes which, if the refractive error is corrected, can gather information efficiently. The next major aspect of the visual system is the integration of the information gathered from each eye into a binocular percept.

Binocular vision

The twelve extra-ocular muscles (EOMs) con-stitute a fascinating tribute to the design of the human sensory-motor system. The actions of these muscles are coordinated with the mus-cles of the lids, intra-ocular muscles and those controlling head movements. The EOMs are innervated by the IIIrd, IVth and VIth cranial nerves. Each eye movement is precisely coor-dinated to that of the other eye via centres and interconnections within the central nervous system.

Evaluation of each athlete's extra-ocular movements and binocular function includes

fixation, speed and accuracy of pursuit and saccadic eye movements and the ability to converge and diverge.

It is recommended that sports vision practi-tioners should apply the principles of visual task analysis so that an athlete's vision is examined not only in the primary position but also at work distances and locations specific to their sport. The cover test may detect whether an athlete has a latent (heterophoria) or manifest (heterotropia) squint, either of which may affect sports performance. In screening binocular function, the cover test should be performed and the deviation measured with the fixation target at all nine positions of gaze. Sports vision practitioners must also be mind-ful of the importance of concomitance when screening athletes' vision. This is most sig-nificant when the condition is of recent onset and is most likely to occur in contact sports. Alphabetical syndromes, such as A or V patterns, may affect sports as disparate as bicycle racing, snooker (billiards and pool) and basketball where the player's head is in a position with the eyes concentrated in upgaze. Such a binocular deviation can lead to erratic performance as general body fatigue becomes a factor. Having the player simulate their active sports position may often uncover a binocular problem not found with the head in the straight-ahead position.

The Brock string test is a simple method of evaluating suppression and accuracy of ocular alignment. This is a cord of approximately 10 feet in length (although it can be much longer) usually with three coloured beads or buttons positioned at various lengths on the cord. One end of the string is attached to a fixed object (wall, doorknob or basketball rim) and the other end is held up the player's nose as shown in Figure 2.4. The subject is instructed to look at the bead at the middle of the string. If both eyes are converged and focused on the bead, the subject should see a double string approaching the bead, meeting at the bead and a double string diverging from that crossing. The ability to perform this test depends on physiological diplopia, which

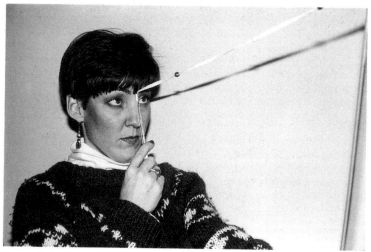

Figure 2.4 The Brock string tilted in the habitual sports viewing position (e.g. upwards in sports such as volleyball, basketball and high jumping)

indicates that suppression does not exist. The accuracy of binocular function is determined by the string meeting at the object of regard (the bead). If the string appears to meet closer than the bead, this is known as exoprojection and if beyond the bead, esoprojection. This may be important in basketball, as esoprojectors tend to see targets closer than they are and therefore may undershoot, while exoprojectors tend to see targets further than they are and therefore overshoot.

The following are some examples of sports from Table 2.1 with high, medium and low demand of ocular-motor skills.

(a) High demand: in boxing, the participant has to make very rapid eye movements to assess the position of the opponent's hands, eyes and body position in order to achieve a successful punch. The hitter in cricket or baseball must be able to make rapid convergence and saccadic fixations. These ocular-motor skills are necessary to track the ball properly and to communicate its relative position in space to the neuromuscular system to position the bat to make contact.

(b) Medium demand: gymnastics makes a medium demand of ocular-motor skills. For example, while vaulting, gymnasts must sprint down a runway and assess their relative position in space by converging and making rapid fixation to determine their exact position relative to the vault itself. This is of medium demand because the speed of movement involved is determined by the gymnast's speed while approaching the box.

(c) Long distance running requires very little fixation other than a very general long distance viewing of the track or path over which the athlete is running. Another example of a sport with a low demand of ocular-motor skill is swimming, especially in long distance events.

Depth perception/stereopsis

While the terms depth perception and stereopsis are similar, they are not entirely synonymous (see Glossary). Monocular individuals may have depth perception which is derived from various clues such as parallax, overlap, shadow, relative target speeds and sizes.

One-eyed athletes would not be disadvantaged in sports such as running and swimming which do not require critical depth perception. However, as mentioned in Chapter 1, athletes with established binocular vision who suddenly lose the sight of one eye may find themselves seriously disadvantaged in many sports which require accurate and rapid stereopsis for successful participation, such as motor racing or skiing (see Table 2.1).

Tests for stereopsis use polaroids or anaglyphic materials which permit slightly disparate points of the observed object to be viewed by each eye of the person being tested. Stereoacuity is expressed as seconds of arc and is the ability to detect the difference between the image presented to each eye and to perceive that as depth.

The design of most tests of stereopsis requires that they be done at the conventional near point test distance of 16 inches (40 cm). Most athletic events that require stereopsis, however, require it beyond this distance. The Howard–Dolman apparatus tests retinal disparity at a distance of 20 feet by aligning pegs but is inappropriate for office and/or on-site testing. There are, if necessary, vectographs that can be projected and separated in slight increments to create retinal disparity and, therefore, may be used to evaluate stereopsis at various distances and direction of gaze. The Mentor BVAT (binocular visual acuity test) has the ability to evaluate stereopsis at 10 feet (3 m) or more and has been modified to make it portable for on-site testing. This test is a television-based system in which a subject views targets through polarized goggles. Stereoacuity is measured in seconds of arc by viewing a diamond configuration of circles and the observer is asked to report which one appears closest.

Fusion may be classified as motor or sensory: the quantity of motor fusion may be evaluated by measuring the prism fusion range and the sensory fusiion quantified in stereopsis terms in seconds of arc. The quality of fusion may be inferred but not evaluated by the existence of signs and symptoms such as headaches, eye strain and evidence of intermittent suppression by formal testing or by observing player effort including frowning or squinting.

The following are some examples from Table 2.1 of sports with high, medium and low demand of depth perception or stereopsis.

(a) High demand: cycling, hitting in cricket or baseball, and blocking a shot in hockey or soccer represent high demands of knowing exactly where the object of regard is in space in order to accomplish or complete the task.
(b) Medium demand: in platform diving and basketball, the player must complete the task by a given position in space and is performed at very high speed.
(c) Low demand: wrestling and weightlifting have been successfully performed by players who have significantly compromised binocular vision and therefore little or no depth perception.

Accommodation

Accommodation is closely linked with the vergence system: focusing on close objects is associated with convergence and relaxing accommodation to fixate in the distance is accompanied by divergence. Tests of the accommodative facility may be accomplished by controlling the vergence demand, for example by using plus or minus lenses to blur test letters, as shown in Figure 2.5. This test determines the accommodative ability relative to vergence at specific distances such as 16 inches or 40 cm.

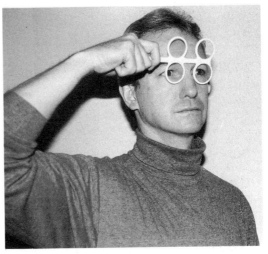

Figure 2.5 The Flipper Accommodation Test comprises pairs of +2.00 and –2.00 dioptre spheres

Accommodative cycles from near to far to near again probably yield the most beneficial information because they mimic the real-life siutation. An example is the operation of a motor vehicle, in which the driver looks from the road to the odometer/speedometer and then back down the road. In this example, one sees that rapid and accurate change must take place in order to assure safe operation of the motor vehicle.

To test accommodation, flipper lenses as shown in Figure 2.5 of +2.00 and −2.00 are used binocularly and monocularly at 16 inches (40 cm). The norms established are 8 cycles per minute binocularly and 11 cycles per minute monocularly. Another test used is the Haynes distance rock test that utilizes a 20/60 (6/18) row of letters for the distance target (6 m) and a 20/40 (6/12) row at near. The test subject calls out the first letter on the distance chart then refocuses to the first letter on the near chart then back to the second letter on the distance then back to the second letter on the the near chart and so forth. The examiner counts the number of correct cycles completed in 30 seconds. The results of this test may be contaminated by poor near–far saccadic fixations.

Example of some sports from Table 2.1 with high, medium and low demand of accommodation are:

(a) High demand: tennis players need to track an approaching ball by quickly focusing and converging as it moves towards them. After striking the ball, the eyes diverge and relax accommodation very rapidly to follow the flight of the ball and the position of the opponent. Another example is table tennis, where the same accommodative convergence and divergence applies.
(b) Medium demand: hurdlers in track and field events must change focus and converge to the exact take-off position to clear the hurdle and then change focus again, very rapidly, to the next hurdle in order to determine their position and modify their stride.
(c) Low demand: in long distance running, swimming and weightlifting the visual information comes much more slowly. Consequently, accommodation is a very low demand ability in such sports.

Mid-chapter recap

The eye health-care professional has now established that the eyes are healthy, the images on both retinas are sharp and accurate, and that those two images are formed into one binocular percept which is held accurately in the visual system at all distances and in all directions of gaze. The next step is to assess what can be done with that information. That is, the visual percept must be analysed, interpreted, and responded to intellectually, verbally, or by motor response.

Visual motor responses

Although visual reaction time (See Appendix 1) is widely used, the term is somewhat of a misnomer because what is actually being measured is the motor response to a visual stimulus. This measurement requires the use of specialized equipment, most commonly in the form of a computerized panel upon which are a number of lights attached to switches. Each of the following tests described herein refers to those available on the Wayne Saccadic Fixator, which is illustrated in Figure 2.6.

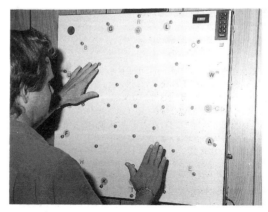

Figure 2.6 The Wayne Saccadic Fixator. (Courtesy Wayne Engineering Co. Inc.)

Eye-hand coordination

Multiple test modalities are available. Sherman (1983) suggests the following protocol: the centre of the saccadic fixator device is placed approximately at eye level. The habitual prescription for sports and normal overhead illumination are used

Part I of the test requires the athlete to press the button next to a red light. After this is done, the light moves randomly to another position on the board and remains there until the athlete hits that button. The number of 'hits' in 30 seconds is recorded as the 'visual proaction time'.

Part II requires the athlete to perform the same task, with the exception that the red light is now programmed to move randomly at the rate of one light per second. If the athlete does not react quickly enough, the light will move to the next position on the board without a 'hit' being recorded. This correct number of 'hits' in 30 seconds is read off the fixator and recorded as the 'visual reaction time'. Gardner (1988) believes that one second as the recommended norm is too long in this 'reactive' stage and recommends 0.75 seconds.

The person administering the test makes the instructions to the test subject very simple and avoids leading the person to any particular action: 'When the light comes on, hit it as quickly as possible and continue to hit as many lights as you can until the test stops.' In addition to the score achieved, the test administrator observes and records if the athlete:

1. Uses both hands to hit the lights or predominantly one. If one, which one?
2. Becomes flustered or upset during the test or stays calm and focused on the task.
3. Fixates on the centre of the target panel such that they demonstrate trust of their 'peripheral' vision (this test predominantly is a central vision task) or moves their head and eyes to search for the light before initiating motor movement of the arms or hands to hit the target. If a lot of eye and head movement is used, the score is likely to be lower and the performance slower than the score and performance of the athlete who maintains a fixed central gaze and consequently 'sees' the whole panel at once.

Early research by Sherman (1983) described what was called the 'sports vision average' (SVA), which is the ratio of the 'reaction' score to the 'proaction' score. For example, the SVA of the player who hit 20 targets on the 'reaction' portion and 30 targets on the 'proaction' portion would be computed as follows:

$$SVA = VR\ score/VP\ score \times 100 = 20/30$$
$$= 0.667$$

This SVA is of value if all players are scoring at the same relative level. However, when testing was done on younger children, it was found that lower scores denoted slower performance and whole numbers yielded the same SVA as scores that were higher and performances that were faster. For example, a 6-year-old boy who scored a 10 'reactive' and 15 'proactive' had an SVA = 10/15 = 0.667, the same SVA as the higher scoring adult in the preceding paragraph. Thus, what appeared to be a solid way to relate performance on this battery had to be re-evaluated. Currently, whole numbers are being used to relate one athlete's performance to another.

A third test that is performed in this portion of the evaluation involves starting the presentation of the lights at a slow pace. For every 'hit' of the lighted target, the processing unit of the panel speeds up the presentation of target (which means that they are displayed for increasingly shorter periods of time). When the player misses two targets in a row, the panel's processing unit begins to slow the presentation of targets, displaying the stimuli for longer periods of time. This allows the player to regain composure. Then the unit speeds up again. This de-challenge/re-challenge feature was developed by one of the authors (J.J.G.) and allows the player to recover and continue. This test can become quite frantic, which can provide an indicator of concentration and coolness under pressure.

Engineers at Wayne Engineering Co. decided to multiply the number of targets hit by the speed of the final target to produce a whole number which they called the Gardner Product. Gardner (1992) emphasizes that the product of a whole number times a speed of light exposure yields a value that can be used only for motivation of the player who is using this instrument for visual motor training and not for evaluative purposes. Players can use the highest Gardner Product as a number to aim for as their training progresses.

A fourth test that may be performed at this portion of the evaluation involves a determination of how quickly a player can move their hand through a distance of 28 inches (72 cm). This distance represents the overall distance from the light at the 9 o'clock position on the Wayne Saccadic Fixator to the light at the 3 o'clock position. Five trials are performed with the right hand and five trials with the left hand. The readings are averaged. Gardner (1988) determined that the average player performs 0.08 seconds faster with the dominant hand versus the non-dominant hand. This may be a function of the accuracy of the movement as opposed to the speed of the movement.

The evaluator needs to be able to assess hand speed from other positions as well. For example, a basketball player's ability to move from the 6 o'clock position to the 12 o'clock position on a panel placed above eye level or an ice-hockey goaltender's ability to perform the same task on a panel placed so that the light at the 12 o'clock position is at the height of the top of the net. Further investigations are needed.

The following sports from Table 2.1 are some examples of high, medium and low demand of eye–hand coordination.

(a) High demand: the goaltender in ice-hockey must have an extremely quick identification of the location of the puck, how quickly it is moving towards him and how to get that information to his hands to make an accurate save or efficiently block the shot.

(b) Medium demand: in cricket bowling the target is fixed and the bowler takes a predetermined number of steps, although many bowlers pick what is called a 'spot'. A spot bowler tries to get himself in a position to release the ball at the same place every time. Therefore, there is a medium demand of eye–hand coordination involved: the bowler and the ball are moving at slow speed relative to other sports.

(c) Low demand: weightlifting and long distance running are examples of sports where there is very little that the eye must interpret in terms of eye–hand coordination.

Eye–body coordination

The final test that we include in the evaluation of the player's visual motor system involves a balance board attached to a light panel (Figure 2.7). This test measures the athlete's ability to change balance in response to a visual stimulus. The test subject is positioned on a board whose dimensions are 18 inches square (46 cm square). This board has four on–off switches on its underside and is raised in the centre approximately 2 inches (5 cm) from the floor

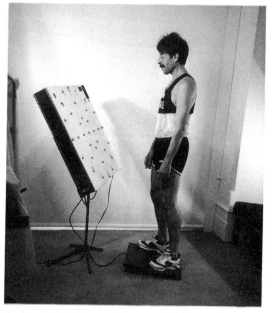

Figure 2.7 Balance board which determines the subject's ability to change balance in response to a visual stimulus

by a block of wood which acts as a pivot point. All switches are in the off position when the subject is balanced evenly on the board. The light panel is 15 feet (4.5 m) away and in this testing mode only four lights will light up – those at the 3, 6, 9 and 12 o'clock positions. As the first light comes on (e.g. at the 12 o'clock position), the subject reacts to the visual stimulus by shifting their body (in this example shifting forward) to unbalance the board and to engage the forward switch on the bottom of the balance board to score a point. The balance position is then resumed ready for the next target light. The speed of the lights can be controlled by the test administrator. During the evaluation phase the lights are usually left on until the proper body shift to depress the 'on' switch has been performed. In this way, it is similar to the 'proactive' phase of the eye–hand evaluation. When the proper on–off switch is depressed, a point is scored (recorded) and the panel lights up another light that the athlete must respond to. There is no foot movement during this test. However, equipment is currently being developed that will require a first step to be made in order to score a point. Certain sports such as gymnastics, skiing, soccer, basketball, ice-hockey and figure skating require rapid and efficient shifting of balance in the legs and feet.

Central peripheral awareness

This skill is tested using a device that requires the player to maintain central fixation on a target and to make a motor response to a light presented in the peripheral visual field. The Peripheral Awareness Tester (see Chapter 8) from Wayne Engineering has a central fixation target with multiple 'arms' that branch out from the centre target. The players are asked to move a joystick that they are holding in the direction of the light that comes on at the end of the 'arm'. Lights are presented in a random sequence. Test distance is crucial (20 inches / 50 cm) since moving further away from the

device will make the task more one of central vision rather than peripheral vision. Conventional visual field units could be used instead if the manufacturers would make a modification to include a measure of the time lag between the target light coming on (stimulus) and the player's responses to that target. That stimulus / response time could be analysed for specific sports / athletes.

The following are examples from Table 2.1 of sports with high, medium and low demand of central peripheral awareness.

(a) High demand: basketball, ice-hockey and football (soccer) require high degrees of central peripheral awareness. In these sports, the player must be aware of the position of his team mates and opponents as they can rapidly change positions relative to one one another and to him. The ball or puck must be focused on centrally while team mates, opponents and the field boundaries must be at a high level of awareness to the player.
(b) Medium demand: baseball and cricket fielders must focus on catching the ball (central) while being aware of baserunner or movement peripherally, while recreational skiers must be aware of where they are going, other skiers, etc.
(c) Low demand: snooker, darts, bowls and target sports require virtually no peripheral awareness.

Visualization

While not a skill that is currently tested, the authors feel that visualization merits mention in a chapter about vision requirements in sport. Visualization is the ability to form a mental visual image of an object not presented to the eyes. Visualization has been called mental rehearsal, the picturing in the 'mind's eye' of an object, a situation, or perhaps an athletic performance. It is a difficult skill to test in the context of this evaluation.

Examples of athletes performing visualization are seen especially in high jump and in figure skating. TV cameras often focus on a figure skater beneath the arena in a holding area where they can be seen to visually rehearse the routine that is about to be performed.

Visualization is a learned skill and can be easily enhanced: the body responds to what the mind harbours. Goal-orientated visualization techniques are used to help develop consistency in athletic performance. If players can be trained to mentally perform properly, they may tend to perform properly in the actual event.

Summary

This chapter has discussed the visual process, beginning with the eyes and following the visual pathway to the brain. There, the input from both eyes is integrated, analysed and responded to via motor responses. The basic tests necessary to evaluate the athlete in these respects are described. Additionally Table 2.1 provides a comprehensive reference source of visual skills and their relative importance in a wide variety of sporting activities.

References

Coffey, B. and Reichow, A. (1990) Optometric evaluation of the elite athlete. *Problems in Optometry*, **2**, 32–58

Gardner, J.J. (1988) The results of testing high school athletes. *American Optometric Association, Sports Vision Section, News and Views*, **8** (2), 19–30

Gardner, J.J. (1992) Vision testing of sports officials. Unpublished manuscript

Garner, A.I. (1977) Visual aid prescribing for the athlete. *California Optometry*, **3**, 18–19

Kirshner, A.J. *Manual for the Oculorotor*, Keystone View, Meadville, PA

Long, G.M. and Garvey, P.M. (1988) The effects of target wavelength on dynamic visual acuity under photopic and scotopic viewing. *Human Factors*, **30** (1), 3–13

Long, G.M. and Penn, D.L. (1987) Dynamic visual acuity: normative functions and practical applications. *Bulletin of the Psychonomic Society*, **25** (4), 253–6

Ludvigh, E. and Miller, J.M. (1958) Study of visual acuity during pursuit of moving test object. I. Introduction. *Journal of the Optical Society of America*, **48**, 799–81

Rouse, M.W., DeLand, P., Christian, R. and Hawley, J.A. (1988) A comparision study of dynamic visual acuity between athletes and nonathletes. *Journal of the American Optometric Association*, **50**, 947–50

Sanderson, F.H. and Whiting, H.T.A. (1978) Dynamic visual acuity, a factor in catching performance. *Journal of Motor Behavior*, **10**, 7–14

Sherman, A. (1980) Overview of research information regarding vision and sports. *Journal of the American Optometric Association*, **51**, 659–65

Sherman, A. (1981) Prescribing for patients who play. *Optometric Management*, **17**, 67–8

Sherman, A. (1983) A method of evaluating eye–hand coordination and visual reaction time in athletes. *Journal of the American Optometric Association*, **54**, 801–2

Sherman, A. (1990) Sports vision testing and enhancement: implications for winter sports. In *Wintersports Medicine* (ed. Casey, Foster and Hixson), F.A. Davis, Philadelphia

Vinger, P. (1985) The eye in sports medicine. In *Clinical Ophthalmology* (ed. T.D. Duane). J.B. Lippincott, Philadelphia

3

Sports for the visually impaired
Ian Fell

Introduction

The Royal National Institute for the Blind (RNIB) survey conducted in 1987 presented impressive evidence suggesting that there were nearly one million people aged 16 years or older in Great Britain who could be registered either blind or partially sighted (Bruce *et al.*, 1991). Further examination of the data shows that 90% of these were over 59 years of age and that, in all age groups, there are significantly more women than men. Their definition of blind or partially sighted was better than 6/24 (20/80) (distance Snellen acuity) but worse than N12 reading ability. Of those of working age, it was estimated that 75% were unemployed at the time of the survey. Of the 25% employed, significantly more were in the unskilled and semi-skilled occupations than would be found in the general population. Even amongst those working, the average earnings were significantly less than the average earnings of the non-disabled working population.

The second volume of the same survey deals with blind and partially sighted children in Britain, in which the projected population of under 16-year-olds in 1991 was 11 500 (Walker *et al.*, 1992). The adult survey goes on to identify interest in outdoor sports, which covers both competitive sport and physical recreations such as walking. Swimming and walking are the most common activities, and that section of the findings concludes with the comment 'although the popularity of sport among younger blind people may surprise many sighted readers, it is at least partly explained by the active sports programmes in schools and also the activities of the many specialist sports organisations for blind people. Sports activity among younger blind people is a success story and as such particularly worthy of support.'

British Blind Sport currently has some 350 individual members and 56 clubs and associations with a total membership of between 3000 and 4000. The National Organization for Visually Impaired (VI) Sportsmen and Sportswomen in the United Kingdom was formed and is run by the visually impaired. Apart from individual members, most VI sports clubs are in membership as are independent sports-specific organizations, such as the Home Country VI Bowls and Golf Associations.

British Blind Sport is responsible for coordinating blind sports activities at national and international level and for negotiating with other national, international and governing bodies of sport. It is also responsible for rule modifications and sight classification in the United Kingdom and takes a major role in the

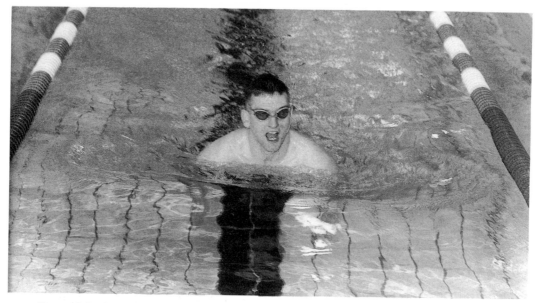

Figure 3.1   Swimming – a very popular sport with the visually impaired. (© Som Raj)

development of new sports for the visually impaired. Within its own structure there are sports-specific committees dealing currently with athletics, archery, bowls, cricket, football, goalball (see Appendix to this chapter), judo, swimming and tandem cycling (see Figures 3.1, 3.2, 3.3).

In essence the information from the RNIB survey has provided British Blind Sport with much information on the size, age, income, sex, bias and social perceptions of the visually impaired population that it should be serving. The brief description of British Blind Sport and its development indicates how far we are from the ideal in the UK. The timing and nature of blind sport development differs from country to country, but as might be expected, progress has been greatest in the more developed countries. Differing attitudes to the blind has also influenced blind sport development and, just as interest in sports differs among the sighted, so does interest vary among the blind from one country to another.

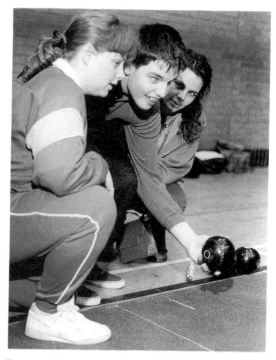

Figure 3.2   A visually impaired boy bowling. (© Nikki Berriman)

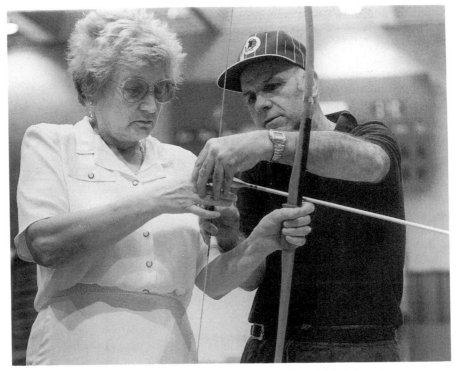

Figure 3.3   A visually impaired woman archer. (© Nikki Berriman)

Origins of visually impaired sport

Physical activities and sport for the general population most likely evolved as a surrogate activity when human evolution meant that man was not exclusively involved in the business of survival. There is no reason to believe that the same instincts were not present in the visually impaired, whose perception was such that they envisaged themselves capable of participating in such activities. In particular, once visually impaired people came together in sufficient numbers, physical activities and sport would seem to be a natural consequence. This tendency was reinforced in the nineteenth century in the early schools for the blind where positive attempts were made by those in charge of these establishments to encourage physical activities as a means of improving mobility.

By the early part of the twentieth century, the social structure of the VI world was such that, for the more fortunate, sport was an important part of the curriculum. High standards were achieved and in the 1920s and 1930s rowing eights were entered from Worcester College for the Blind at Henley Regatta, the premier British rowing event. Since its inception during the First World War, St Dunstan's, the British and Commonwealth association for war-blinded, included sport and recreation amongst its varied activities. Although there is limited documented evidence, it is clear that sport for the blind was sufficiently advanced in the 1930s for athletics competitions to be organized between Scotland and England.

The period following the Second World War saw further development of sport in the schools for the blind. In parallel, sport for those with motor disabilities was developing, mainly as a therapeutic agent. People with traumatic spinal cord injuries were surviving longer with a far better quality of life, and sport was increasingly used as part of their clinical management. In fact the rate of progression was such that it was the people with motor disabilities who were at the forefront of international disabled sport. At the same time, sport for the visually impaired was developing, and a feature of the past three decades has been the growth of blind sports clubs providing young adults with the opportunity to continue the sports they had participated in when at school. The vast majority of these clubs were created by blind sportsmen and sportswomen themselves in stark contrast to many of the blind societies of an earlier age. It was a case of 'of the blind' rather than 'for the blind'.

Modification of sports and sports equipment for the visually impaired

Blind men and women are exposed to sports peculiar to their own countries in a similar manner to their sighted counterparts. It is quite understandable, therefore, that those sports which become dominant for the blind in each country will be derived from those of interest to their sighted counterparts. As a general principle, a sighted sport is taken and modified as little as possible in order that blind people can compete. As a sport evolves, the modifications are merely a consensus of those involved, but as a sport becomes established nationally and internationally, the wording of its rules becomes much longer and more precise. Occasionally, a sport has been developed by the visually impaired which has no non-disabled counterpart. For the reader interested in how this sport of goalball is

played, there is a synopsis of the game in the Appendix to this chapter and derived from the International Blind Sports Association (IBSA) regulations for international goalball. According the the foreword of these regulations, the game was invented in 1946 by an Austrian, Hanz Lorenzen, and a German, Sett Reindle, in an effort to help in the rehabilitation of blinded war veterans. However, similar games had evolved in other countries prior to this date although usually with a lighter ball. It came to prominence internationally at the Paralympics in Canada in 1976 and the World Games in Austria in 1978. Although there was no need to modify a parallel sighted sport, this has not prevented the IBSA goalball committee from re-defining its own rules and regulations.

Modifications may be made to the rules or to the equipment. As an example, in international swimming the principal modification is the tapping of swimmers by coaches as they come to the end of the pool enabling the swimmer to organize their turn. Another example, from athletics, is the use of a guide runner or runners. The guide runner is linked to the blind runner by a short tether ensuring that the blind runner can negotiate the bends and maintain a straight line in between as well as coping with overtaking or being overtaken. In lawn bowls, a string is laid from the mat to the opposite side of the green and once the jack is bowled it is realigned at that distance on the string, giving the blind bowler direction.

There have been many suggestions for more sophisticated equipment to enable the visually impaired to compete in sport, particularly with the general advances in electronics. However, those responsible for defining rules have to bear in mind that, for a sport to be accessible to the blind, modifications need to be easily obtained, reliable and relatively inexpensive, particularly for the visually impaired in Third World countries. Modifications of rules or equipment are not always the complete answer. Taking the example of the guide runner, three issues arise that have occupied those organizing track events for some time. First, guide runners are mandatory for those runners with no sight, and are allowed for those with very little sight. Competing with a guide runner requires two lanes for each entrant so, in order to have at least four runners in such a race, competition requires at least an eight-lane track. Secondly, there is a strong feeling that a guide runner may improve the performance of a runner, presumably by dragging him or her round the track! Although this fear is illusory, the rules are written so that any guide runner leading the competitor would be disqualified. Finally, with the improvement in performance of visually impaired runners, finding a guide runner of adequate standard has become an increasing problem, as the guide runner needs to be able to perform at a higher level than the visually impaired competitor. The latter needs to train and race with their guide runner, but as performances improve, it becomes increasingly difficult to find guide runners who can afford to disrupt their own training programmes. One answer to this has been to introduce a relay of guide runners. This at least means that each individual guide would not necessarily have to be capable of out performing the visually impaired competitor.

Taking up sport

Considerable confusion exists amongst sighted people as to how the visually impaired learn sporting skills. The simplest way to understand the issue is to consider how a sighted person becomes competent in a particular sporting activity. Initially they are exposed to the sport as a child or an adult. Generally they learn the rudiments of the sport by watching others. As an example, many soccer supporters are familiar with the intricacies of the sport but may well not have done more than kick a football about in the street.

Assuming sufficient interest to want to take part, it is possible to try to emulate what has been observed. Probably many golfers, tennis players or bowls players are initially self-taught. Alternatively, sports can be taught, and this is particularly the case in schools or in sports where the individual is aspiring to higher levels of competition. It is at this point that the coach enters the picture: a person with a good understanding of the sport, its techniques and tactics, together with an appreciation of the physiological and psychological requirements of the athlete. Perhaps most important for the coach are the abilities to analyse and compare performances and to be able to teach and motivate players.

However, as a sighted individual gains competence in a particular sport, the ability to observe other players is of paramount importance. Although the process of learning a skill is predominantly visual, this need not necessarily be the case. Instead of watching how someone carries out a particular manœuvre, a blind person will use touch to follow the movement patterns of an activity. A coach will endeavour to manipulate the aspiring blind sportsperson to teach the appropriate patterns of movement. As a process, it is slower than in the sighted world, but though slower, it can often be as effective. As Clive Spencer, senior physical educationalist at RNIB New College Worcester, UK, says: 'We get there in the end, it just takes a bit longer.'

This requirement for one-to-one coaching, together with the difficulty of following movement patterns in real time, is probably the major difficulty for the visually impaired, particularly those with little useful vision. Other skills that are more difficult to develop are spatial orientation and an understanding of what others are doing. For instance, a track runner needs general information about the performance of other competitors and specific information during a race. A golfer needs to know his or her position during play in relation to the green and the various hazards between his or her position and the pin.

It is not surprising that the younger visually impaired are generally more successful than older people at gaining expertise in sport. However, there is another group of visually impaired sportspeople whose problems are rather different. These are individuals who have competed in sport, often at high levels, and who have subsequently lost most or all of their sight. Here the issue is more one of general rehabilitation, and those who are successful in developing general skills are quite likely to return to their sporting interest and re-acquire high levels of skill. It is often a question of believing in the possibility.

One bar to many visually impaired sportspeople is persuading clubs and coaches that their objectives are realistic. Very often, the coach approached will have had no experience of working with the visually impaired. Providing the coach is willing to learn, then there is a reversal of roles with the visually impaired person teaching the coach how to interpret visual information and pass it on to them. There is an important role here for national VI sports organizations in liaising with governing bodies of sport and providing written information, videos and seminars for them and their coaches.

To summarize, for anyone to teach any skills to a visually impaired person, they need to be able to communicate effectively in a non-visual fashion while recognizing that whatever useful vision that person retains should be used when feasible. In addition, a knowledge of the rules of the sport together with any modifications required by the visually impaired participants is also needed.

The international scene

Serious international Sport for the visually impaired began in the 1970s as part of international competition involving a range of disabilities. At this stage, those disabled with spinal cord damage were organized internationally under the aegis of the International Stoke Mandeville Games Federation (ISMGF). The International Sports Organisation for the Disabled (ISOD) was developed as an umbrella organization, but in practice became the international body for amputees, the visually impaired, those with cerebral palsy and 'les autres' in parallel to the ISMGF. Although the visually impaired were involved in the Disabled Olympics of 1976 and 1980 through the auspices of ISOD, it was not until 1981 that the International Blind Sports Association (IBSA) was formed in Paris. From 1981 onwards, a policy of regional championships reinforced quadrennial Olympics and by the second half of the decade World Championships were held in Sweden in 1986 and The Netherlands in 1990. The IBSA defined international modifications to the international rules and thereby gave recognition to an increasing list of sports which could be played at international level. At present sports recognized by IBSA and the International Paralympic Committee (IPC) are: athletics, swimming, tandem, judo, powerlifting, wrestling, winter sports, lawn bowls and chess together with three sports not played outside the disabled world: goalball, torball and showdown. In addition golf, water skiing and sailing take place unofficially at international level.

Disabled sport generally, and visually impaired sport specifically, is in a state of change. With the formation of IBSA in 1981 and the Cerebral Palsied International Sport and Recreation Association (CPISRA) a few years earlier, an International Coordinating Committee (ICC) was created to coordinate the international disability sports organizations for the purposes of multidisability international events such as the Paralympics. In the late 1980s a rival organization, the International Paralympic Committee (IPC) was formed which superseded the ICC after the Barcelona Paralympics in 1992.

As has already been indicated, development of visually impaired sport has varied in degree and timing in different countries. An analysis of activities in different European countries produced a wide variety of different sports played, and wide variations in the way in which visually impaired sport was funded. Some thirty-two sports and activities were identified with athletics, swimming, tandem cycling, goalball and judo being the most popular. As far as funding was concerned, Denmark, who topped the list at that time, was spending seventeen times as much per visually impaired sportsperson as the USSR, which was bottom of the list. Funding sources varied, but most countries fell into one of two groups: primarily government funded or those raising their funds privately.

Problems for the visually impaired taking part in sport

It is possible to identify a range of issues that create problems for visually impaired men and women taking part in sport at all levels and in all countries.

Acceptance by society

For the visually impaired person to be able to participate in the sport of their choosing, access to training facilities similar to those available to the rest of the sporting world is essential. Where such facilities are limited, as in less developed countries, the attitude of society to the visually impaired may limit effective access to available facilities. Even in the UK, where facilities are less limited, the understanding and acceptance of those non-disabled who work in sports centres or coach in specific sports is variable. There are staff in sports centres and coaches who are still

hostile to the idea of the visually impaired being involved in sport, although the main problem tends to be ignorance rather than prejudice. To give an example, for the visually impaired person to train regularly at a sports centre they need to locate a suitable centre and become familiar with its layout. In addition, advice and coaching are necessary in order for them to reach their full potential. They may also need facilities for a guide dog, to travel to, and train at, other venues and also bear the associated cost of the sport. If competing, they will be very lucky indeed if there is a VI sports club close by and therefore will probably have to travel a considerable distance, even when competing 'at home'.

Society in general determines facilities and attitudes and the deterioration of public transport in developed countries since the 1960s has been a big disadvantage for the visually impaired. Attitudes are changing for the better in many countries, but all too frequently the staff at sports centres do not understand the needs of the visually impaired and their guide dogs and many coaches remain unwilling or incapable of assisting the visually impaired.

Finance is inevitably an issue, and while in some countries there is generous government funding of sports activities for the disabled, in others, the cost of anything other than major competition is carried by the individual. Since the visually impaired are more likely to be unemployed than employed and even if they are employed it is at the lower end of the salary scale, they are at a disadvantage compared to the non-disabled.

The size of the sporting visually impaired population

In developed countries the number of visually impaired people who are involved in sport under retirement age is quite low. Consequently the density of those with visual impairment is not very great, except in populous areas. Where they look to a VI sports club as their solution, they may have to travel some considerable distance. For instance, in the UK there are clubs in London and Coventry but none in between – a distance of 160 kilometres. In developed countries with small overall populations this can lead to a situation where the development of a specific visually impaired competitive structure presents problems. This is particularly the case for less popular sports. A number of solutions have evolved in different countries and in different sports.

Mixed disability sports

This seems to work satisfactorily in those sports involving a team in which the participants have different functions or where the priority is participating rather than competing. Proposals for interdisability competition based on banding or handicapping have received mixed responses. Imagine a parallel situation in, say, golf, where club competitions are often played on a handicap basis. It would be difficult to persuade top golfers that entrants could compete in circuit tournaments on a handicap basis, particularly with the money that is at stake. When visually impaired people do not have easy access to a sports club for the visually impaired, then this solution may have to be accepted.

Mixed disability sports clubs

The advantage of these is mainly where the total number of disabled persons is small. They do not alter the basic problem of insufficient visually impaired competitors to make up the numbers.

Non-disabled sports clubs

The current British Blind sport view is that non-disabled sports clubs are the natural

progression for some people and some sports. This already occurs in archery, athletics, bowls, golf, judo, swimming and tandem to varying degrees and is not unique to the UK. It is of course dependent on the willingness of these clubs to take visually impaired members.

Competition with the non-disabled

This is more difficult if there is a requirement to incorporate modifications to the national and international rules of the sport. For instance, in tandem time trialling, there is no need for rule modification, whereas for archery, a special sighting device is needed. National and international governing bodies tend to be conservative in nature and understandably are unwilling to modify the rules of their sport if they feel that this would disadvantage the non-disabled. However, where modifications are minimal and clearly do not disadvantage the non-disabled it seems that, with time, this process will be the solution for the better visually impaired competitor in some sports. One major advantage is that those people with partial sight who, for social reasons, do not see themselves as part of the visually impaired world, are able to retain that relationship in their sporting activities more easily.

Sports such as cricket and soccer seem destined to remain separate games for those with and without visual disabilities. In the former, the rules for the game, as played by the visually impaired in the UK, change the game significantly and the rules, as played in Australia and New Zealand, change the game to an even greater extent. Five-a-side soccer, as played in the UK, is not greatly modified but serious competition between those with severe visual impairment and non-disabled players is generally too one-sided. Again, on the International front, the rules used by the visually impaired in the main footballing countries vary considerably. Attempts are being made to standardize these in order to introduce international visually impaired competition, but so far with limited success.

Sight classification of the visually impaired

In the UK, blind sport has traditionally been played by those people interested in sport who found themselves a part of blind society, for example, war-blinded servicemen and women involved with St Dunstans or blind children with special schools. Given the extreme variability present in the selection of children for special education, it was perhaps not unreasonable that the usual distinction made was that an individual was either totally or partially blind. (There was the added assumption that everyone in a special school came within one or the other of these categories.)

Today, with the intense competition at both national and international levels, the International Blind Sports Association (IBSA) have laid down a three-class system based on either visual acuity and/or field of vision. The three classes are B1, B2 and B3 and all assume best corrected vision where appropriate in the better eye.

Class B1 is defined as: 'No light perception in either eye up to light perception, but inability to recognize the shape of a hand at any distance or in any direction.'

Class B2 is defined as: 'From ability to recognize the shape of a hand up to a visual acuity of 2/60 (0.6/20) and/or visual field of less than 5 degrees.'

Class B3 is defined as: 'From visual acuity above 2/60 (0.6/20) to visual acuity of 6/60 (2/20) and/or a visual field of more than 5 degrees and less than 20 degrees.'

Problems of classification

The human instinct to classify and order, while understandable, can sometimes trans-

fer a problem rather than solve it. In classifying competitors, the underlying assumptions are that above a certain level of sight, individuals should be excluded from competition and that within the classification bands, the better the sight the better an individual will perform, all other things being equal.

The immediate result of the IBSA classification was that a number of better-sighted competitors who had hitherto competed in 'blind' sport were excluded from serious visually impaired international competition. This disenfranchisement has presented problems which have been partially resolved in some sports. For instance, in cricket, which is played nationally but not internationally as far as the UK is concerned, the old division of totals and partials has been retained and peer pressure used to ensure that those with comparatively good sight do not distort fair competition. In bowls, as far as the English National Association of Visually Handicapped Bowlers (ENAVHB) is concerned, a B4 class has been instituted with an acuity range of 6/60 (20/200) to 6/24 (20/80). ENAVHB have also dropped that part of the classification system relating to limited field of vision, arguing that for a sport like bowls, limited field of vision is of little importance, given the nature of the game.

There has been much discussion in many countries about classification. Proposals that have emerged which may influence future developments include changing the upper limit of the present B3 class, changing the number of classes and classifying competitors for specific sports. As soon as classification was taken seriously, some athletes looked to play the system. All competitors taking part in international events are required to attend with their sight classification card which gives the competitor's name, date of birth, medication (if applicable), nationality, right and left eye acuity and field, with and without best correction. It is signed by the national tester and the appropriate class indicated. At any international event an IBSA tester re-tests and confirms or alters the classification. The test is, of course, dependent on the honesty of the competitor as well as the integrity of the tester. Competitors often believe that to be classified B2 rather than B3 gives them an advantage and some testers understandably sympathize with those who are just above the B2 upper limit. Even with the safeguard of testing at international competition, the time needed to test perhaps 200 competitors is quite considerable and the same problems of the honesty of the competitor exist. Perhaps a system of random tests, plus tests on medal winners would be more effective.

Accusations of substituting sight classification cards are not unknown. This occurred in the European Athletics Championships in 1987, and although the accusation was dismissed, it is clear that the system must be meticuluously observed by competition organizers. The most useful development that could occur would be the development of a rapid and inexpensive system of testing together with a foolproof system of enforcement. It is quite clear that, if financial reward for visually impaired athletes goes the way of those in non-disabled sport, these problems will become as acute as those of performance enhancing drugs.

Some countries, such as Spain, would like to remove the B3 class altogether and retain just B1 and B2. Others see this as creating an even greater devisive effect on their visually impaired populations. The proposal would reduce costs, particularly for international competition, even if team sizes remained constant since when classes compete separately, this presently means that six 1500 m track events would run as opposed to the four that would be the case with just B1 and B2 men and women. Others have commented on the problem of those who are at the bottom of B2 class and have suggested that there should be a complete reclassification: NPL to P of L, P of L to 1/60, 1/60 to 3/60, and 3/60 to 6/60. The difficulty here is that there would be four classes in B2 with the associated logistical problems. Additionally,

the greater the number of classes, the fewer competitors there would be in each class.

Certainly one of the most interesting proposals is sport-specific classification. Reverting to the ENAVHB modifications, it would seem quite reasonable not to classify a person with normal acuity but limited field for bowls or archery but to classify them for football.

The future

Some future changes are predictable, while others are more speculative. It seems certain that even more sports will become part of the visually impaired repertoire, particularly in those developing countries where the social and economic structure is expanding. In many countries, including the UK, the higher profile of disabled sport will increase the pressures on government and associated organizations to increase their financial support to the national governing bodies of visually impaired sport.

Perhaps the major debating point at present is the organization of Paralympic, world and regional competition. This debate can be summarized as 'disability-specific versus multidisabled'. The current situation is that the International Paralympic Committee, (IPC) organizes the Paralympics through their member organizations in each country. The IPC also defines modifications to international rules for all disabilities and the classification systems for all disabilities for the Paralympics. The IPC would also claim these roles for world championships and there are those who would like the IPC to take responsibility for regional championships. If successful, it would seem to sound the death knell for the disability-specific organizations, at least internationally. Even as it is, the overlapping functions of classification and rule definition seem unnecessary.

There are two particular problems that arise from the multidisabled approach to international competition. The first is that numbers are restricted, resulting in successful countries being unable to take all the competitors to international events that they would wish. For instance, in 1992 the organizers of the Barcelona Paralympics restricted the UK team to 228 competitors and support staff for all disability individual sports. This restriction excluded 44 visually impaired competitors and support staff whose performances outweighed many of those who were present from other countries. Clearly, this problem is much less likely to arise if events are disability-specific. The second problem relates to media coverage of disabled sport. While this varies from country to country, multidisabled games receive greater media coverage and have a higher profile than disability-specific games. This, in turn, makes fund raising easier, but has the disadvantage that the media tail can wag the disability sport dog. While not being a major problem with the visually impaired, this tends to mitigate against the severe motor disabled such as the severely cerebral palsied, since the media prefer disabled sport to look reasonably 'normal'.

Those countries who would prefer to continue with the disability-specific approach, probably do so as a consequence of the history of their own VI society. It is natural that in countries where the visually impaired have been educated separately from those with other disabilities, their sportsmen and women look to separate development with the longer-term goal of integration into non-disabled sport where possible. The reverse is equally natural for those countries who have a history of mixed disability societies. What is not clear at present is what the final outcome will be.

Some authorities in the UK and other countries believe that the visually impaired should be educated in their local schools as opposed to specialist schools. This presents British Blind Sport and the integrated visually impaired with serious problems. Even if local authorities provided the resources to ensure effective integration, there is no longer the concentration of visually impaired that was found in specialist schools, and exactly the same problems have now arisen as occur with those visually impaired who are of post-school age. It would seem sensible that, for those who are interested in sports which are not easily carried out with the non-disabled, local authorities should accept the responsibility for providing a regional sports facility. If this was done in cooperation with VI sports organizations, then much less difficulty would be experienced in identifying the whereabouts of those young visually impaired people interested in sport. Likewise those teachers in schools where visually impaired pupils are integrated would gain a far wider experience of what was feasible and what was available in VI sport.

Perhaps the future will question the whole philosophy of elite disabled sport. Why should society establish parallel international sporting championships for defined disabled groups? Carried to its logical conclusion, we should look to provide equivalent opportunities for all who are similarly disadvantaged in elite sport. Should we not classify high jumpers by height? After all, a 1.5 m tall man is never going to take part in an Olympic high jump final.

Why should the visually impaired expect the media to present these events as on a par with those of the non-disabled? A person involved in VI sport, may well enjoy the Paralympics VI track and field events, but since performances are likely to be no better than non-disabled club performances in many countries, are the visually impaired not deluding themselves when they expect the same enthusiasm from the general population?

This chapter began by posing the question as to how far sporting development has answered the needs of the visually impaired population in the UK, a question equally valid for other countries. A report produced by BBS in 1991, which was based on questionnaire responses from its membership, recognized that resources expended on grass roots development should be given priority over elite sport development. This response from members in part reflects the fact that, by definition, the majority of members are grass roots sportspeople. However, it also reflects that visually impaired sportsmen and women are at last becoming aware of the numbers of visually impaired people in the population and the need to address the issue at a national level. The sooner nationally coordinated initiatives are developed by the visually impaired, the sooner societies will answer the challenges of reports such as the RNIB Needs Surveys.

Appendix: the game of goalball

Many sports may be suitably modified in order that visually impaired people can participate. Goalball, however, is different in that it is a sport that was developed for and played exclusively by the visually impaired (IBSA, 1992).

The regulations for goalball as defined by IBSA parallel the regulations for any other sport, be it sport for the disabled or not. Thus the regulations provide precise information regarding both rules and tournament regulations at differing levels. Over the years, the rules have been modified and clarified but it is noticeable that as fast as this occurs, the consequences of these changes have resulted in further modifications and refinement.

The rules of the game cover the court and equipment, contestants, officials, conduct of the game, infractions, penalties, free throws and disputes. The tournament regulations cover sanctioning, facilities and equipment, accommodation, referees, finances, qualifying standards, conduct of tournaments, games protocol and, inevitably, protests.

The game is played between two teams of three players with a maximum of three substitutions for each team. The game is conducted in a sports hall within an 18 × 9 metre rectangular court divided into two halves by a centre line. A goal extends across the whole of the court at either end and is 1.3 metres high. Each half of the court is further divided into thirds by two further lines creating a team area nearest the goal, a landing area in which a thrown ball must touch the ground on its way to the opposing goal and a neutral area adjacent to the central line. All lines are raised to provide tactile orientation for the players. All players wear eyeshades that totally exclude light thus bringing all competitors to the same visual level.

The game consists of two seven minute halves and the clock runs only during play so that the length of a match may be considerably longer. Provision is also made for extra time and if necessary a shoot out. Other factors that increase the length of a match are time outs which may be called by officials for offences, injuries, substitutions or displacement of shades. Additionally, up to three 45 second time outs may be requested by the coach of either team.

To control and record the game there are ten officials; two referees, four goal judges, and four other officials concerned with timing, shooting and scoring.

The objectives of the game are to score goals against the opposing team and to prevent the opposing team from scoring. Players should remain within their own half. The ball used weighs 1.25 kg and contains bells, thus the game calls for considerable acoustically initiated agility. The game is also profoundly influenced by the tactics, not only of the competitors but also of the coaches. Although coaches are penalized for direct coaching, tactical play comes to the fore with the use of advice during time outs, via substitutions and at half time.

Readers interested in the detailed regulations of goalball or any other IBSA recognized sport can obtain these from the International Blind Sports Association Secretariat, 42 rue Louis Lumiere, 7502 Paris, France.

References

Bruce, I., McKennell, A. and Walker, E. (1991) *Blind and Partially Sighted Adults in Britain: the RNIB Survey,* HMSO, London

Fell, I. (1991) The IBSA Europe Survey. In *Participation* (ed. R. Smith), Wencelle Publications, Croydon

International Blind Sports Association (1992) *Handbook,* IBSA, Madrid

Walker, E., Tobin, M. and McKennell, A. (1992) *Blind and Partially Sighted Children in Britain: the RNIB Survey,* HMSO, London

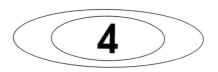

Eye injuries in sport
Nicholas P. Jones

The epidemiology of sports injury

Eye trauma provides a substantial and important part of the work of the ophthalmologist. On average, one patient in every ten seen has sustained an eye injury. In addition, the majority of eye injuries probably never reach a medical doctor; they are minor, are shrugged off and heal themselves. Of those which reach a hospital emergency department, only a small proportion (about 2.3%) are sustained during sport (McEwen, 1989). Glynn *et al.* (1988), in Massachusetts, found the incidence of sports-related eye injury to be as low as 61 per 100 000 population per year. However, of greater importance are the severe injuries, those which require medical or surgical treatment after admission to hospital. On average, an injured patient attending an emergency department has about a 2% chance of requiring such admission (Jones *et al.*, 1986). For eye injuries sustained during sport, this chance rises to 27% (Jones, 1988). The message is clear; in the overall view, eye injury in sport is very uncommon. When it does occur, it tends to be serious and can lead to permanent visual damage.

Estimations of the frequency and distribution of eye injury in sport are influenced by many parameters. Different countries, and different regions within countries, will have sports of varying popularity. Some sports are multinational, others entirely confined to one country, or even a small part of it. The statistics for cricket injuries in the USA are unimpressive, as are those for baseball in Australia. There are seasonal variations in incidence, especially for outdoor sports, and the rapidly increasing popularity of sport worldwide renders each published statistic almost out of date by the time it reaches print. In 1968 in the UK, 4.2% of injuries admitted to hospital were sustained during sport (Lambah, 1968). By 1976 this had risen to 7.0% (Canavan *et al.*, 1980), in 1988, 25.1% (Jones, 1988) and, most recently, 42% (McEwen, 1989). This latter survey identified sport, for the first time, as the most common cause of severe eye injury in the UK.

The management of a severe eye injury by the ophthalmologist is often a matter of damage limitation. Visual loss is frequently permanent. The great majority of eye injuries are preventable, and this is true for sport as in any other field. To understand the need for prevention, there follows a detailed account of sports eye injury; of the physical forces involved; of the injuries sustained by the eye, and the effects that these may cause; of the immediate and secondary treatment of such injuries. The matter of greatest importance in relation to sports eye injury is **prevention**. This can be approached by proper coaching into safe play, by modifying regulations, and perhaps most importantly by proper eye protection, which is dealt with elsewhere in this book (see Chapter 5).

The sports involved

Racquet sports

All racquet sports have in common a very high-velocity projectile. Overall the squash ball is probably the fastest moving, with measured velocities of 60 m/s but the tennis ball (50 m/s), badminton shuttlecock (55 m/s) and racquetball ball (45 m/s) are all capable of similar velocities and therefore carry substantial kinetic energy. The projectile is struck by a strung racquet which is swung in a wide arc around the player. Both racquet and ball can therefore cause injury.

In tennis singles, eye injury is rare. In doubles, however, since two players occupy the same space on court, the risk of racquet injury exists. Also in doubles, where it is common for one player to stand at the net, there is a risk of eye injury from a smash, and retinal detachments have been reported (See Lanfreund and Freilich, 1976), amongst other injuries. Such reports are, however, anecdotal.

Squash racquets has a much higher risk of eye injury. In a survey of eye injury in sport, squash was considered to be the most dangerous (Barrell et al., 1981), in terms of the risk of significant eye injury per unit time playing the sport. The play is fast, and both players are within the same space. The causes of eye injury in this game are quite consistent. Most are caused by the ball (Kennerley Bankes, 1985), and the classical risk situation is a player caught at the front of the court, turning to watch the progress of his shot, being hit by his opponent's next stroke. About one-quarter of squash eye injuries are caused by the racquet. There is greater risk of severe injury in such incidents. Players of unrefereed games are known to underuse the obstruction rule

and are more likely to attempt a stroke near their opponent's body. The corner of the court is also a high-risk area, where the follow-through of the racquet may strike the unseen opponent standing behind.

Singles badminton is not associated with eye injury, for the same reasons as single tennis. Mixed doubles provides most injuries (Kelly, 1987). Some are sustained when the player at the net is struck by a smash. Many experienced players will hold the racquet in front of the face in this situation, held in readiness for a stroke, and doubling as a face protector. Others are caused by the partner's racquet. Typically one player is at the net while the other is at the back of the court and a high stroke is played, which both players attempt to return. The incoming player (usually the man) smashes and his follow-through hits the upturned face of his partner (usually the woman). Injuries of this sort are quite avoidable by better positional play. In response to a cleared shot, most experienced players will return to sides, rather than front and back. Both of these classical badminton injuries are largely avoidable by basic coaching in safety and technique.

Racquetball, played on a squash court with a ball similar to but larger than a squash ball, and a shorter racquet with a larger head, is becoming increasingly popular, especially in North America. While some of the same risk factors as squash are present, the game is slower and injury appears to be less frequent. It has however become clear that the racquet is of the right length to strike the player himself in the face, if the follow-through is uncontrolled (Doxanas and Soderstrom, 1980).

Overall, in the USA and Europe, racquet sports together account for a significant proportion of injuries (McEwen and Jones, 1991) (about half of all sports eye injuries in the UK) and are clearly the most amenable to prevention by wearing eye protection. In this context, Canada and the USA are years ahead of the UK and Europe: the Canadian Standards Association (1982) and the American Society for Testing and Materials (1988) have had standards for eye protectors in squash for several years. At the time of writing, neither the British Standards Institution nor the Comité Européen Normalisation have yet developed a standard.

Large ball sports

While this category contains a huge variety of sports, many have aspects in common which put the eye at risk. Most of these sports are fast-moving team games, and usually involve handling of the ball. The ball itself is the cause of only a few injuries. A hard shot striking the head distorts the ball enough to allow partial penetration into the orbit, but such injuries are uncommon. Far more important are the physical clashes with opponents' hands, elbows, feet, or sometimes fists. Competition for the ball involves fast-moving hands near faces. In these circumstances fingers can hit eyes accidentally, or perhaps deliberately (see below). Such injuries are typically seen in rugby, basketball and water polo. It should be noted that although Canadian and American football involves the use of considerable head protection, the use of wire facemasks does not prevent the penetration of fingers (Helveston, 1987). Some large ball sports will clearly benefit from the widespread use of eye protectors, and this is becoming commonplace in basketball, which is now the most common sport in the USA to cause an eye injury, followed by baseball. In others such as soccer or rugby, eye protectors are not feasible and visors mounted in helmets would clearly be impossible without destroying the style of the game. In the UK at present, soccer is responsible for more eye injuries than any other sport (MacEwen, 1987). While accidental collisions and mistimed headers will always occur, the apparently increasing proportion of deliberate injuries should be the main target of some concern. Soccer has been found to generate more such injuries than other sports, and some cases have led to successful prosecution

(Grayson, 1990), even though internal disciplinary action may not have been taken.

Bat and stick sports

Ice-hockey, field-hockey, baseball, golf and cricket may be very different sports, but share certain characteristics. The projectile is small, hard, unyielding and travels at high velocity when struck by a stick or club. Golf is set aside because the ball is only struck when static. Moreover the risk of eye injury to an opponent by the club itself is clearly very low and should be completely avoided by courteous and sensible play. Injuries caused by a flying ball are rare but are obviously serious and have caused loss of the eye on several documented occasions (Portis et al., 1981). The old rubber-wound golf ball core has been replaced by the new solid-core golf ball; this has fortunately removed the temptation to dissect the interior of the ball. Several instances of exploding latex cores from the old type of ball have resulted in serious eye injury. This phenomenon is likely to disappear completely with the old ball.

The story of eye injuries in Canadian ice-hockey is an important lesson in prevention (Pashby et al., 1975; Pashby, 1977, 1979, 1987). In the 1970s the statistics on eye injuries sustained at this sport gave cause for great concern. Sixty per cent of high school hockey players had sustained eye or facial injury at some time. Over a period of years, Pashby and others of the Canadian Ophthalmological Society documented an unacceptable level of injury, with 15% of those eyes injured becoming legally blind (Pashby et al., 1975).

Over a period of years the incidence of eye injury fell precipitately (Pashby, 1977, 1979). First, a widespread public education campaign raised the level of awareness of eye injury and led to the more frequent use of head and eye protectors, the quality of which was enhanced by regulations of the Canadian Standards Association (CSA, 1982). The rules of hockey were changed to outlaw the raising

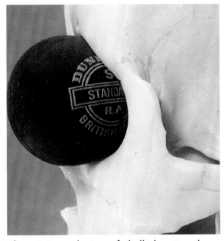

Plate 1 Lateral view of skull showing the ease of penetration of a squash ball into the orbit.

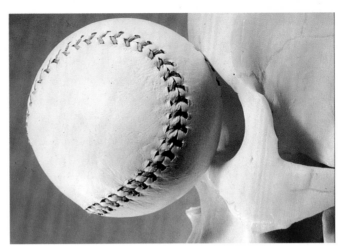

Plate 2 The raised seam on a baseball, cricket or rounders ball may complicate an injury by shearing forces and subsequent abrasion or laceration.

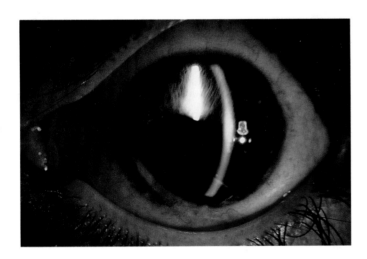

Plate 3 The result of a penetrating injury – there is a corneal scar below, and the pupil is drawn downwards after the loss of iris tissue. The lens was lost during the injury.

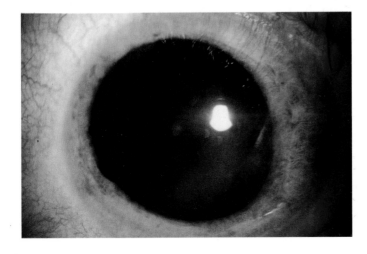

Plate 4 An abnormal anterior segment after blunt injury. The pupil is abnormally dilated because of neurological damage, and is (permanently) irregular in shape. The iris is stained yellow by blood previously in the anterior chamber.

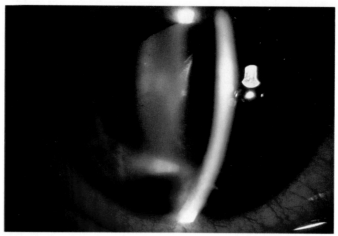

Plate 5 A hyphaema; blood in the anterior chamber after a severe blunt injury

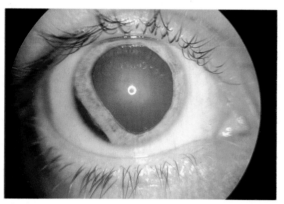

Plate 6 An iris dialysis; the iris has become disinserted from its normal attachment to the ciliary body.

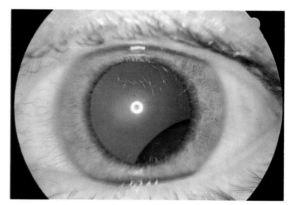

Plate 7 Dislocation of the lens.

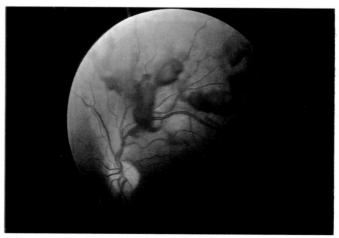

Plate 8 Vitreous haemorrhages after blunt injury.

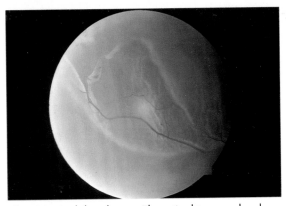

Plate 9 Retinal detachment. The retinal tear can be clearly seen at top of picture.

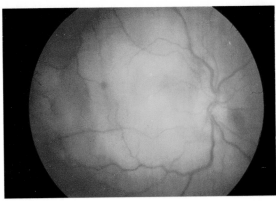

Plate 10 Retinal oedema (commotio retinae) after a blow from a football.

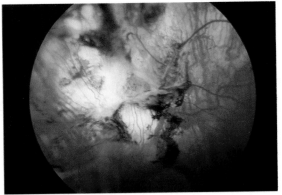

Plate 11 Choroidal and retinal scarring following a complicated posterior segment injury.

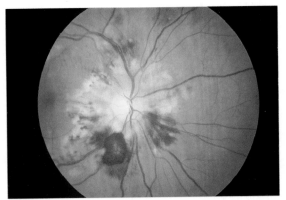

Plate 12 Purtscher's retinopathy; severe retinal haemorrhage and ischaemia (demonstrated by fluffy white 'cotton-wool spots' after a crush injury to the chest.

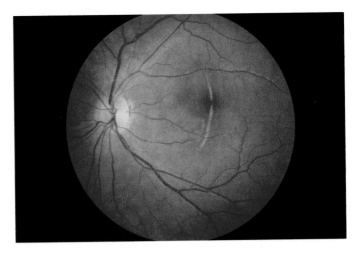

Plate 13 A choroidal rupture following a tennis ball injury. The rupture crosses the fovea.

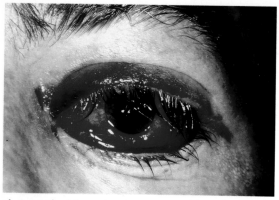

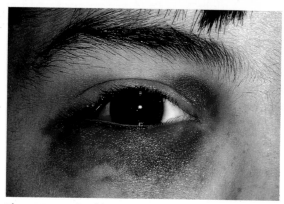

Plate 14 The left eye has been 'gouged' by a finger during a game of rugby. The eyelid bruising, conjunctival haemorrhage and oedema, hyphaema, low vision and soft eye are accompaniments to a rupture of the sclera.

Plate 15 An orbital haematoma, or 'black eye'. A significant eye injury may also be found.

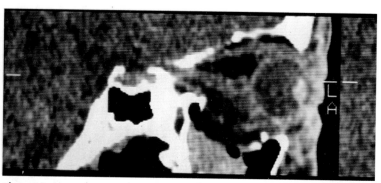

Plate 16 A computerised tomogram of an orbit after blunt injury. There is a blowout fracture of the orbit floor, which is now largely absent, and the maxillary sinus is opaque with blood.

SQUASH AND BADMINTON
EYE SAFETY TOP TEN

- Protect your eyes - wear sports safety glasses
- Play safe - know the rules of your sport and become a skilful player
- Never wear glass-lensed spectacles for sport
- Avoid lensless goggles - balls and shuttlecocks can penetrate them
- Always follow the ball or shuttlecock. Don't leave it too late before you look behind. That's how eye accidents happen
- Sports eye injuries can be blinding - get expert medical help fast
- In squash never crowd in close to your opponent
- In badminton keep your racket head up when playing close to the net
- In squash, if your opponent obstructs your shot don't play it. Ask for a let
- Watch out! Shuttlecocks can shoot through torn or loosely tied nets

 Royal National Institute for the Blind Eye Safety

Sponsored by optrex

 SUPPORTED BY SPORTS COUNCIL

Royal National Institute for the Blind, 224 Great Portland Street, London W1N 6AA. Tel 071-388 1266

Plate 17 An example of concise, useful safety information for players of squash and badminton, for the use of sports centres and clubs (Courtesy of RNIB).

of the stick above shoulder height, and protection was made mandatory for juniors. The level of eye injury in this sport in Canada and the USA is now dramatically lower than twenty years ago. Similar problems are associated with (illegal) high sticking in field-hockey yet injuries appear to be much rarer.

Cricket, that most sedate of pastimes, might be a surprising inclusion in the catalogue of eye injury. However, the ball may travel at over 40 m/s and the use of head and eye protection for batsmen and close fielders is by no means universal. Batsmen may be hit directly in the face by the ball, or it may glance off their bat into their eye, an especial risk when hooking the short-pitched ball or sweeping the overpitched leg-side delivery. The angle of approach here gives rise to the risk of globe rupture (Jones and Tullo, 1986). Fielders at short leg and silly mid-off increasingly wear helmets, but this should become universal. The wicket-keeper may also be at risk from the ball, or even from the flying bails when the wicket is struck. Injuries have also been described in indoor cricket. Polycarbonate visors or face cages are not always fitted to cricket helmets. If they were, and helmets were always used in high-risk situations, eye injuries would be avoided entirely.

Combat sports

Combat sports, which may be armed or unarmed, aim to cause or simulate injury. The martial arts occasionally give rise to eye injury. Accidents occur even in non-contact bouts, and severe injuries have been reported after a poorly aimed face kick in semi-contact karate. The unarmed combat sport that has received most attention is boxing. Both eye injury and brain injury are common in this sport. Giovinazzo et al. (1987), in examining the eyes of seventy-four boxers who were applying for the renewal of a licence to box in New York State, found eye injuries in 66%, and eye injuries considered to be vision-threatening in 58%.

The sport of boxing is clearly based upon the intent to injure, with loss of consciousness of the opponent being the most prestigious objective, yet efforts by medical organizations to investigate the frequency and severity of injuries have not met with universal approval from the boxing fraternity. The Report of the UK Board of Science and Education Working Party (1984) identified the dangers of eye injury and chronic brain damage, but was met with vigorous resistance from boxers and their organizers. The frequency of retinal injury in professional boxers is undisputed by those ophthalmologists who are commonly approached after such injuries. Media publicity of boxers injuries is, however, frequently transient and confined to high profile champions. The recent disappearance of a heavyweight champion from the European scene after a severe eye injury received little publicity and is all but forgotten. The underlying trend of severe injury is sadly masked by inadequate documentation.

That boxing is a dangerous sport is denied only by the most rabid enthusiast. The honest will reveal that they are well aware of this fact, and it is partly that which encourages their voyeuristic fascination in watching the prizefighter become bloodied. If boxing is to continue as a sport, then every effort must be made to ensure that ocular injuries are reduced to a minimum. The opinion of one eminent ophthalmologist (McLeod, 1992) that prophylactic laser treatment to boxers' retinas might help towards such an aim, has been vigorously opposed because this would amount to tacit medical approval of the sport. Other measures can however be taken. The use of thumbless boxing gloves, though unpopular amongst boxers, is felt to reduce the risk of eye injury greatly as it is the thumb which is thought most easily to cause ocular damage. All boxers should routinely undergo ophthalmic examinations at stated intervals, and high risk groups such as those who have undergone treatment for a retinal injury or have had previous intra-ocular surgery should be required to have an examination after every bout. Stringent records of eye injury should be maintained by the organizers of boxing, both amateur and professional.

The armed combat sports require body protection. Inevitably, failure of either the weapon or of the protection may occur. In 1982 a broken fencing blade passed through the facemask of an international fencer and penetrated the orbit and brain (Crawfurd, 1990). The orbital injury was incidental as the accident proved fatal. Two similar injuries, both fatal, occurred when bamboo splinters penetrated the facemask, eye and brain after a kendo *shi-ai* shattered. Apparently adequate facial protection cannot be considered infallible.

War games began their meteoric rise in popularity in the 1980s. A team game, the objective is to simulate a military operation, using body and face protection. The players carry projectile weapons simulating firearms of various types, but capable of discharging a small paint-filled pellet at high speed. The paint, on striking the body of an opponent, provides an indelible record of a 'hit'. Eye protectors and face masks may mist over during such vigorous exercise, and may be removed temporarily for cleaning. Some participants decide not to wear them at all. Inevitably eye injuries sustained in this way have regularly been reported (Easterbrook and Pashby, 1985; Mamalis *et al.*, 1990). Such injuries are usually severe and most lead to profound permanent visual loss.

Other sports

The overwhelming majority of eye injuries tend to arise in only a few sports. In the UK, soccer and the racquet sports together account for the majority of injuries. In the USA, basketball and baseball together do the same. At the other end of the spectrum are anecdotes of injuries which are rare enough to be considered extremely unfortunate. Such accidents include penetrating eye injuries by fishhooks (Bartholomew and MacDonald, 1980) and by ski poles or tree branches while skiing (Rousseau *et al.*, 1987). Aquatic sports in indoor pools have been associated with chemical eye injury after inappropriately large quantities of disinfectants had been put into the water. The classical example of an inappropriately-designed eye protector was a swimming goggle which had a sharp rim. On being lifted off the face after a swimming session, the goggle could slip out of wet fingers and back into the eyes. A number of penetrating injuries were sustained in this way (Jonasson, 1977).

There is no sport which is entirely free from risk of injury. Though some risk is accepted by all sports participants, this should always be tempered by proper education of the risks: by courteous and safe methods of play; by minimization of those risks wherever possible; and when such risks cannot be minimized, by the use of properly designed, fitted and maintained eye protection.

Factors affecting the type of injury

Ocular exposure and the point of impact

Only a small part of the eye is directly accessible to injury, the majority of the globe being protected by the bony orbit. The degree of protection offered by the orbit depends upon several factors. First, the size of the eyeball. The average axial length is about 24 mm, but in high myopes can be 28 mm or more. Ocular prominence, and therefore greater accessibility to injury, is therefore affected by refraction (assuming an orbital cavity of fixed volume).

The orbital volume does, however, vary, as does its shape and its relationship to the face. The smaller the orbital volume, the greater the ocular exposure for an eyeball of given size. This is of particular significance in some Mongoloid races where a combination of flattish face, myopia and smaller orbital volume can greatly increase ocular exposure. In contrast, some racial skull characteristics can greatly increase the ocular protection afforded by the supraorbital ridges (brows). These features also distinguish the sexes – males tend to have more prominent supraorbital ridges and correspondingly greater ocular protection.

To a projectile of any significant size, a well-protected eye essentially presents only one aspect. With greater exposure as above, much of the anterior half of the ocular sphere is at risk of direct injury, depending on the direction of gaze at the time of injury. The point of impact on the globe can significantly affect the resultant ocular damage, for a variety of reasons. First, the ocular surface coats have known weak points. The thinnest point of the sclera is at the insertion of the four rectus muscles, about 7 mm behind the limbus. Direct injury can rupture the globe. Secondly, the immediate post-trauma oscillations of the globe can vary depending upon the point of impact. Thirdly, the intra-ocular hydrostatic effects of an external blow will vary for the same reason.

The direction of approach

The greater the degree of natural ocular protection, as explained above, the less the likelihood of a projectile making its way into the orbit and causing ocular damage. Likewise, the more oblique the angle of approach to the orbit, the less likely it is to penetrate. However, the orbital walls are not symmetrical around the eye. The greatest protection is afforded by the supraorbital ridge and nasal side, the least inferolaterally. It is for this reason that a projectile approaching from below and to the temporal side is most likely to cause severe ocular damage, up to and including a ruptured globe, as has been described for instance after a mistimed hook at cricket (Jones and Tullo, 1986).

The kinetic energy of the projectile and the force exerted on the eye

The energy carried by a moving projectile is calculated by:

$$E = 1/2mv^2$$

where m is the projectile mass and v its velocity. The velocity thus has proportionately a much greater influence on kinetic energy than its mass. All (if the projectile is small and only hits the eye) or some (if the face and orbit absorbs part) of this energy may be imparted to the eye over a variable area. The smaller the area over which the energy is imparted, or the 'sharper' the projectile, the greater the likelihood that penetration of the eye will occur, with its attendant complications. Energy imparted over a larger area will result in a 'blunt' injury.

The projectile size and its malleability

Assuming a spherical projectile, which is common in many sports, then the larger the object, the greater its radius of curvature and the 'flatter' its leading surface. Bearing in mind that the orbital walls offer some protec-

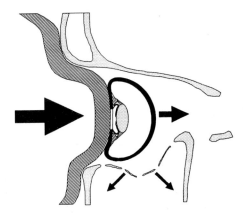

Figure 4.1 A hollow sphere (football) striking the face and orbit. Surface deformation allows local protruberance, and therefore access to the orbital space. Compression of the eye, and blow-out fracture is seen in this instance

tion against injury, then a large diameter object such as a soccer ball is less likely to cause ocular damage than a smaller one, for example a squash ball, assuming that all other parameters are equal. However, many balls used in sport are capable of considerable deformation because they are hollow and air-filled. High-speed photography has demonstrated the ability even of hard objects such as golf balls to deform on impact. Squash balls can very easily penetrate orbits (Plate 1) yet so can footballs, which can bulge and therefore cause eye damage, especially if underinflated (Figure 4.1). Solid balls such as baseballs or cricket balls are much less capable of deformation on impact.

Surface, shearing and rotational effects

The above paragraphs have assumed a projectile which is perfectly spherical, smooth-surfaced and presents a non-rotating surface to the eye. In the majority of instances this is of course not the case. Many objects have rough surfaces, for instance the raised seam on a cricket or baseball (Plate 2), the half-buried strings on a squash racquet. These surface irregularities are very likely to exert tractional forces, especially where the projectile is rapidly rotating. In addition to the simple anteroposterior forces described above, these other forces may result in greater tissue damage in the form of surface abrasion, laceration, eyelid avulsion and contusion. In rare circumstances, surface irregularities alone may be responsible for a penetrating eye injury.

Intervening objects

The ideal intervening object is a well-fitted, well-designed, tried and tested protector. In this circumstance ocular damage can be eliminated. Unfortunately, too many injuries occur because adequate protection is not worn. In some instances, inappropriate spectacles were being used. A blunt injury of moderate severity can with great ease be converted into a blinding penetrating injury by wearing spectacles with glass lenses. Spectacles with unstrengthened glass lenses should never be worn in sport where there is a risk of high-velocity injury, where polycarbonate is the material of choice (see Chapter 5).

Many sportspeople wear contact lenses for visual reasons, wrongly believing that these also have a protective effect. This is not the case. At best, contact lenses will do no additional damage in the event of a sports injury and at worst, a fractured rigid lens may lacerate or penetrate the eye. Furthermore, dislodged or lost contact lenses, especially the rigid corneal variety, may cause problems and also interrupt play.

The spectrum of eye injuries in sport

Sharp or penetrating injury

There are two ways in which the eyeball can be opened by an injury. The first, direct entry by a sharp object, is dealt with here. The second, globe rupture, is an indirect injury caused by generalized pressure on the eye.

Fortunately, penetrating injury is rare in sport. Direct entry of a sharp object into the eyeball is not a feature of most sports injuries. There are occasional reports of penetration by darts or fishhooks (the latter providing an interesting surgical challenge in their removal). The fracture of spectacle lenses or frames is a notorious complicating factor in what may otherwise have been a recoverable blunt injury.

Penetration into the eye, via cornea, sclera or both, gives rise to a mixture of complications. Any such injury carries with it the risk of intra-ocular infection, a potentially devastating sequel. If uvea is prolapsed, particularly from posterior segment penetrations, the rare but blinding disease of sympathetic ophthalmia is also a risk. Intra-ocular foreign bodies, such as splinters of spectacle lenses, can cause immediate and, if retained, progressive damage and must be surgically removed. The physical disruption of the cornea often renders it postoperatively irregular and scarred. Laceration or avulsion of the iris or part of it is frequent (Plate 3) and penetration of the crystalline lens will require immediate or delayed intervention to remove the resultant cataract. The long-term vitreoretinal complications that may ensue are a particular concern. In very severe penetrating injuries of this sort, the eye may be blinded or may require removal.

Blunt injury of the anterior segment of the eye

Superficial injuries of this sort result in a subconjunctival haemorrhage or a painful corneal abrasion. Regarding more serious intra-ocular damage, it is convenient to consider the eyeball in the anatomically distinct anterior and posterior segments for this purpose. A blunt injury directed onto the cornea

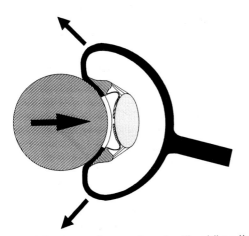

Figure 4.2 A small, round projectile strikes the eye. Anteroposterior compression results in equatorial expansion (arrows) causing intraocular traction and rupture. The anterior chamber is compressed and the crystalline lens is pushed posteriorly

will immediately compress the globe anteroposteriorly (Figure 4.2). The intraocular pressure rises precipitately as the cornea is flattened. In certain circumstances the cornea touches the crystalline lens, squeezing the iris and pupil between them, which may leave a permanent brown impression on the anterior lens capsule, known as Vossius' ring. The anterior chamber is centrally compressed and therefore the aqueous humour is pushed peripherally. The resultant forces impinging on the pupil often cause a series of ruptures in the sphincter pupillae and pupil edges, leaving tell-tale notches in the normally smooth round pupil outline. As the peripheral anterior chamber deepens, great tension on the peripheral iris occurs, which is its weakest point. Tractional ruptures of iris nerves and blood vessels may occur, the former being responsible for sluggish pupil reactions and a partially dilated or irregular pupil (Plate 4), the latter for hyphaema (bleeding into the anterior chamber) (Plate 5).

If enough tension is put on the peripheral iris it will disinsert from its attachment to the ciliary body (Plate 6). Such an iris dialysis is not possible to correct surgically and will lead to long-term optical effects. If a dialysis does not occur, then a rupture into the ciliary body itself may occur instead. By allowing the iris/ciliary body attachment to fall posteriorly, this injury will deepen the anterior chamber, either locally or generally. Such injury (known as angle recession) reflects profound damage to the anterior chamber drainage angle, which may well manifest itself as glaucoma at a later date, though it is likely that 150° or more of an otherwise healthy angle has to be injured in this way before glaucoma will occur. Figure 4.3 shows a cross-sectional representation of iris dialysis and angle recession.

The hyphaema that is such a common accompaniment to blunt ocular injury may cause immediate or long-term problems. The massive load of erythrocytes can stretch the drainage function of the anterior chamber angle to its utmost, especially if already compromised by the same injury. A rise in

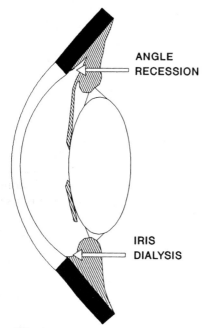

ANGLE
RECESSION

IRIS
DIALYSIS

Figure 4.3 A cross-section of the ocular anterior segment, illustrating the anatomical position of both angle recession (posterior displacement of iris/ciliary body junction) and iris dialysis (disinsertion from ciliary body)

intraocular pressure is therefore a common accompaniment to hyphaema, and requires strict supervision and treatment by both topical and systemic medication. In most instances the hyphaema will reabsorb and any secondary glaucoma may settle. In some instances, however, the hyphaema may fill most or all of the anterior chamber, either directly after the injury, or after a secondary haemorrhage which may occur at any time between two and seven days later. Large hyphaemas with high intraocular pressure are a particular problem. If left to their own devices, blood pigments can be hydrostatically forced into the corneal stroma, giving corneal bloodstaining which can permanently affect vision. Surgical evacuation of blood from the anterior chamber may be necessary to prevent this complication from arising.

Contusional injury of the crystalline lens may cause a cataract of rapid onset. Such a 'concussion cataract' is often stellate in shape and occasionally disappears over a period of days or weeks. More often though it remains or progressively develops, necessitating surgical intervention. A more severe injury may disrupt the suspensory ligament of the lens, either partially or completely. The lens may become displaced partially or totally (Plate 7), and may be mobile, with all the attendant optical problems that that implies.

Blunt injury of the posterior segment of the eye

The initial blow to the eye causes anteroposterior compression. Some have suggested that the crystalline lens may touch the retina in these circumstances. Whether or not that is true, it is certain that the eyeball is capable of very substantial distortion, while still maintaining its overall integrity (Figure 4.2). It is in the few milliseconds after injury that the globe, in oscillating back to its proper shape, creates internal tractional forces which can be particularly disruptive.

The vitreous humour in the young person is strongly attached to retina around the optic disc and macula, along blood vessels and at the vitreous base, which straddles the anterior retina and pars plana of the ciliary body. Tractional forces are particularly important along the vitreous base. The entire base can become detached over a considerable length, hanging down into the eye as a 'buckethandle'. Often the detachment of the vitreous base carries the peripheral retina with it. This peripheral disinsertion, or dialysis, may not be obvious directly after the injury but may present later with retinal detachment. Such peripheral vitreous disruption causes traction on retinal blood vessels and consequent vitreous haemorrhage (Plate 8), seen by the patient as large floaters.

It is always wise to look for retinal tears after a blunt eye injury. They are not uncommon and may be treated prophylactically with the argon laser to prevent retinal detachment which may otherwise arise. Once a detachment has arisen (Plate 9), surgical intervention is necessary.

A heavy blow on the eye sends considerable hydraulic pressure waves posteriorly. As with any such travelling wavefront, maximum damage will occur at the interfaces where the contiguous tissues have very different densities. An interface of particular significance is that between vitreous and retina. The resulting retinal injury causes cell death, oedema and haemorrhage to occur in a patch which is often at the posterior pole. The retina looks pale and is thickened (Plate 10). This condition is known as **commotio retinae**. Visual acuity may be immediately affected, and the prognosis for visual recovery must remain guarded. The retinal oedema and haemorrhage will recover, but the underlying damage to retinal photoreceptors and pigment epithelium may cause considerable retinal scarring (Plate 11) and permanent visual loss.

The phenomenon of indirect ocular injury should be mentioned here as it predominantly affects the retina. Any severe crushing injury to another part of the body can, either by suddenly raised vascular pressure or by embolization of fat, cause dramatic retinal damage consisting of intraretinal and preretinal haemorrhage and ischaemia (Plate 12). This picture of Purtscher's retinopathy is seen only in severe crush injuries, which are rare in sport, but for completeness the condition is included here. In addition head injuries which involve certain areas of the brain may result in abnormalities of eye movements or field of vision defects.

The anteroposterior compression of an eye during the injury (Figure 4.2) will stretch the choroid, that delicate, friable, vascular tissue that lies between retina and sclera. Ruptures of the choroid are an occasional sequel. The resultant, often dramatic, subretinal haemorrhage will clear, sometimes over a period of months, to reveal an arcuate choroidal rupture, typically with the optic disc at its centre of curvature (Plate 13). It is unfortunate that such choroid ruptures seem to have a pre-

dilection for the temporal retina, and occasionally cross directly underneath the fovea, with no recovery of central vision. Even when healed, choroid ruptures may cause problems in the distant future, by growing neovascular membranes from their disrupted edge which may cause further subretinal haemorrhage, analogous to disciform maculopathy in age-related macular degeneration.

The sclera, a tough collagenous meshwork, is the strongest part of the eye yet also has its breaking point. A blunt injury of sufficient force to cause rupture of the sclera is a severe injury indeed, yet such injuries do occur, especially in sport (Plate 14). The rupture is usually posterior and the loss of intraocular contents into the orbit is manifested by an extremely soft eye with considerable subconjunctival haemorrhage and oedema. Often a total hyphaema is present. These signs, in an eye which can detect light and no more, are poor prognostic indicators and generally such eyes are unsalvageable.

Injury to the eyelids, orbital contents and bones

Any blunt injury of sufficient force may be associated with lacerations of the periorbital and eyelid skin that will need suturing. Substantial subcutaneous haemorrhage will lead to a 'black eye' (Plate 15) which in itself is painful and may force the eyelids closed. Haemorrhage may also occur behind the eyeball, in the orbital fat, involving the extraocular muscles or underneath the orbital periosteum. Such injuries can cause proptosis, and it is particularly important to monitor visual acuity and pupil function in these circumstances, in order to assess possible progressive damage to the optic nerve. Extraocular muscle haematomas may also temporarily cause double vision because of restricted ocular movement. It is important to distinguish this from diplopia caused by orbital fracture (see below).

Penetrating injuries of the orbit are rare but have been described in sport. The injury entails an object (of necessity reasonably long and thin) penetrating the orbital septum and entering the orbit around the side of the eyeball, either through eyelid or conjunctival fornix. Such injuries have been caused by ski-poles during a tumble, but the human finger is also well designed to fit the space. Sports requiring fast-moving hand-to-ball contact, such as basketball, may inadvertently cause fingers to be thrust into the orbit. Apart from the above injuries, the optic nerve itself may be contused or even disinserted from the eyeball. Vision does not recover in these circumstances.

The bony orbital margins are very strong, yet the internal orbital walls, for reasons of low weight, are very thin, especially in the medial wall (the lamina papyraceae or papery layer) and floor. A blow to the eye propels it backwards into the orbit (Figure 4.1), a conical space of ever-decreasing dimensions. The resultant increase in intra-orbital pressure may hydraulically 'blow out' one or two orbital walls, into the ethmoid sinus (medial wall) or maxillary sinus (floor) (Plate 16). It is also likely that direct sudden pressure on the inferior orbital margin (rather than the eye itself) can buckle the orbital floor and cause it to snap-fracture, simulating a blow-out.

As a result of a blow-out fracture of the orbit floor, the infra-orbital nerve may be contused or severed. The resultant numbness of the skin of the cheek and upper teeth on that side is one of the cardinal signs of blow-out fracture, as is proptosis after blowing the nose. The abnormal connection between sinuses and orbit means that any retrograde air pressure will push air into the orbit and protrude the eye. The resultant subcutaneous gathering of air gives an unmistakable crepitant sensation. The lack of support for the eyeball may, as time passes, cause it to sink downwards and backwards, giving an unacceptable cosmetic result. Orbital tissues may become comminuted within the fracture, restricting eye movement and causing double

vision and pain, especially when looking upwards.

Most orbital fractures are small and visual function settles without the need for intervention. However, it may be necessary to operate to disimpact orbital contents from the fracture and to insert a false silastic orbit floor which remains permanently in situ. The surgery aims to improve the cosmetic appearance and to enlarge the field of binocular vision, which may remain permanently restricted after blow-out fracture.

Occasionally the orbital rim itself is fractured, for instance in a tripod fracture of the zygoma. Such fractures may require surgical repositioning and are the territory of the maxillofacial surgeon. An ocular injury involving the orbital rim fracture denotes considerable force, and a particularly careful search should be made for signs of scleral rupture.

Eyes at particular risk of injury

In certain circumstances, pre-existing eye conditions can enhance the danger of eye injury. They are reduced vision in one eye which predisposes the player to injury, and pre-existing ocular weakness.

Reduced vision predisposing to injury

Ocular or neurological disease giving rise to poor visual acuity or a constricted visual field can reduce visual awareness and make an injury more likely. For instance, any person with monocular vision or grossly decreased vision in one eye (perhaps because of previous injury) will have disordered or absent binocular vision. Though, with experience, visual environmental clues can compensate to a degree, in a dynamic situation as is encountered during many sports, calculations in time and space can be affected. The possibility of collision must therefore be worsened.

Similarly, in conditions reducing visual field, such as chronic glaucoma, peripheral vision may be patchy or absent, narrowing the visual environment and decreasing the reaction time available for injury avoidance. Although people with significantly decreased visual acuity may not attempt fast-moving sport which carries a significant risk of injury, it is not uncommon for low myopes to choose to participate without spectacles or contact lenses, thus increasing their chances of injury.

Pre-existing ocular weakness

Pre-existing ocular weakness can greatly increase the severity of an injury which to a normal eye would have been sustainable. Such weakness can be natural or acquired. High myopia predisposes to severe injury for several reasons. First, the sclera tends to be thinner and therefore more susceptible to rupture. Secondly, the axial length of the eye is greater, giving more ocular exposure and therefore susceptibility to injury. Thirdly, high myopes have a predisposition to retinal degenerations which may lead to post-traumatic retinal tears and subsequent retinal detachment. It is also possible that myopes may have undergone refractive surgery (see below).

Previous intraocular or surface ocular surgery may permanently weaken the integrity of the eye. In these circumstances a blunt injury which would otherwise be tolerated with minor damage, might lead to rupture at the site of the previous surgical wound. In some cases, expression of intra-ocular contents including lens implants has occurred. Surgical management is likely to be fraught, and a poor outcome, sometimes leading to removal of the eye, can result. Cataract surgery of any type is the most common predisposing operation (though small-incision sur-

gery is less likely to be associated with severe injury). Glaucoma drainage surgery or corneal grafting may equally weaken the eye. Refractive keratotomy for myopia or astigmatism is known to grossly weaken the cornea and has been associated with postoperative globe rupture. Excimer laser treatment is much less likely to weaken the eye, but thins the cornea by up to 150 μm. The risks after retinal detachment surgery are less well defined. In some circumstances, effective retinal reattachment operations can enhance retinal adhesion so that further injury does not cause re-detachment. Further injury does, however, remain a considerable risk after such surgery, which usually requires the permanent insertion of silastic explants around the eye.

Retinal degenerations (with or without myopia) are quite common. They may predispose to retinal tear formation after even relatively minor blunt injury. In some circumstances tear formation goes on to produce retinal detachment which will require surgery if blindness is to be avoided.

The patient with one good functional eye is not only at greater risk of injury, but has more to lose after uniocular trauma. Any patient with unilateral poor vision from whatever cause (including amblyopia) should be considered high-risk for injury. Injuries to only eyes do occur, in sport and elsewhere. They are a tragedy.

Protection of the at-risk eye is one of the most important aspects of sports opthalmology and is the responsibility not only of the player, but of his optometrist and ophthalmologist. The subject of protection should be discussed with every patient acquiring a new spectacle prescription, and for every patient after intra-ocular surgery. The increasing number of older patients who participate in sport (and who are more likely to have undergone intra-ocular surgery) makes this of paramount importance. It is not merely good practice; it is becoming increasingly clear that it is perceived as a medicolegal responsibility of practitioners to identify risks of injury and to offer advice on protection.

The law and eye injury

In English law, the legal principle of *volenti non fit injuria* relates to injury in sport. The principle essentially states that, in participating in a sport where there are well-known and identified risks intrinsic to the game in its proper mode of play, the participant tacitly accepts that risk. Thus if during a game of rugby a player sustains an accidental eye injury during play which is within the rules of the sport, there is no case against the 'offending' player, nor for any form of compensation.

Deliberate injury in sport is a phenomenon difficult to quantify. In several surveys of sports eye injuries, a significant proportion were considered to be deliberate. The distinction between 'overenthusiastic' play and assault is a blurred one. The player elbowed in the eye by an opposing soccer player while both were trying to head the ball may find it difficult to judge on which side of the boundary the event lies (as indeed may the referee).

There are, however, events which occur on the sports field which are by no means covered by the principle of *volenti non fit injuria*. The soccer player does not, in participating in the game, accept the risk of a punch in the face in an off-the-ball incident, neither does the rugby player accept the risk of being 'gouged' in the eye by an opposing player during a scrummage. Such injuries are, legally, *assault and battery*. They may equally have been committed on the street during a brawl. The fact that they took place in a sports venue is irrelevant. The legal precedents for both civil and criminal prosecution have been set, in addition to whatever internal disciplinary arrangements each sport has at its disposal.

Eyes have been blinded or removed after injuries sustained during sport as a result of an assault. In English law this level of injury constitutes *grievous bodily harm* (Offences Against the Person Act, 1861), and if convicted, a sentence of up to five years imprisonment can be passed. If the prosecution can prove that the level of injury sustained was the deliberate intent of the assailant (for example, it was the intention, in gouging the eye of the rugby player, to blind him) then the crime of *grievous bodily harm with intent* carries a much greater penalty. No such charge has yet been answered for an injury on a sports field, but those who recklessly and violently abuse the rules of their sport are increasingly being pursued by both internal disciplinary proceedings and by the law.

The treatment of eye injuries in sport

First aid

Most injuries in sport occur in the heat of the action. Though it will be apparent that an injury has occurred, it may be some time before the circumstances of the injury and its cause become clear, especially in the context of team sports. On a squash court the fact that a ball or racquet has struck the eye is immediately obvious. The player surfacing from a loose maul in rugby with a blunt injury may not be so clear as to the cause, and sometimes the history is hidden because the injury was deliberate. The exact cause of the injury may not be identified. The first-aider is therefore sometimes denied the accurate history which will give an idea of the physical forces involved in the injury.

In most significant sports eye injuries, the trauma will be blunt and will give rise to immediate pain and visual disturbance. A formal assessment of vision will not yet be possible, yet bruising and swelling may shortly become obvious. At this stage several questions should be answered.

Is the player fit to continue?

In the context of most sports sessions, any significant injury is likely to lead to curtailment of the game for that player, which is usually the wise choice. In the context of a major team game the decision might not be so easy. In general, any sportsperson affected by an eye injury leading to significant immediate visual loss, double vision or visible hyphaema should not continue to play. It should be borne in mind that corneal abrasions may be at greater risk of infection if play continues; that hyphaemas may be exacerbated (sometimes severely) by continued activity; that diplopia may compromise future safety in the game or may be a sign of additional head injury; and that any major blunt injury will require the attention of an ophthalmologist and that delaying this attention must be weighed in the balance against the importance of continuing the game.

What immediate measures are necessary?

Having chosen to discontinue the sports session, immediate treatment may be valuable. Blunt injury may cause significant subcutaneous haemorrhage and oedema, both of which can be limited by mild pressure and/or a cool compress. A painful corneal abrasion may be treated with a sterile topical anaesthetic agent (guttae benoxinate or proxymetacaine for instance) for the purposes of enhancing examination by a doctor. At this stage the following examination should be performed.

1. Rough visual assessment (using newspaper, wall sign, fingers etc.).
2. Pen-torch or natural light examination of cornea and anterior segment. The sports physician should be equipped with pen-torch and fluorescein.

Any corneal abrasion, hyphaema, diplopia or significant visual loss requires same-day attention at a hospital casualty department or by a doctor with ophthalmological experience.

Is immediate treatment of any use?

Clearly the removal of minor foreign bodies is a common requirement on the sports field. Apart from this, the immediate management of sports eye injuries tends to focus on decreasing discomfort if possible and preventing further damage until proper assessment and treatment can be carried out. Anaesthesia as above has been suggested. The abraded, bruised eye may be more comfortable under a pad. For clearly severe injuries, the temptation to give a drink should be avoided, and food should not be taken. There is a possibility that surgery on the same day may be necessary, which would be delayed by food or drink. If there is any suggestion that a penetrating injury might have occurred, it is essential that no pressure is applied to the eye. A protective shield or cartella is a standard disposable in casualty departments; those responsible for sports medical supervision would be wise to have one available to offer adequate protection to such an eye.

The greatest service that a team doctor or physiotherapist can do for a sportsman with an injured eye is to learn to tell the trivial from the serious; to remove the sportsman from play immediately if it is serious; to alleviate discomfort and prevent further injury; and to ensure rapid and appropriate attention by those with greater expertise and better equipment.

Casualty treatment

If the injury is severe enough to warrant hospital attendance, the following should be standard practice.

1. A formal history is taken, including an accurate account of the incident causing the injury, some estimate of vision prior to the injury, any previous or predisposing eye problems which might complicate the injury and a brief medical and drug history.
2. An accurate assessment of visual acuity is made using a Snellen chart. This is essential, not only for medical, but for medicolegal reasons.

3. The anterior segment and the pupil reactions are examined with a pen-torch. Fluorescein drops should always be instilled to help detect any corneal epithelial abnormality when viewed with a blue light.
4. The eye movements should be examined in the nine cardinal positions of gaze. The red reflex is examined with the ophthalmoscope. If possible the optic disc and macula are examined.

A corneal abrasion is treated by topical antibiotic prophylaxis and temporary mydriasis (dilatation of the pupil) is achieved with either homatropine 1% or cyclopentolate 1% eye drops, instilled once only. If there is significant visual loss, traumatic intraocular inflammation or hyphaema, a distorted pupil or an abnormal red reflex, then the patient must be referred to an ophthalmologist. If an eyelid laceration is involved, then a penetrating injury should be eliminated. Any laceration involving the eyelid margin should be sutured by an ophthalmologist.

Treatment by the ophthalmologist

The ophthalmologist follows the same principles of examination and treatment as the casualty officer. Following accurate visual assessment, the eye is examined with the slit-lamp which can reveal more subtle intraocular changes. The intraocular pressure is measured; it is often raised when a hyphaema is present and this may require the use of ocular hypotensive agents. Intraocular inflammation may require topical steroid treatment. The iris and pupil are examined with care and, if safe, the pupil should be dilated at this stage for a proper retinal examination, especially of the peripheral retina. Immediate surgery will be required for penetrating injury. Hospital admission may also be required for large hyphaemas with secondary glaucoma or other severe manifestations of blunt trauma.

The management of blunt eye injury, whatever the cause, is essentially a process of damage limitation rather than restoration.

Both immediate and delayed surgical intervention may be necessary which may entail prolonged inpatient or outpatient supervision. Immediate surgery to repair a penetrating injury may be required. Further surgery to treat retinal detachment or cataract is occasionally needed.

Late sequelae of eye injury

If a penetrating injury has occurred, it is likely that some degree of permanent corneal distortion, scarring and irregular astigmatism will result. The eye may, in ideal conditions (such as Snellen acuity testing), attain a reasonable visual acuity. Contrast sensitivity will, however, be reduced and the eye is likely to function worse in adverse lighting conditions, with haloes and dazzle effects. In this circumstance, appropriate contact lens fitting may be of considerable benefit. Permanent loss of iris tissue or iris dialyses often also follow a penetrating injury, and the use of a painted contact lens may be of both cosmetic and functional benefit.

Blunt injury typically causes neurological damage to the iris. In the early stages this is manifested as a dilated pupil with a sluggish reaction, but this may go on to become permanent so that accommodative miosis may not be possible. Accommodation itself may also suffer, because of direct ciliary body trauma, damage to suspensory ligaments or both. Near vision may therefore suffer considerably in an injured eye. This may be amenable to optical correction, as it will be after the removal of a traumatic cataract. This unilateral 'presbyopia' in a young person may be very inconvenient and may be present despite normal Snellen acuity.

Injury prevention

The ophthalmological experience of the treatment of eye injuries repeatedly shows that the whole exercise is one of damage limitation. Once the accident has happened, it is already too late. Prevention, in this field, is overwhelmingly better than attempts at cure and should receive much attention. Other causes of eye injury have been dramatically reduced because of sensible prevention measures. Occupational eye injuries, once by far the most important cause of ocular trauma in the UK, have been pursued by legislation and widespread ocular protection so that now only a few severe injuries are seen (MacEwen, 1989). Road accidents, once the producer of a constant stream of lacerated faces and eyes, have, by the introduction of seat belt legislation and laminated windscreens, largely been eliminated as a cause of severe eye injury.

The value of a strategy for injury prevention in sport has already been shown by the success story of Canadian ice-hockey. In essence, the problem must first of all be identified and quantified. Common features of injuries must be recognized, obvious areas of prevention explored and tackled by straightforward methods. A simple change in style of play, or of the sport's regulations, may in itself make a huge difference. To all those beginning a sport, the rules of safety should be explained by coaches who know not only the technicalities of the sport, but its danger zones too. Where eye protection is felt to be needed it should be encouraged, readily available within the purse of the average player, fitted with prescription lenses if necessary, and worn properly.

Education of sports players

Various misconceptions amongst sportsmen and women are partly responsible for injury. Perhaps the most unwise attitude is that 'it will never happen to me'. This maxim is disproved with depressing regularity, and those sportspeople who, having sustained a significant injury, make the mistake of assuming that their turn has passed, are occasionally unlucky enough to be injured again. The risks of injury should never be exaggerated, and if education into these risks causes people to stop playing, then it has failed. A realistic approach, stressing the positive steps that can be taken to reduce the low but significant risk of injury, is essential.

The assumption that injury in sport is largely a problem of the novice is grossly mistaken. This misconception is often heard, but has no data whatever to support it. Loran (1992), in surveying injuries in squash, found that novices probably have a greater risk of injury per unit time than experts, but the latter tended to spend much more time in their sport. Overall, the accomplished regular player had a greater risk of eye injury if protectors are not worn.

All sports participants should look to the national and local organizers of their sport to disseminate useful information about safety. All sports centres should regard it as their responsibility to obtain and display useful and constructive information about sports safety (Plate 17), stressing a few salient points for each sport. Coaches of novices should start with safe techniques and the avoidance of dangerous situations. All too often, coaches, though experts in technical teaching, are unaware of the main problems leading to eye injury.

Style of play and sports legislation

The encouragement of safe play may in itself be inadequate. Instructions can be ignored, sometimes wilfully. In this circumstance, a change in the law of the sport may be most productive. In ice-hockey, for example, the practice of high sticking (raising the stick above shoulder level) has now largely been stopped, and the incidence of head injury has been substantially reduced.

Eye protection

In certain sports it is clear that the risk of eye injury cannot be minimized simply by safe coaching and technique. Where possible, if the risk justifies it, the use of eye protection should be recommended. The particular risks of the sport and the kinetic energies involved should be considered in devising an appropriate protector, which may also have to incorporate head and face protection. The use of such protection should be widely encouraged, or made mandatory in certain circumstances (for juniors for instance) if the risk is felt to be high. Again, the national organizers of sport should have a leading role to play.

Conclusion

Sport of one kind or another is played regularly by millions. The numbers of injured may appear high but should be placed into perspective. Even in sports with a relatively high risk of injury, the average player participating regularly over a period of many years will probably have a better than even chance of not sustaining a significant eye injury during that playing career. Many players will say that they have never suffered an eye injury, and neither have any of their close acquaintances. This is the main reason given for choosing not to wear eye protection. The same argument can be used for severe road accidents, yet very few choose to leave off their seatbelt regularly. It is a matter of appreciation of the risks and sensible judgement. The author, experiencing the down side of sports eye injury with great regularity, would always recommend to err on the side of safety rather than convenience. Play sport by all means, but play safe.

References

American Society for Testing and Materials (1988) F803–38 *Standard Specification for Eye Protectors for Use by Players of Racquet Sports*, ASTM, Philadelphia

Barrell, G.V., Cooper, P.J., Elkington, A.R., MacFayden, J.M., Powell, R.G. *et al.* (1981) Squash ball to eye ball: the likelihood of squash players incurring an eye injury. *British Medical Journal*, **283**, 893–5

Bartholomew, R.S. and MacDonald, M. (1980) Fish hook injuries of the eye. *British Journal of Ophthalmology*, **64**, 531–3

Board of Science and Education Working Party Report on Boxing (1984). British Medical Association, London

Canadian Standards Association (1982) CSA P400-M1 *Racquet Sports Eye Protectors*, CSA, Ontario

Canavan, Y.M., O'Flaherty, M.J., Archer, D.B. and Elwood, J.H. (1980) A 10-year survey of eye injuries in Northern Ireland: 1967–76. *British Journal of Ophthalmology*, **64**, 618–25

Crawfurd, A.R. (1990) The medical hazards of fencing. In *Medicine, Sport and the Law* (ed. S.D.W. Payne) Blackwell, Oxford

Doxanas, M.T. and Soderstrom, C. (1980) Racquetball as an ocular hazard. *Archives of Ophthalmology*, **98**, 1965–6

Easterbrook, M. and Pashby, T.J. (1985) Eye injuries associated with war games. *Canadian Medical Association Journal*, **133**, 415–17

Giovinazzo, V.J., Yannuzzi, L.A., Sorenson, J.A., Delrowe, D.J. and Cambell, E.A. (1987) The ocular complications of boxing. *Ophthalmology*, **94**, 587–96

Glynn, R.J., Seddon, J.M. and Berlin, B.M. (1988) The incidence of eye injuries in New England adults. *Archives of Ophthalmology*, **106**, 785–9

Grayson, E. (1990) Sports medicine and the law. In *Medicine, Sport and the Law* (ed. S.D.W. Payne), Blackwell, Oxford

Helveston, E.M. (1987) Football. In *Sports Ophthalmology* (eds L.D. Pizzarello and B.G. Haik), Charles C. Thomas, Springfield, Ill.

Jonasson, F. (1977) Swimming goggles causing severe eye injuries. *British Medical Journal*, **275**, 881

Jones, N.P. (1988) One year of severe eye injuries in sport. *Eye*, **2**, 484–7

Jones, N.P., Hayward, J.M., Khaw, P.T. Claoue, C.M.P. and Elkington, A.R. (1986) Function of an ophthalmic 'accident and emergency' department: results of a six month survey. *British Medical Journal*, **292**, 188–90

Jones, N.P. and Tullo, A.B. (1986) Severe eye injuries in cricket. *British Journal of Sports Medicine*, **20**, 178–9

Kelly, S.P. (1987) Serious eye injury in badminton players. *British Journal of Ophthalmology*, **71**, 746–7

Kennerley Bankes, J.L. (1985) Squash rackets: a survey of eye injuries in England. *British Medical Journal*, **291**, 1539

Lambah, P. (1968) Adult eye injuries at Wolverhampton. *Transactions of the Ophthalmology Society (UK)*, **88**, 661–73

Loran, D. (1992) Eye injuries in squash. *Optician*, **204**, 18–23

MacEwen, C.J. (1987) Sport associated eye injury: a casualty department survey. *British Journal Ophthalmology*, **71**, 701–5

MacEwen, C.J. (1989) Eye injuries: a prospective survey of 5671 cases. *British Journal of Ophthalmology*, **73**, 888–94

MacEwen, C.J. and Jones, N.P. (1991) Eye injuries in racquet sports. *British Medical Journal*, **302**, 1415–416

McLeod, D. (1992) Ocular injuries from boxing: what about prophylactic laser coagulation of boxers' retinas? *British Medical Journal*, **304**, 197

Mamalis, N., Monson, M.C., Farnsworth, S.T. and White, G.L. (1990) Blunt ocular trauma secondary to 'war games'. *Annals of Ophthalmology*, **22**, 416–18

Pashby, T.J. (1977) Eye injuries in Canadian hockey Phase II. *Canadian Medical Association Journal*, **117**, 671–8

Pashby, T.J. (1979) Eye injuries in Canadian hockey Phase III. Older players now at risk. *Canadian Medical Association Journal*, **121**, 643–4

Pashby, T. (1987) Eye injuries in Canadian amateur hockey still a concern. *Canadian Journal of Ophthalmology*, **22**, 293–5

Pashby, T.J., Pashby, R.C., Chisholm, L.D.J. and Crawford, J.S. (1977) Eye injuries in Canadian hockey. *Canadian Medical Association Journal*, **113**, 663–74

Portis, J.M., Vassallo, S.A. and Albert, D.M. (1981) Ocular sports injuries: a review of cases on file in the Massachusetts Eye and Ear Infirmary Pathology Laboratory. *International Ophthalmology Clinics*, **21**, 4

Rousseau, A.P., Amyot, M. and Labelle, P.F. (1987) Winter sports: hockey and skiing. In *Sports Ophthalmology* (eds L.D. Pizzarello and B.G. Haik), Charles C. Thomas, Springfield, Ill.

Seelanfreund, M.H. and Freilich, D.B. (1976) Rushing the net and retinal detachment. *Journal of the American Medical Association*, **235**, 2723–6

UK Board of Science and Education Working Party (1984) Report.

Further reading

Jones, N.P. (1989) Eye injury in sport. *Sports Medicine*, **7**, 163–81

Pizzarello, L.D. and Haik, B.G. (eds) *Sports Ophthalmology*, Charles C. Thomas, Springfield, Ill.

Vinger, P.F. (1985) The eye and sports medicine. In *Clinical Ophthalmology*, vol. 5 (ed. T.D. Duane), Harper and Row, Philadelphia

5

Eye protectors for sport
Michael Easterbrook

The purpose of this chapter is to illustrate that eye protection is available for almost all recreational and professional sport. A player has never lost an eye while playing squash, racquetball, badminton or tennis while wearing a certified eye protector designed for sport or a protector that met Canadian and American impact standards.

Polycarbonate

Approximately half of the population wear eye glasses (Keeney *et al.*, 1972): polycarbonate is a modern plastic with superior impact resistance for all projectiles compared with streetwear (CR39) plastic and crown glass. For a small object such as 1/8–1/4 inch steel ball fired at high velocity, polycarbonate has approximately ten to twenty times the impact resistance of normal streetwear CR39 plastic used in usual prescription glasses. For larger objects, polycarbonate is extremely resistant to breakage. Davis (1988, 1994) could not break a polycarbonate lens with a 40 lb steel plate dropped from 1 m (3 ft). Vinger (1985/1994) has confirmed the marked difference in impact resistance between polycarbonate glass, high index plastics and standard streetwear (CR39) spectacle lenses with golf, lacrosse and tennis impacts.

The significant difference to impact of hardened safety glass, streetwear (CR39) prescription or non-prescription plastic and polycarbonate to a BB gun pellet (round 1–2 mm diameter pellet) is demonstrated in figures 5.1–5.3. Polycarbonate lenses have surface qualities at least as good as the usual allyl resin lenses and come close to the surface quality of the finest glass lenses. The material

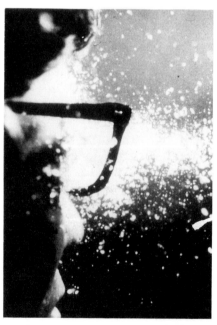

Figure 5.1 Streetwear hardened safety glass shattering with a BB pellet

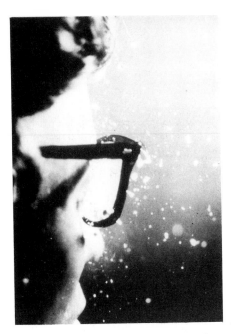

Figure 5.2 CR39 plastic lens fracturing with a BB pellet

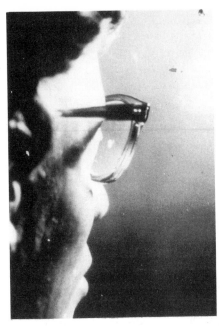

Figure 5.3 Polycarbonate lens withstanding a BB pellet

has excellent resistance to high temperatures and coated lenses are inert to most solvents. Polycarbonate is available for players who do not require prescription and for most players who are myopic and/or astigmatic.

Standards for eye protectors

Many streetwear eye wear glasses will break on impact in many sports because the energy levels exceed their impact resistance. In Canada between 1978 and 1986, twenty-one sports players sustained serious eye injury when their prescription lenses (hardened glass or plastic) shattered (Easterbrook, 1987). It is imperative that standards be written which are *performance* standards: it is up to the manufacturer to design a protector that meets these performance standards. Certification of such equipment to this standard is then carried out by the manufacturers. Sports regulatory bodies, such as the United States

Squash Racquets Association, have mandated the use of such equipment that meets these standards. It would be the wish of sports vision practitioners and all involved in eye care, that governing bodies should legislate against uncertified protection which gains access to the market place. In Canada only eye protectors and helmets which meet with Canadian Standards Association standards for hockey are allowed to be sold in the country.

The American National Standards Institute (ANSI) has published standards for some years in the field of eye protection. Z80 gives standards specifications for prescription ophthalmic lenses and frames, contact lenses, lens solution and sunglasses (Keeney, 1984). ANSI standard Z86 has been written for scuba diving masks (American National Standards Institute, 1986) and Z90 for protective head gear for sports including bicycling (American National Standards Institute, 1990).

In 1898 the American Society for Testing and Materials (ASTM) was formed: this is a non-profit-making, non-governmental, non-manufacturing body which was developed to produce voluntary standards which are arrived at as a consensus of all interested parties. It is the largest of 400 standards organizations in the United States. In 1968 the ASTM F-8 Committee in Sports Safety Standards was formed, originally to address the increase in head and neck injuries in American football. The ASTM F-8 now has committees for publishing standards in many sports including gymnastics, golf, archery, wrestling, fencing, trampoline, fitness sports, racquet sports, hockey and baseball (Vinger, 1985/1994). These ASTM committees consist of volunteers (producers, users, consumers, those representing the general public interest), who are representative of those in the community who are interested in the development of protective devices for a particular sport. These standards are *performance* standards, which relate to certain specifications such as the visual field performance, impact resistance or distribution of forces of each device. In comparison, design standards are concerned with design elements which may or may not relate to performance. ASTM eye safety sub-committees usually arrange the testing of protective devices against specific squash balls, racquets and hockey pucks for example, in an attempt to simulate real game conditions.

Revisions of standards are required on a regular basis. It would be ideal to have an international standard for all eye protectors in sport. Canada and the United States are working towards similarity in standards in hockey and racquet sports, which may provide a prototype for international standards.

Headforms

Eye guards are tested on headforms. The Canadian Standards Association has developed a new headform (available in different sizes) based on the physical measurements of thousands of heads. These head forms are better proportioned, particularly in the eye area, than the Alderston headform, previously used in the United States (Vinger, 1985/1994).

Table 5.1 772 Racquet sports injuries reported in Canada, 1976–1993 (44 blind eyes)

Year	No. injuries	% racquetball/Squash	% Badminton	% Tennis
1982*	90	73	13	14
1983	87	59	22	19
1984	115	58	16	26
1985	82	50	33	17
1986	83	39	33	28
1987	68	36	38	26
1988	46	39	46	15
1989	62	35	47	18
1990	40	35	55	10
1991	35	23	40	37
1992	33	24	52	24
1993 (to June)	31	23	55	22

* CSA Standard was published in 1982.

Protective devices for specific sports

Racquet sports

Since 1982, 772 racquet sports eye injuries have been recorded in Canada (Table 5.1). Our experience has demonstrated that:

1. Experience does *not* protect squash and racquetball players.
2. Eye glasses, when they are hardened glass or plastic, do not protect a squash or racquetball player and may break, producing severe ocular injury.
3. Open eye guards are of no use and may contribute to ocular injury.

These observations are based on many studies (Easterbrook 1978, 1980, 1981, 1982, 1985, 1988a, b, 1989, 1990 a, b, c, 1992, 1993).

Handball

The first eye protector designed for racquet sports was a lensless, rubber covered, wire eye guard (Figure 5.4). This eye guard did not prevent hyphaema and retinal tears; consequently the United States Handball Association Board of Directors voted in 1988 that all players were required to use a one-piece lens, polycarbonate eye protector when participating in nationally sanctioned events (Vinger,

1985/1994). No injuries have been reported in any handball player wearing such a lensed polycarbonate protector.

Badminton

The Badminton shuttlecock is a projectile which fits into the orbit perfectly (Figure 5.5). It is apparent that the open eye guard will not prevent this from happening (Figure 5.6). Table 5.1 demonstrates the relative increasing incidence of badminton as a cause of ocular injury from racquet sports in Canada. With the inclusion of badminton as an Olympic sport, the resurgence in the interest in badminton has been accompanied by an increase

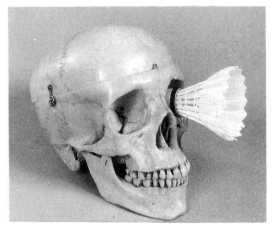

Figure 5.5 Badminton shuttlecock fitting into the orbit

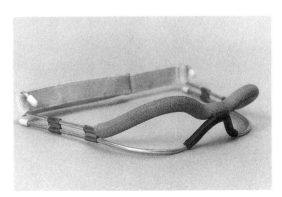

Figure 5.4 Lensless wire open eye guard, first used in handball

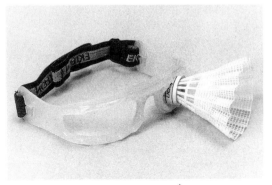

Figure 5.6 Open eye guard not preventing penetration of a shuttlecock

in ocular injury, particularly in doubles. At the 1992 Olympics in Barcelona one badminton player was recorded as hitting the shuttlecock at 187.5 mph (Badminton Association, personal communication). Dr Paul Vinger at Tufts is presently testing squash protectors against the 5.5 gram shuttlecock. Although no standards have been written for badminton, we are presently recommending that eye protectors which meet FA 803 ASTM impact standards (American Society for Testing and Materials, 1988), which are for squash and racquetball, are also used for badminton. No injury with a polycarbonate lens in badminton has been recorded to date.

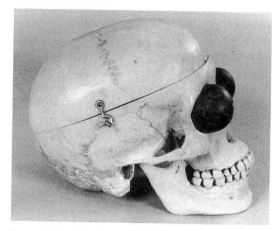

Figure 5.7   70 plus squash ball in the right orbit; yellow dot international ball in the left orbit

Tennis

In tennis, ocular injuries usually occur at the net in doubles matches. They may also be the result of a mis-hit off one's own racquet. Occasionally a spectator is injured in tennis. Although the incidence of tennis injuries is low, particularly in singles, sports vision practitioners are currently recommending that tennis players, especially in doubles, should wear polycarbonate lenses in a sports frame designed for racquet sports. No injury has been recorded in tennis with players using such a protector.

Squash

Squash is a significant cause of ocular injury (Figure 5.7) and injuries have been recorded in almost all countries which play squash.*

*There is a wide literature on this subject. The reader is directed to the following references: Barrell *et al.*, 1981; Bell, 1981; Berson *et al.*, 1978; Blonstein, 1975; Diamond *et al.*, 1982, 1984; Doxanas and Soderstrom, 1980; Easterbrook, 1978, 1980, 1981, 1982, 1988a, 1988b, 1989, 1990a, 1990b, 1990c, 1992, 1993; Easterbrook and Cameron, 1985; Fowler *et al.*, 1980; Ingram and Lewkonia, 1973; Jones 1989, 1993; Keates *et al.*, 1978; Kennerley Banks, 1985; Maberley, 1981; MacEwen and Jones, 1991; Moore and Worthley, 1977; North, 1973; Pashby, 1992; Pashby *et al.*, 1982; Rose and Morse, 1979; Vinger, 1980, 1981a, 1981b, 1985/1994; Vinger and Easterbrook, 1983; Vinger and Toplin, 1978.

Clemett and Fairhurst (1980) demonstrated that a dedicated squash player has the odds of 1 in 4 of a serious eye injury if he plays once or twice per week for 25 years.

In the United States squash eye protection has been promoted since 1976. In September of 1983 the United States Squash Racquets Association became the first national body to require that eye protection, which meets or exceeds ASTM F803 standards, be worn by all participants in national championships. Subsequent to this, the USSRA has made the wearing of polycarbonate lens eye guards mandatory.

The first eye guards designed for racquet sports were polycarbonate, but they were

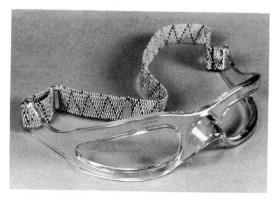

Figure 5.8   Polycarbonate open eye guard

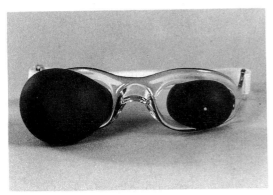

Figure 5.9 Racquet ball and soft squash ball penetrating an eye guard

Table 5.2 Injuries sustained by 80 athletes wearing open eyeguards

Injury		
Lid haemorrhage		11
Lid lacerations		3
Corneal abrasions		10
Iritis		8
Hyphaemas		56
Mechanism of injury		
Ball		77
Racquet		3
Ball penetrated eye guard		69
Eye guard displaced		11

Eye guard	Squash	Racquetball
Protec	14	22
Ektelon	1	15
Rainbow	5	2
Voit	2	13
Solari	1	2
Champion	1	–
Duraguard	0	2
	24	56

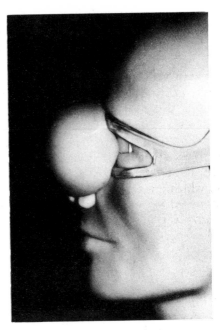

Figure 5.10 Compressible racquet ball funnelled into the orbit

open guards (Figure 5.8) and therefore readily penetrated by a squash or racquet ball (Figure 5.9). In squash 60% of injuries are caused by the ball and 40% by the racquet. Some players have told us that eye injury has been pre-vented by these eye guards when struck by a racquet, but in racquetball, where 95% of the injuries are caused by the ball, these open eye guards are not effective. In addition, because they are polycarbonate they may *increase* the risk of injury (Table 5.2), because of the funnelling effect of the unbreakable eye guard when struck by the compressible squash or racquetball ball (Figure 5.10). In 1980 CSA, and subsequently ASTM, formed committees on eye protection in sport. Work was commissioned whereby Dewey Moorhouse and Pat Bishop, using high speed film, demonstrated that the open eye guard was readily penetrated by the squash or racquet ball at speeds of even 50 mph. A polycarbonate protector did prevent eye contact when tested under these experimental conditions (Figure 5.11).

In Canada, CSA designs performance standards and performs testing. In the US the ASTM writes the standards, but individual laboratories do the testing. In testing eye protectors for sport the eye guard is placed on a headform (Figure 5.12) and then squash, racquetball and tennis balls (Figure 5.13) are shot at different speeds to test whether eye contact is made. These are performance, not design standards. In squash and racquetball the balls are projected at 90 mph directly at the lens and from the side, which specifically tests the hinge, if a hinge is present. Table 5.3 demonstrates ball speeds in the different racquet sports.

For those without a prescription, the initial bubble eye guards (which are also used in basketball) will prevent eye injury (Figure 5.14), however some players find that these

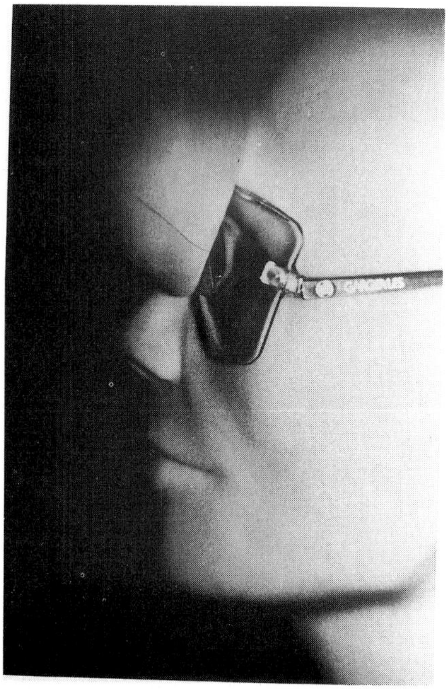

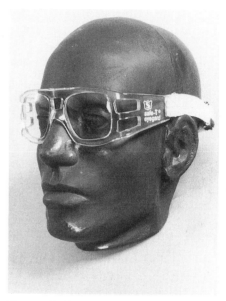

Figure 5.11 Polycarbonate lensed protector preventing eye contact. (Courtesy of M. Elman)

Figure 5.12 Eye guard placed on headform for testing

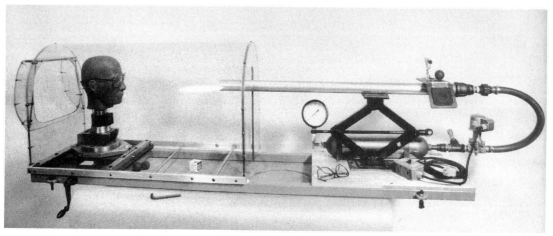

Figure 5.13 Testing of eye guards by projecting squash, racquet and tennis balls

Table 5.3 Ball and racquet velocities in different sports

	Speeds (m.p.h.)
Racquetball	
Ball	85–110
Racquet	85–90
Squash	
Ball	130–140
Racquet	95–110
Tennis	
Ball	90–110
Handball	
Ball	60–70
Badminton	
Shuttlecock	130–135

Source: C.A. Morehouse, ASTM

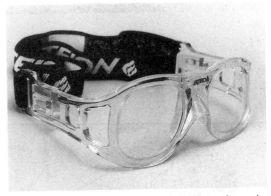

Figure 5.15 Ektelon lensed polycarbonate protector, available as prescription or non-prescription

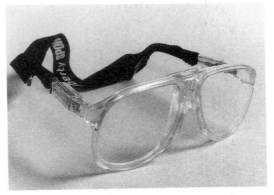

Figure 5.16 Liberty lensed polycarbonate protector, available as prescription or non-prescription

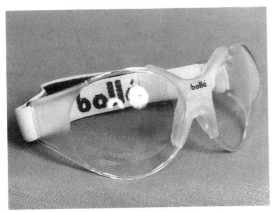

Figure 5.14 Polycarbonate bubble eye guards used by racquet and basketball players

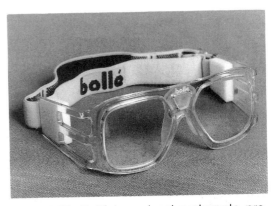

Figure 5.17 Bollé lensed polycarbonate protector, available as prescription or non-prescription

are not well ventilated. For those players who wear a prescription lens there are many products on the market (Figures 5.15–5.18, see also Figure 5.23). These are eye protectors which are designed for racquet sports with a posterior lip and contain polycarbonate prescription or non-prescription lenses. Several companies have designed non-prescription polycarbonate eye guards with anti-fog coats, which have been very popular with squash

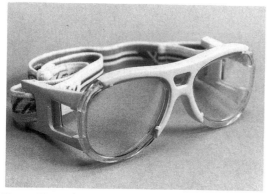

Figure 5.18 Liberty lensed polycarbonate protector, available as prescription or non-prescription

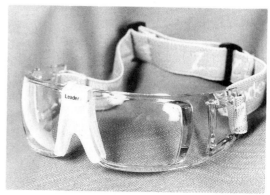

Figure 5.21 Leader non-prescription polycarbonate racquet sports protector with non-fog coat

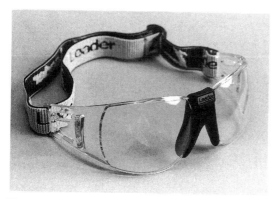

Figure 5.19 Leader non-prescription polycarbonate racquet sports protector with non-fog coat

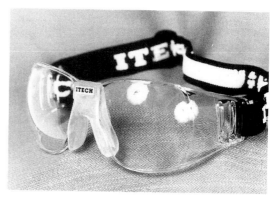

Figure 5.22 I-Tech non-prescription polycarbonate racquet sports protector with non-fog coat

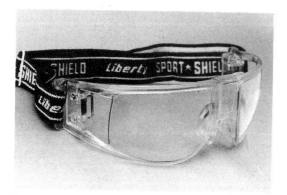

Figure 5.20 Liberty non-prescription polycarbonate racquet sports protector with non-fog coat

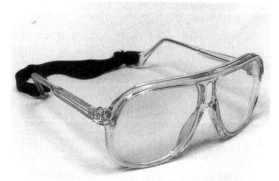

Figure 5.23 Action Eyes (Black Knight) non-prescription or prescription polycarbonate racquet sports protector with non-fog coat

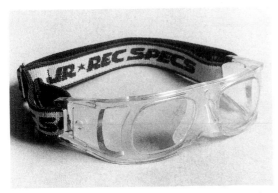

Figure 5.24 Eye guard designed for junior players: smaller frames

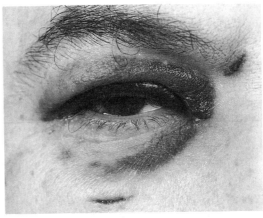

Figure 5.26 Skin lacerations, but no eye damage – this can be considered a 'save'

and other racquet players (Figures 5.19–5.23).

Eye guards have also been specifically designed for junior players (Figure 5.24). These are smaller protectors which contain a polycarbonate lens. Most junior players, at least in squash, are required to wear an eye guard, as a novice 10-year-old who has never struck a squash ball may be capable of striking the ball at 80 mph.

Figures 5.25 and 5.26 demonstrate one experienced squash player whose eye was saved when he was struck head-on with the hard doubles ball at a speed probably in excess of 120 mph. Although there were cuts around the skin, his eye was saved because he was wearing a polycarbonate eye lens in an eye protector designed for racquet sports.

Fashionable lenses are seen commonly worn by baseball, racquet and cricket players

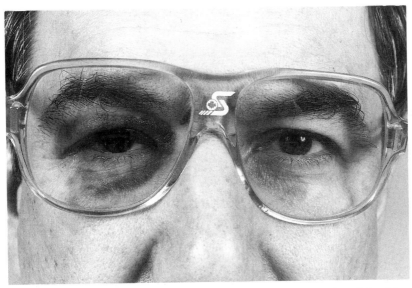

Figure 5.25 Experienced squash doubles player struck by a hard doubles ball

Table 5.4 Sports eye protectors*

I. Protectors into which a 3 mm prescription polycarbonate spectacle lens may be inserted

Liberty Sport, Liberty Optical Company (Mark Donovan)
380 Verona Avenue Newark, NJ 07104 (800) 444–5010; (201) 484–3446: fax (201) 484–3446

Junior Rec Specs, small	45 ❏ 15	R, S, T, H
Junior Rec Specs, large	51 ❏ 17	R, S, T, H
All Pro Rec Specs, small	54 ❏ 17	R, S, T, H
All Pro Rec Specs, large	59 ❏ 17	R, S, T, H
Sportgoggle 2	57 ❏ 20	R, S, T, H
Sport-Lok, small	57 ❏ 14	R, S, T
Sport-Lok, large	60 ❏ 14	R, S, T
Pro Guard Rec Specs	61 ❏ 18	S, T, H

Black Knight USA (Robert Morgan)
5355 Sierra Road San Jose, CA 95132 (800) 535–3300; (408) 923–7777; fax (408) 923–7794

Action Eyes	59 A
Action Eyes	54 A

Eagle Eyewear, Inc. (John Bartolotta)
P.O. Box 486 Whitehouse, NJ 08888 (908) 236–9300

REP 1, small	45 ❏ 14 ED 51
REP 1, large	50 ❏ 17 ED 55
REP 2	52 ❏ 20 ED 59

Rem. Los Angeles London (Mike Hundert)
9301 Laurel Canyon B1 Arieta, CA 91331 (800) 423–3023; fax (818) 504–3950

Sports Goggle 1	small, large, extra large
Sports Goggle 2	small, medium, large, extra large
Sports Goggle 3	62.3 ❏ 20
Sports Goggle 4	52.7 ❏ 19

II. Plano moulded protectors (for emmetropes or contact lens wearers)

Black Knight USA
Sight Guards

Leader Sports Products Inc. (Guy Fortin)
60 Lake Shore Road Essex, NY 12930 (800) 847–2001
New Yorker
Albany
Dallas
Optivue
Maxum

III. Plano goggle-type moulded protector (may be worn over streetwear spectacles)

Leader Sports Products, Inc.
Vizion II

---

* Tested either by independent laboratory or manufacturer to ASTM F803 or CSA racket sport eyewear standards.
  List may be incomplete and is subject to change.
R, racquetball; S, squash; T, tennis; H, handball. No letter, specific racket sport not stated by manufacturer.
Data collected by Tom Woods, Michael Easterbrook and Paul Vinger. Tests not certified by authors.

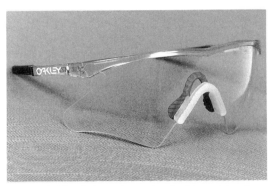

Figure 5.27 Polycarbonate fashionable flexible lenses, used by some racquet players, baseball players and cyclists

(Figure 5.27). These lenses are polycarbonate, but are quite flexible and therefore may produce some skin laceration. No injury to the eye has been recorded with these lenses to date. They are presently being tested to see if the flexibility of the lens will permit eye contact when struck by a squash and racquetball ball.

Table 5.4 lists eye protectors that manufacturers have stated meet ASTM F803 impact standards.

Australia also has a standard for racquet sports (Standards Association of Australia, 1992) which covers lenses and eye guards. Britain has no standard, although an investigation is being carried out into this.

Hockey

Ice-hockey

Before the use of widespread eye and face protectors, 37%–67% of the total injuries in hockey were to the head and face, the face receiving the majority of head injuries (Vinger, 1985/1994). The documentation of blinding injuries started when Pashby and the Canadian Ophthalmological Society reported 478 eye injuries in the 1972–1973 season, with 33 Canadian youngsters becoming legally blind in amateur hockey games in the 1974–1975 season (Pashby *et al.*, 1975). With use of

certified full-face protectors the number of eye injuries reported in 1993 was 29 with 2 blind eyes. None of these injured players was wearing a full-face protector. Two-thirds of hockey eye injuries are due to the stick and the remainder are due to the puck. Since most injuries are accidental the only means of prevention is protective equipment. Rules designed against high sticking and to reduce fighting help, but because of the accidental nature of the injury, the majority of eye and facial injuries would persist despite rule changes (Vinger, 1985/1994).

Hockey face protectors are now worn by millions of North American hockey players. The CSA in Canada and the Hockey Equipment Certification Council (HECC) have approved face guards for hockey, which may either be wire (Figure 5.28) or full-face with polycarbonate (Figure 5.29).

In an attempt to encourage older recreational players to wear eye protection an international standard has been written concerning the half visor (Figures 5.30, 5.31).

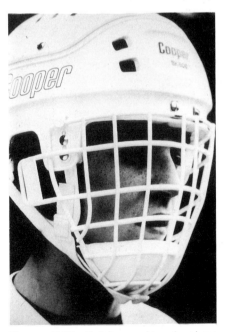

Figure 5.28 Full-face wire hockey protector, CSA and HECC approved

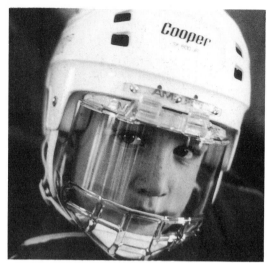

Figure 5.29 Full-face polycarbonate protector, CSA and HECC approved

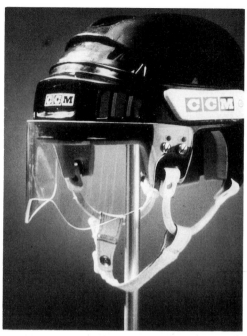

Figure 5.31 Half-visor polycarbonate

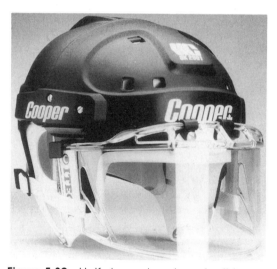

Figure 5.30 Half-visor polycarbonate; this protector will stop most sticks and pucks

Recently a Japanese–Canadian recreational player lost an eye when a stick came between his face and such a protector, which was apparently worn in its correct position.

Another recreational player using a referee's version of the half visor also lost his eye from a high stick. Although the half visor will not stop all such injuries, it should reduce most injuries from the stick and almost all injuries from a puck. Apart from these two injuries with the half visor, there has been no blinding injury recorded in hockey to a player wearing a certified full-face polycarbonate or wire face protector.

Although the National Hockey League (NHL) in 1992 made the use of helmets optional, no player in the NHL to date has removed his helmet. At the recent Team Physicians Meeting of the NHL a resolution requesting that the league make helmets and visors mandatory was passed unanimously.

Street- and floor-hockey

The energy levels in street-hockey and floor-hockey are probably less than in ice-hockey. Consequently eye protection may be possible with the protectors that meet the standards for racquet sports (Vinger, 1985/1994). However, the injury rate is sufficient that a minimum requirement should be mandated for all organized amateur and school play and highly encouraged for unorganized play.

Field-hockey

Global ruptures produced by an opponent's stick have been recorded in field hockey (Vinger, 1985/1994). Although the incidence of injury appears low, an argument can been made for field-hockey players to wear at least polycarbonate eye protectors designed for racquet sports.

Soccer

Soccer is a well-recognized cause of ocular injury (Burte *et al.*, 1983; Orlando, 1988). The exact mechanism of injury is unknown. Likely causes are deformation or underinflation of the ball. The question is – can sports eye protectors presently used in racquet sports prevent such injuries? Current regulations of soccer prevent the use of any guards as they may, themselves, cause injury to the wearer or any other player.

Basketball

Approximately one in ten college players sustain an eye injury per year (Vinger, 1985/1994), of which the majority are corneal abrasions, but blow-out fractures are not uncommon. Zagelbaum and Hersh (1992) reported 50 injuries in one year through a survey of the National Basketball Association. Many players are now wearing eye protectors because of the risk of corneal abrasion and/or blow-out fracture (Figure 5.14). No injuries have been reported in basketball to a player wearing polycarbonate lenses.

Baseball

Because of the enormous number of people playing baseball in the United States, face protectors that meet ASTM 910 attached to approved helmets are strongly recommended for little league batters and base runners (Figure 5.32).

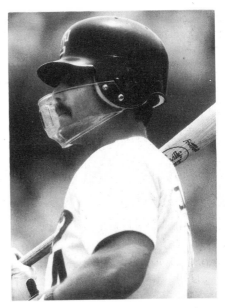

Figure 5.32 Polycarbonate protector attached to a helmet, ASTM approved; this protector will prevent eye injury

Lacrosse

In the men's game international rules now require a vertically barred face guard to prevent eye penetration as a lacrosse ball, smaller and harder than a baseball, can reach speeds of 90 mph.

In the United States the Women's Lacrosse Association permits mouth guards and the voluntary use of eye guards, but is adamantly opposed to the concept of helmets and face guards, as worn by the men. Fractured orbits and hyphaema have been well recorded in unprotected women lacrosse players: most of the injuries are accidental, with two-thirds caused by the stick and one-fifth by the ball (Lapudus *et al.*, 1992). In 1991, Wendy Piltz in Australia prospectively recorded head or face contact in 22% of players, at least once per game (Vinger 1985/1994). At one point, the United States National Women's Lacrosse team refused to play the Australians unless the Australians removed helmets and face masks that they felt necessary for their protection (Vinger, 1985/1994)!

The vast majority of eye guards that pass the racquet sports standard ASTM F803 do not give adequate eye protection for the higher momentum lacrosse balls (Vinger, 1985/1994). An ASTM committee will be established which will address the task of developing adequate head and face protection to eliminate all lacrosse head, tooth and face injuries.

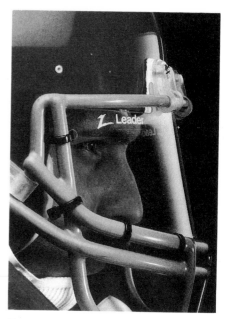

Figure 5.33 Polycarbonate protector for North American football

Cricket

Indoor and outdoor are cricket a concern for eye injuries. In Australia, ruptured globes, retinal detachments, hyphaemas and lid lacerations have been caused by the very hard 5½ oz ball (Jones and Tullo, 1986). To date no standards have been developed for testing eye guards against a cricket ball, however many cricket batsmen now wear protective head gear and eyewear. No testing has been carried out on these devices to date.

American football

Football face guards have effectively caused an 80–85% reduction in facial injuries (Figure 5.33). Polycarbonate eye guards are available which prevent penetration by the opponents fingers and elbows.

Boxing

The incidence of eye injuries in boxers increases with the number of fights and the number of losses (Vinger, 1985/1994; Giovinazzo *et al.*, 1987; Sinett, 1988). Boxing injuries can be reduced by wearing a protective helmet with lateral face guard, thumbless gloves and the early detection and treatment of eye injuries, specifically retinal holes.

Wrestling

Wrestling is not recommended for one-eyed athletes. Vinger (1985/1994) reports the case of a 12 dioptre myopic teenager who lost the vision in one eye from a giant retinal tear which occurred while wrestling. He then continued to wrestle, only to lose the remaining eye the following year from a giant retinal tear, also secondary to a wrestling injury.

Water sports

Polycarbonate swimming goggles can be used, particularly for the one-eyed athlete in sports such as water polo (Figure 5.34). The most common injuries are facial lacerations and broken fingers. However, eyes have been lost (Paceli, 1991). Eye injuries can occur from elbows, fingers or the ball, which is thrown at speeds in excess of 40 mph.

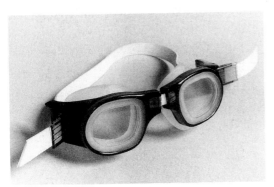

Figure 5.34 Polycarbonate eye guards for water polo

Fishing

Fishing injuries, particularly from hooks, are usually serious and can result in enucleation (Aiello *et al.*, 1992). Spectacles, preferably with polycarbonate lenses, offer excellent protection and should be worn at all times by anglers.

Golf

Golf injuries are uncommon, but golf balls can produce very serious injuries. Most injuries are caused by the ball and occasionally by the golf club. The only sports resulting in more enucleations are incidents involving BB gun pellets, arrows and darts (Vinger, 1985/1994). The high enucleation rate is explained by the size and consistency and high speed of the golf ball and club, both of which can fit within the bony orbit. Laboratory tests against projected golf balls have shown racquet sports eye protectors will *not* protect the one-eyed golfer (Vinger, personal communication).

Cycling

Many cyclists complain of irritation from wind, sun and flying debris, particularly when moving at high speed, high altitudes and/or in competition. Many fashionable polycarbonate eye protectors are available and are now being worn by many recreational and professional cyclists (see Figure 5.27).

Skiing

Cross-country skiers, particularly those travelling through woods, should wear a polycarbonate eye protector. Ski poles are the commonest cause of injury in skiers. Good ultraviolet absorbing goggles offer adequate protection from snow blindness. Polycarbonate lenses have a far higher impact resistance than ordinary plastic lenses and are the only goggles or sunglasses recommended for skiers.

Shooting and fencing

Polycarbonate lenses have sufficient impact resistance to prevent most frontal accidental injuries in shooters, but integral side shields and head bands are necessary to obtain proper side protection in fencing. An ASTM committee on fencing safety has been established following two fatal injuries occurred in fencing: one was the penetration of a face mask with a broken foil resulting in intracranial injury through the orbit (Vinger, 1985/1994).

BB guns and air rifles

Approximately 1300 eye injuries occur per year from BB and air gun pellets in the United States (Vinger, 1985/1994). BBs are round pellets, approximately 1–2 mm in diameter. Shooting BBs is popular in North America. Despite major advances in surgical techniques the majority of eyes perforated with such pellets suffer permanent visual loss, many resulting in enucleation. Eye protectors providing total protection are now available. The use of protective goggles, which several manufacturers package with the firearm, would prevent ricochet injuries to the user. The

National Rifle Association has committed its certified instructors to a strong initiative in the area of air gun safety, with training programmes and material.

War games and paintballing

In North America there are approximately 1 million war game players who are usually teenagers and young adults. Compressed air guns are used to shoot a gelatine-coated pellet containing dye at 205 mph outdoors and 170 mph indoors (Figure 5.35). Severe eye injuries have been recorded in war games participants in North America. Seventeen blind eyes were reported in a series of 44 injuries; in no case was a visor being worn (Easterbrook *et al.*, 1985; Easterbrook and Pashby, 1988). Recommended ways to decrease injuries include eye guards at all times, banning alcohol, forbidding head shots,

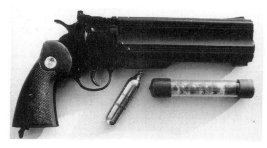

Figure 5.35 Gelatine pellet, CO_2 cannister and war games gun

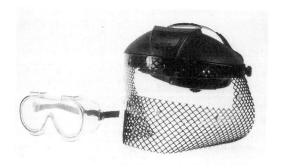

Figure 5.36 Two types of war games protectors

duels and quick draws. Plastic goggles are worn and should be firmly fixed to the head as soon as the player is given a gun (Figure 5.36).

Although these eye guards are not polycarbonate, to the author's knowledge no injury has been reported in a player wearing protective eye wear. However, it must be emphasized again that polycarbonate is the optimal material.

The one-eyed athlete

A person is functionally one-eyed when the loss of the better eye would result in a significant change in lifestyle due to poor vision in the remaining eye. In North America many states do not allow a player seeing less than 20/40 to drive. The inability to drive interferes significantly with the range of jobs available to children when they became adults.

It is far more dangerous to play a racquet sport without an eye protector than to play hockey with a full-face mask. High schools and universities should specify that the one-eyed athlete wears sports eye protectors that meet ASTM or CSA racquet sports standards for all sports with risk of eye injury, for all games. These protectors should be worn under the face mask of those sports that require a face mask, i.e. hockey, American football and lacrosse. Face protectors should be used for baseball batting and base running, ice-hockey, women's lacrosse (already required for men's lacrosse) and field-hockey. For daily wear off the field one-eyed players should wear polycarbonate lenses mounted in a sturdy streetwear frame to protect the good eye.

Vinger recommends that the only sport absolutely contraindicated for the effectively one-eyed is boxing, since the risk of serious injury is so high and there is no effective eye protector. The functioning one-eyed should also be discouraged from wrestling and the martial arts, even though the incidence of eye injury is low. Good eye protectors, which are guaranteed to remain on the player at all times are not available in these sports.

Contact lenses

Soft contact lenses provide no protection to an athlete. Patients with rigid corneal lenses have an increased risk of eye injury because the lens may break, thereby possibly lacerating the cornea and/or producing a corneal abrasion. Any contact lens wearer involved in racquet sports or hockey should wear an eye protector that meets the impact standards in that sport over their lenses.

Refractive surgery and the athlete

Refractive surgery is dealt with in detail in Chapter 7. Radial keratotomy (RK) structurally weakens the eye and Vinger reported at the International Ophthalmology Congress in 1994 that 24 eyes ruptured after RK; although many of these received only slight trauma, enucleation was necessary in many of these patients due to the extent of the injury. Any athlete who has had radial keratotomy must be informed that the eye is structurally weakened and they must wear appropriate certified, polycarbonate eye protection. Excimer laser refractive surgery appears to be a safer technique from the point of view of subsequent injury.

Conclusion

Eye injuries in sport are common. Excellent polycarbonate protection is available for almost all sports: appropriate notices such as that in Figure 5.37 should be posted at every court and rink or wherever sport is played.

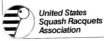

The **Rules of Squash** *require* Protective Eye Guards. Your eyes are important to us and you. Play Safely!

Let the Games Begin!

United States Squash Racquets Association

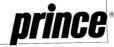

Figure 5.37 Safety posters such as this should be posted at every court, rink and place of play

The use of polycarbonate certified protection or protectors that meet impact standards set in Canada, the United States and eventually internationally should be encouraged by all who love sport.

References

Aiello, L.P., Iwamoto, M. and Taylor, H.R. (1992) Perforating fishhook injury. *Archives of Ophthalmology*, **110**, 1316

American National Standards Institute (1986) Z86 *American National Standard Recommendation for Divers*, ANSI, New York

American Society for Testing and Materials (1988) F803–88 *Standard Specification for Eye Protectors for Use by Players of Racquet Sports*, ASTM, Philadelphia

Barrell, G.V., Cooper, P.J., Elkington, A.R. *et al.* (1981) Squash ball to eye ball: the likelihood of squash players incurring an eye injury. *British Medical Journal*, **283**, 893–5

Bell, J.A. (1981) Eye trauma in sports: a preventable epidemic (Editorial). *Journal of the American Medical Association*, 246–56

Blonstein, J.L. (1975) Eye injury in sport. *Practitioner*, **215**, 208–9

Berson, B.L., Passoff, T.L., Nagelberg, S. and Thornton, J. (1978) Injury patterns in squash players. *American Journal of Sports Medicine*, **6**, 323–5

Canadian Standards Association (1982) CSA P400–M1 *Racquet Sports Eye Protectors*, CSA, Ontario

Clemett, R.S. and Fairhurst, S.M. (1980) Head injuries from squash: a prospective study. *New Zealand Medical Journal*, **92**, 1–3

Davis, J.K. (1988) Perspectives on impact resistance and polycarbonate lenses. In *Prevention of Ocular Sports*

Injuries (International Ophthalmology Clinics) (ed. P. Vinger), Little, Brown, Boston, pp. 215–18

Davis, J. (1994) Clinical ophthalmology. In *Clinical Ophthalmology* (eds T.D. Duare and E.A. Jaeger), Harper and Row, Philadelphia

Diamond, G.R., Quinn, G.E., Pashby, T.J. and Easterbrook, M. (1982) Ophthalmologic injuries. *Clinics in Sports Medicine*, **1** (3), 469–82

Diamond, G.R., Quinn, G.E., Pashby, T.J. and Easterbrook, M. (1984) Ophthalmological injuries: primary care. *Clinical Office Practice*, **11** (1), 161–74

Doxanas, M.T. and Soderstrom, C. (1980) Racquetball as an ocular hazard. *Archives of Ophthalmology*, **98**, 1965–6

Easterbrook, W.M. (1978) Eye injuries in squash; a preventable disease. *Canadian Medical Association Journal*, **118**, 298–305

Easterbrook, W.M. (1980) Eye injuries in racquet sports: a continuing problem. *Canadian Medical Association Journal*, **123**, 268

Easterbrook, W.M. (1981) Eye injuries in racquet sports. *International Ophthalmology Clinics*, **21**, 87–119

Easterbrook, W.M. (1982) Eye injuries in squash and racquetball players. *Physician and Sports Medicine*, **10**, 47–56

Easterbrook, M. (1987) Protection in racquet sports update. *Physicians Sportsmedicine*, **15**, 180

Easterbrook, M. (1988a) Ocular injuries in racquet sports. In *Prevention of Ocular Sports Injuries (International Ophthalmology Clinics)* (ed. P. Vinger), Little, Brown, Boston, **28**, 232–7

Easterbrook, M. (1988b) Assessing ocular trauma in atheletes. *Canadian Journal of Diagnosis*, **5**, 43–9

Easterbrook, M. (1989) Keeping an eye on sports – retinal injuries. *Current Therapy*, **2**, 21–33

Easterbrook, M. (1990a) Eye protectors in racquet sports. In *Current Therapy in Sports: 2* (eds J. Torg, R.P. Welsh and R.J. Shepherd), B.C. Decker, Philadelphia, pp. 356–62

Easterbrook, M. (1990b) Standards for protective eye guards. In *Sports Medicine and Health* (eds G.P.H. Hermans and W.L. Mostend), Excerpta Medica, Amsterdam, pp. 1101–6

Easterbrook, M. (1990c) Prevention of eye injury in badminton. In: *Sports, Medicine and Health* (eds G.P.H. Hermans and W.L. Mostend), Excerpta Medica, Amsterdam, pp. 1107–10

Easterbrook, M. (1992) Getting patients to protect their eyes during sports. *Physician and Sports Medicine*, **20**, 165

Easterbrook, M. (1993) Eye injuries in sports: prevention and cure, *Canadian Journal of Diagnosis*, pp. 77–89

Easterbrook, M. and Cameron, J. (1985) Injuries in racquet sports. In: *Sports Injuries: Mechanisms, Prevention and Treatment*. (eds R. Schneider *et al.*), Williams and Wilkins, Baltimore, pp. 553–64

Easterbrook, M. and Pashby, T.J. (1985) Ocular injuries in war games. *International Ophthalmology Clinics*, **133**, 415

Easterbrook, M. and Pashby, T.J. (1988) Ocular injuries and war games. *International Ophthalmology Clinics*, **28**, 222

Editorial (1973), A ball in the eye. *British Medical Journal*, **2**, 195–6

Fowler, B.J., Seelenfreund, M. and Newton, J.C. (1980) Ocular injuries sustained playing squash. *American Journal of Sports Medicine*, **8**, 126–8

Giovinazzo, V., Yannuzzi, L.A., Sorenson, J.H. *et al.* (1987) The ocular complications of boxing. *Ophthalmology*, **94**, 582–96

Ingram, D.V. and Lewkonia, I. (1973) Ocular hazards of playing squash. *British Journal of Ophthalmology*, **57**, 434–8

Jones, N.P. (1989) Eye injury in sport. *Sports Medicine*, pp. 163–81

Jones, N.P. (1993) Eye injury in sport: incidence, biomechanics, clinical effects and prevention. *Journal of the Royal College of Surgeons of Edinburgh*, **38**, 127–33

Jones, N.P. and Tullo, A.B. (1986) Severe eye injuries in cricket. *British Journal of Sports Medicine*, **20**, 178

Keates, R.H., Easterbrook, M. Vinger, P.F. *et al.* (1978) Eye protection for athletes (roundtable). *Physician and Sports Medicine*, **6**, 44–60

Keeney, A.H., Fintelmann, E. and Estlow, B. (1972) Refractive corrective and associated factors in spectacle glass injury. *Archives of Ophthalmology*, **88**, 2

Keeney, A.H. (1984) Ophthalmic standards: ANSI provides room for participation. *Argus*, **4**, February

Kennerley Bankes, J.L. (1985) Squash rackets: a survey of eye injuries in England. *British Medical Journal*, **291**, 1539–40

Lapudus, C.S., Nelson, L.B., Jeffers, J.B. *et al.* (1992) Eye injury in lacrosse: women need their vision less than men? *Trauma*, **32**, 555

Maberley, A.L. (1981) Retinal detachments and athletic eye injuries. *British Columbia Medical Journal*, **23**, 70–3

MacEwen, C.J. and Jones, N.P. (1991) Eye injuries in racquet sports. *British Medical Journal*, **302**, 1415–16

Moore, M.C. and Worthley, D.A. (1977) Ocular injuries in squash players. *Australian Journal of Ophthalmology*, **5**, 46–7

North, I.M. (1973) Ocular hazards of squash. *Medical Journal of Australia*, **1**, 165–6

Orlando, R.G. (1988) Soccer-related eye injuries in children and adolescents. *Physician and Sports Medicine*, **16**, 103

Paceli, L.C. (1991) Water polo's benefits surface. *Physician and Sports Medicine*, **19**, 119

Pashby, T.J. (1992) Eye injury in Canadian sports and recreational activities. *Canadian Journal of Ophthalmology*, **27**, 226–9

Pashby, T.J., Bishop, P.J. and Easterbrook, M. (1982) Eye injuries in Canadian racquet sports. *Canadian Family Physician*, **23**, 967–71

Pashby, T., Pashby, R.C., Chisholm, L.D.J. and Crawford, J.S. (1975) Eye injury in hockey. *Canadian Medical Association Journal*, **113**, 663

Rose, C.P. and Morse, J.O. (1979) Racquetball injuries. *Physician and Sports Medicine*, 7, 73–8

Sinett, D.J. (1988) Ocular injuries in boxing. *International Ophthalmology Clinics*, **28**, 242

Standards Association of Australia (1992) AS/NZS 4066 *Eye Protection in Racquet Sports*, Standards Association of Australia, Sydney

Vinger, P.F. (1980) Sports-related eye injury: a preventable problem. *Survey of Ophthalmology*, **25**, 47–51

Vinger, P.F. (1981a) Sports eye injuries: a preventable disease. *Ophthalmology*, **88**, 108–13

Vinger, P.F. (1981b) The incidence of eye injuries in sports. *International Ophthalmology Clinics*, **21** (4), 33

Vinger, P. (1985, revised edn 1994) The eye and sports medicine. In *Clinical Ophthalmology* (ed. T.D. Duane. Harper and Row, Philadelphia, pp. 1–51

Vinger, P. and Easterbrook, M. (1983) Prevention of eye injuries in racquet sports (Editorial). *Journal of the American Medical Association*, **250**, 3322

Vinger, P.F. and Toplin, D.W. (1978) Racquet sports: an ocular hazard. *Journal of the American Medical Association*, **239**, 2575–7

Zagelbaum, B.M. and Hersh, P.S. (1992) Major league basketball. Presented at American Academy of Ophthalmology annual meeting, Dallas, 1992

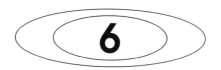

6

Light and lighting

W. Neil Charman and Caroline J. MacEwen

This chapter is in two parts. The first, by Neil Charman, is concerned with the subject of lighting for sport. The second part, by Caroline MacEwen, considers the ways light can damage the eye during sport.

1. LIGHTING FOR SPORT

Introduction

Most major sports originated in the days before cheap and effective artificial lighting was available. They thus relied on daylight and would be interrupted or abandoned when this faded due to heavy overcast skies or the setting of the sun: indeed cricket is still largely constrained in this way. Reliance on daylight also meant that players and spectators usually had to be exposed to the vagaries of the weather, so that many sports were necessarily seasonal in nature. Only exceptionally were outside sports continued into the hours of darkness with the aid of lanterns, for example ice skating on the frozen Thames in the seventeenth century. Very occasionally enclosed window or torch-lit indoor areas were built to satisfy the sporting interests of the wealthy, such as Henry VIII's sixteenth-century real tennis court at Hampton Court or the seventeenth-century indoor riding school of the Marquis of Newcastle at Bolsover in Derbyshire, England.

The advent of gas and electric lighting in the early and late nineteenth century respectively offered new opportunities. For many years the benefits were largely felt by table-top sports which made relatively modest lighting demands. The Edwardian gentleman's billiard room and the town centre snooker or pool hall are typical of this era, although gas and electric-lit indoor skating rinks began to show the wider potential for artificial lighting. It was, however, only in the period after the Second World War that the demands for sporting facilities created by greater affluence and leisure time, combined with advances in lighting technology, led to the widespread adoption of artificial lighting in many areas of sporting endeavour. The commercial pressures of television, with its insatiable appetite for live sport at peak evening viewing times, have led to further improvements in artificial lighting at major sporting venues. In principle, many of today's sports facilities could be used for 24-hours a day throughout the year.

In this section the pertinent characteristics of the visual system and some lighting terms are first briefly outlined. The relevant properties of daylight are then discussed. Artificial lighting is considered next and the section concludes with a discussion of such topics as the possible advantages of using yellow-tinted or polarizing spectacles or goggles.

Basic concepts

The electromagnetic spectrum

Visible light is a form of electromagnetic radiation which is only exceptional in comparison to the rest of the electromagnetic spectrum, which extends from gamma to radio waves, in that it is capable of stimulating the human visual system. Neighbouring the visible wavelengths are the ultraviolet (UV) and infrared (IR) regions. When considering the possible damage effects that these different wavelengths of **non-ionizing radiation** can have on ocular structures, it is conventional to further subdivide the UV into UV-C (100–280 nanometres (nm)), UV-B (280–320 nm) and UV-A (320–400 nm). The IR is divided into

IR-A (760–1400 nm), IR-B (1400–3000 nm) and IR-C (3000 nm–1 mm) (Sliney and Wolbarsht, 1980, see Figure 6.1). The energy of any photon is inversely proportional to its wavelength, so that photon energies are highest at the shortest UV wavelengths.

Visual performance at different light levels

The retina contains two types of light receptor, rods and cones designed to function best at low (scotopic) and high (photopic) light levels respectively. It is therefore not surprising to find that the variation in the eye's sensitivity to different wavelengths (the relative luminous efficiency) is different at low and high light levels (Figure 6.2). At scotopic light levels peak sensitivity moves towards shorter wavelengths and sensitivity to red wavelengths falls to a low level, this change being known as the Purkinje shift. Note that, whatever the source and light level, energy outside the band from about 380–720 nm contributes negligibly to the sensation of vision and hence is wasted for lighting purposes.

Although absolute sensitivity to light is best under the dark-adapted, scotopic conditions

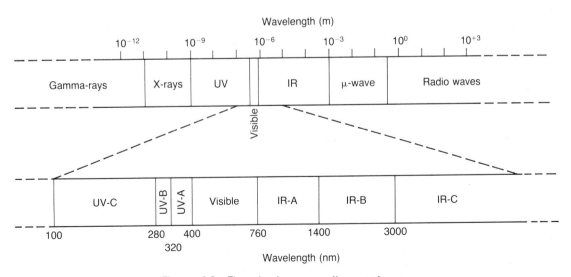

Figure 6.1 The electromagnetic spectrum

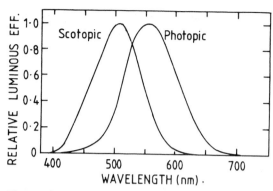

Figure 6.2 The spectral sensitivity of the eye at low (scotopic) and high (photopic) light levels

of rod vision, almost all the aspects of visual performance that are relevant to major sports, such as visual acuity, colour vision, contrast sensitivity, depth perception and movement detection, improve as the illumination is raised to the photopic levels of light-adapted cone vision. Effectively the higher light fluxes involved convey more information to the visual system and hence allow enhanced performance. Examples of these light-dependent changes are shown in Figure 6.3. It can be seen that performance progressively improves as the light level is raised from scotopic levels, to reach a more or less constant level once photopic conditions have been achieved. At very high levels of illumination (not shown),

performance may begin to decline again due to glare (see below).

In most sporting contexts, particularly for fast ball games, it is desirable that light levels are at, or very near to, the photopic levels at which optimal visual performance is achieved. A further reason for using photopic levels is that colour is widely employed in sports to distinguish teams, targets and other important objects in the playing area and it is the essentially photopic retinal cone receptors that are responsible for colour vision rather than the scotopic rods. Even at photopic levels, however, about 8% of males and less than 1% of females have defective colour vision: nearly a quarter of colour defectives report difficulties with sporting activities. Typical problems include confusion between the colours of the opposing teams, losing orange golf balls in the grass and mistaking red for brown snooker balls (Steward and Cole, 1989).

Photometric definitions and units

Photometric units and general lighting concepts are fully discussed in a wide variety of texts (e.g. Cayless and Marsden, 1983; CIBSE, 1984; IES, 1984; Murdoch, 1985; Pritchard, 1990; Lyons, 1992; Schiler, 1992). For the

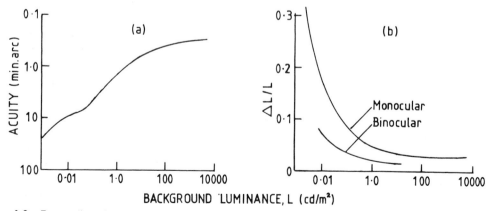

Figure 6.3 Examples of changes in visual performance with light level. *a*, Visual acuity for Landolt 'C' targets. *b*, Luminance discrimination in which a target of luminance $L + \Delta L$ must be distinguished against a background of luminance L

present purposes it is important to note the following terms.

Luminous flux (Φ) is the radiant flux (power) from the source, weighted for the spectral sensitivity of a standard eye (Figure 6.2 – usually the photopic curve is assumed). It can thus be thought of as being the time rate of flow of luminous energy. The metric unit is the lumen. Obviously the greater the luminous flux that a source emits, the more the light that is available for illumination purposes. Since it costs money to provide the power for any lamp and control of costs is usually a major consideration, our sources should produce as much luminous flux for each watt of electricity as possible. Thus the **luminous efficacy** (lumens/watt) should be high. A source which produced 1 watt of radiant energy at 555 nm (the peak of the photopic luminous efficiency function, Figure 6.2) for each watt of electrical power would produce 675 lumens, i.e. its luminous efficacy would be 675 lumen/watt (Pritchard, 1990). Real lamps producing a wider spectrum of light must have lower luminous efficacy than this, partly because not all electrical energy will be converted to radiant energy and partly because luminous efficiency is lower for all other output wavelengths. It can be seen that lamps which produce a broad spectrum of light extending into the blue and red, for which the eye is relatively insensitive, will tend to have a lower luminous efficacy (but better colour characteristics) than those which produce most of their radiation near 555 nm.

Intensity (I) describes the light emitted by a source in a particular direction. In practice, light sources frequently emit varying amounts of light in different directions (for example a spotlight gives a very limited beam and floodlights are also designed to be strongly directional). The intensity is the luminous flux per unit solid angle in a specified direction (lumens/steradian or candelas).

The **illuminance** (E) quantifies the light falling on to a surface, i.e. the luminous flux incident per unit area (lumens/metre^2 or lux). The illuminance is one of the most important

parameters when specifying lighting requirements for particular sports or other activities. Usually the light falling on a horizontal surface is specified, i.e. the horizontal illuminance.

The **luminance** (L) refers to the light being emitted from or reflected by a surface, i.e. it is a measure of the intensity of the light emitted per unit area in a given direction (candelas/metre^2, cd/m^2). Obviously the luminance of surfaces or objects in sports is likely to be dependent upon the illuminance falling upon them and their reflection characteristics. Roughly speaking, vision will be operating in the scotopic region if the surfaces being viewed have luminances between absolute threshold (10^{-6} cd/m^2) and 10^{-3} cd/m^2, and vision will be photopic at luminances above about 3 cd/m^2. Between the scotopic and photopic regions lies the mesopic region, where the visual system is in transition between the full rod and full cone regimes (cf. Figure 6.2).

Although we shall not be concerned with detailed calculations, it is of interest to note the useful inverse-square law relationship between the intensity of a source (I) in a particular direction and the illuminance (E) that it produces on a surface at distance (d) from the source and whose normal makes an angle Θ with that direction. The relationship is $E = I \cos\Theta / d^2$. Obviously as long as light only reaches a surface directly from an array of sources (a situation that holds approximately in the case of exterior floodlit pitches) we can find the resultant illuminance at any point by summing the inverse-square law contributions of all the individual sources (see e.g. CIBSE, 1990, Appendix 2). In indoor installations substantial amounts of light are reflected from the walls and other internal surfaces of the building to reach the playing area indirectly and the inverse-square law is less useful.

Another helpful relation links the luminance (L) of diffuse reflecting surfaces which are lit to an illuminance (E). We find $L = \rho E / \pi$, where ρ is the reflectance of the surface

(ρ is unity for a perfect white diffuser and less than one for all other surfaces). Although in practice the reflecting characteristics of real surfaces are never truly diffuse, this relation gives a useful approximate idea of the likely luminance levels when the illuminance takes a specified value.

Photometric measurements

If we are to assess the quality of sports lighting systems, we need to be able to measure their photometric characteristics. Although detailed measurements are probably the preserve of the lighting engineer, a simple illuminance meter, as found in a camera, for example, can give a very helpful indication of whether illuminance levels meet accepted recommendations. In such meters, some form of light-sensitive (e.g. photo-emissive, photovoltaic, photoconductive) cell generating a light-dependent current is coupled to a suitably calibrated meter, often with switched ranges to enable a wide range of illuminance levels to be measured (British Standards Institution, 1968, BS 677; Illuminations Engineering Society (IES), 1984, section 4; Lyons, 1992, Appendix E). The important feature is that the spectral sensitivity of the cell, as modifed if necessary by a suitable colour filter, should match the photopic spectral sensitivity of the eye. As we would like our readings of horizontal illuminance to include light incident from all directions above the horizontal, a cosine-corrected cell is preferred in which the flat surface of the cell is covered with an approximately hemispherical window. In the absence of a purpose-built illuminance meter, rough values of both illuminance and luminance can be deduced from the readings of ordinary photographic light meters (Long and Woo, 1980; Smith, 1982).

Glare

One other aspect of lighting installations that is of major importance is the **glare** that they produce. Glare can be defined as 'the discomfort or impairment of vision experienced when parts of the visual field (e.g. sky or lamps) are excessively bright in relation to general surroundings' (IES, 1974; CIBSE, 1984, 1990). Glare can merely cause visual discomfort (discomfort glare) or may actually impair ability to see detail (disability glare). Glare effects diminish as the angle of each offending source (or its reflection) increases with respect to the line of sight. Thus glare from, for example, floodlights can be reduced by mounting them as high as possible. This mounting arrangement also tends to improve the uniformity of the horizontal illuminance across the playing area, albeit at the possible expense of more awkward maintenance and some reduction in the illuminance of vertical surfaces. Glare effects are further reduced if the luminance of the background surrounding the glare sources is increased: this can be achieved in indoor sports halls by finishing the walls and ceilings in light colours.

Daylight and Sport

Basic characteristics

Daylight has the obvious merit of costing nothing and of providing relatively high levels of illumination for a substantial fraction of the day. Since we have evolved under daylight conditions, our judgement of colours is best under light of a similar spectral composition (Figure 6.4). It can be seen that in the visible region of the spectrum the spectral power (watts/nm) of daylight is roughly constant across the visible spectrum. The presence of significant amounts of ultraviolet light (wavelengths less than about 380 nm) in sunlight may pose hazards to the eyes of participants in sports in environments where there is a combination of strong sunlight with highly reflecting ground surfaces, such as snow: these are discussed below.

As already noted, daylight has the disadvantage that it is subject to pronounced

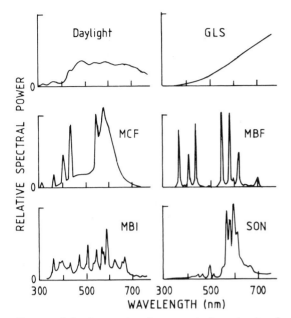

Figure 6.4 Approximate spectral output of various light sources: daylight; GLS – tungsten incandescent lamp; MCF – high-efficacy fluorescent tube; MBF – high-pressure mercury discharge lamp; MBI – high-pressure metal halide discharge lamp; SON – high-pressure sodium discharge lamp

diurnal, seasonal and climatic variations. Figure 6.5 illustrates these for a clear, English sky when the contribution of direct sunlight is excluded (US data are given in IES, 1984, section 7). In direct sunlight, illuminances may rise above 100 000 lux, high enough to cause discomfort unless sunglasses are worn.

Fortunately, because the visual system adapts very successfully to gradual changes in illumination, slow diurnal variation of the type shown in Figure 6.5 is no problem. Difficulties, however, arise in fast ball games such as cricket when abrupt darkening occurs due to rapidly moving heavy cloud, or the illuminance falls slowly to too low a level. Similar adaptational difficulties may arise when a fast motor vehicle is driven from bright sunlight into a much darker tunnel, although these may be reduced by providing a gradation of illuminance at the tunnel entrance and exit, for example by having increased artificial lighting in these areas, or using vehicle head lights.

In an interesting series of experiments it has been shown (Campbell *et al.*, 1987; Rothwell

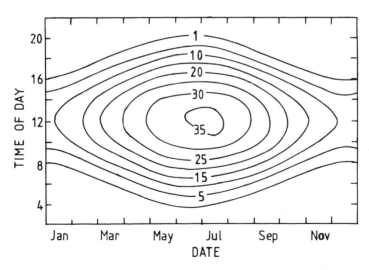

Figure 6.5 Variation in daylight illuminance with time of day and date in the London area, UK. Direct sunlight has been excluded. The contours are labelled in units of 1000 lux. The marked seasonal variation becomes less important for locations nearer the equator

and Campbell, 1987; Perry *et al.*, 1987) that conditions start to appear gloomy when white surfaces have a luminance of about 250 cd/m^2 (i.e. at an illuminance of 800 lux for a perfect white diffuse reflector). Below this level visual reaction times start to rise above their normal value of about 160 ms, by about 33 ms for each log unit of decreasing light level. Campbell and his colleagues point out that when a batsman faces a fast bowler bowling at 90 mph (110 km/h) the reaction time corresponds to the ball travelling some 6 yards and each increment of 33 ms corresponds to a further 1.5 yards. Thus the batsman's time to register the trajectory of the ball is severely eroded at low light levels and the decision 'bad light stops play' is fully justified.

Control of contrast and glare in daylight

In most outdoor sporting situations little can be done to control natural daylight or its effects on the objects that it illuminates. It is, however, possible to improve the contrast of the ball in ball games by suitable choice of the colour of the ball itself and of the background against which it must be detected. Examples are the use of white sightscreens against which the batsman in cricket views the bowler's delivery of the red ball, and green screens behind the baselines in tennis to give a contrasting background to the white or yellow ball. Such screens have the further advantage of eliminating distracting movement in the background. Regular ball replacements in games such as tennis not only ensure that the elastic properties are unimpaired but also help to eliminate the loss of visual contrast that might occur as balls get dirty. Marshals and officials can be made more obvious by wearing fluorescent jackets and judicious use of colour on stairs, passageways and exits can improve crowd control and safety.

It is worth noting that in outdoor ball games occasional glare from the sun is inevitable when high balls are to be caught or struck, particularly when the sun is low in the sky. Thus it may not be reasonable to expect artificial lighting systems to be totally free of glare. It is helpful if the design of outdoor playing areas is such that pitches are orientated north–south rather than east–west. This will minimize the chance that low sunlight shines directly into, for example, a batsman or goal-keeper's eyes.

Use of daylight for interiors

Daylight can, of course, also be used to provide interior lighting in sports halls and swimming pools for much of the day. From the point of view of lighting efficiency and safety it is better that roof lights or clerestories be used (screened if necessary to prevent breakage) rather than side windows. Side windows do have the advantage of providing a psychological link with the open air and may be justified if they provide an attractive view, in spite of possible problems with cleaning and condensation: trees and shrubs are recommended to help to minimize glare originating from over-bright areas of sky. Careful design is necessary, since glare from windows reflected from the choppy surface of a swimming pool may reduce the ability of life guards to see swimmers who are in difficulty below the surface (Lynes, 1968; IES, 1974, 1981). Safety can be improved by having underwater artificial lighting from the longer sides of the pool, the luminaires being either recessed into the sides of the pool or, preferably, placed behind watertight 'portholes' (CIBSE, 1990; CIE, 1984).

Artificial lighting

General considerations

It is evident that while sports lighting's original purpose was to serve the needs of the participants and officials, it is now also frequently called upon to meet the requirements of spectators and television as well. In many instances the latter may necessitate higher levels of lighting than would be required for players alone. Colour TV demands both high levels of illuminance (up to a few thousand lux) and that attention be paid to the spectral characteristics of the light sources (e.g. Davies et al., 1972; CIE, 1989; CIBSE 1990). For these reasons, sports lighting guides (Lumsden et al., 1974; IES, 1974; IES, 1981; CIBSE, 1990) often recommend for each sport successively increasing levels of lighting for purely recreational, club competition and national or international competitive use, as spectator numbers rise and the probability of TV coverage increases (see below).

In general the needs of the various groups involved demand that 'the lighting system provides suitable brightness and colour contrasts over the playing area, sufficient light at all points, correct distribution of light and adequate control of glare' (IES, 1974; CIBSE, 1990). By contrast here, we mean the relationship between the luminance or colour of the player, ball or other feature against its background. Contrast is usually easier to control indoors than outdoors, since the light-reflecting characteristics of the floor, wall and ceiling surfaces can be manipulated much more easily than outdoor backgrounds. The light reflected by grass, for example, is dependent not only on the incidence angle of the light but also upon such factors as whether the grass is wet or recently cut, whereas an indoor playing surface will have constant characteristics. For this reason, the behaviour of outdoor lighting installations cannot be calculated exactly and some empirical adjustment is always necessary.

It is usual to first design the installation so that the horizontal illuminance or light falling on the playing area has acceptable uniformity and is at the required level for the particular sport. Uniformity on and above the playing area is particularly important for ball games, otherwise the ball may appear to accelerate or decelerate as it passes between light and zones, making it difficult for players to the trajectory. The illuminance on vertical surfaces such as the players themselves is obviously also important but it is usually suggested that adequate horizontal illuminance from a well-designed lighting system will also ensure adequate vertical illuminance. This may not always be true, for example in badminton where the fast-moving shuttlecock must be seen well above the normal horizontal line-of-sight of the players (Bradley, 1992).

Obvious problems arise in multi-purpose sports halls where different sports have somewhat different requirements. An overhead lighting installation which is well suited for football may give rise to complaints of glare from badminton players when playing overhead shots. Methods for predicting the subjective impression of discomfort glare from floodlighting schemes have been developed (Tekelenburg et al., 1982; Van Bommel et al., 1983; CIE 5–04) and have been found useful in practice (Hargroves et al., 1986).

Types of lamp

In the early years of sports lighting, wide use was made of conventional tungsten-filament incandescent lamps, since these are relatively inexpensive, have only low levels of mains-related flicker, give acceptable colour rendition and are easy to install. However, they have the disadvantage of relatively low luminous efficacy (Table 6.1), so that running costs are high. Tungsten halogen lamps, which may have built-in reflectors, have enhanced efficacy and somewhat longer lifetimes. For interior use, tubular fluorescent lamps have substantially better luminous efficacy and can give good colour rendition: since there tends to be a relatively low brightness ratio between fluorescent luminaires and the surrounding ceiling they also have good glare characteristics. The various types of high-pressure discharge lamp, some with phosphor coatings, generally have good efficacy but many

Table 6.1   Characteristics of some lamps used in sports lighting*

Lamp type	Wattage	Luminous efficacy (lm/watt)	Life (h)	Colour characteristics
Tungsten	Up to 2000	8–18	Up to 2000	Acceptable
Tungsten halogen	Up to 2000	20–25	2000–4000	Acceptable
Tubular fluorescent	Up to 125	65–100	Up to 15 000	Depends on phosphor Generally acceptable
High-pressure mercury	Up to 2000	35–55	Up to 24 000	Poor (blue–green)
Metal halide	70–3500	65–85	Up to 12 000	Acceptable
High-pressure sodium	50–1000	90–130	15 000	'Golden' colour

* The values are representative only: full details can be obtained from manufacturers.

of them give rather poor colour rendition unless they are used in mixed installations with incandescent lamps: floodlights using metal halide lamps give a good compromise between efficacy and colour characteristics. The spectral characteristics of these various sources are illustrated in Figure 6.4. Discharge lamps operating on a normal mains AC supply have a basic 100 Hz fluctuation in output. To avoid stroboscopic effects due to this flicker, the equipment for discharge lamps should be balanced over three phases, with adjacent lamps being connected to different phases. There tends to be an inverse relationship between the initial cost of a lamp and its running cost.

In floodlighting, the lamp is combined with a reflector to give a strongly directional beam. Compact sources with paraboloidal reflectors give a symmetrical beam, whereas linear lamps in trough reflectors give a fan beam. More subtle asymmetric intensity distributions designed to minimize glare can be obtained with suitable selection of source and reflector design (IES 1974; Lumsden et al., 1974; IES, 1981, 1984; Cayless and Marsden, 1983; CIBSE, 1990).

Recommended lighting levels and designs of installation

Detailed recommendations for particular sports are found in the lighting guides (Lums-den et al., 1974; IES, 1974; IES, 1981, sections 2 and 13; CIE, 1978, 1979, 1983a, 1983b, 1984; CIBSE, 1990). The lighting levels increase with the visual demands made by the sport: important factors are the size, speed, contrast and likely trajectory of any ball, shuttlecock, puck or field-sport missile. Typical recommended illuminances for modest installations range from 30 to 2000 lux (see Table 6.2).

In large stadia for sports such as football, athletics or baseball, however, much higher levels may be required, depending upon the number of spectators and their maximum distance from the centre of the playing area (Figure 6.6), as well as TV requirements. As can be seen, it is usual to increase lighting levels as the number of spectators and their maximum distance from the centre of the playing area increase: floodlights can be mounted either on towers or on the roof of the stands, provided that the stand is robust enough and the design is such that this arrangement does not cause excessive glare for spectators. Where large crowds are involved, lighting is necessary for safety as well as for the observation of the event and an adequate emergency lighting system is always required for evacuation purposes in the event of failure of the main lighting system (CIBSE, 1990).

The requirement for uniformity of illuminance means that most outdoor installations usually consist of a limited number of flood-

Table 6.2   Some typical recommended values of illuminance*

Sport	Illuminance (lux)		
	Recreational	Club and county	National/international
Athletics (outdoors)	50	200	
Badminton	300 (100)	400 (200)	500 (300)
Baseball	165† (150)	550 (700)	1650 (1500)
Basketball	300 (100)	500 (300)	750 (500)
Billiards and snooker	750 (300)	750 (500)	1000 (500)
Bowls (outdoor)	100 (50)	200 (100)	
Bowls (indoor)	300	400	500
Boxing	300	1000 (1000)	2000 (5000)
Cricket (indoor)	400	500	1000
Cycling (indoor)	300	500	750
Ice-hockey (outdoor)	(100)	(200)	(500)
Ice-hockey (indoor)	250 (200)	750 (500)	750 (1000)
Lawn tennis (outdoor)	180 (100)	360 (200)	500 (300)
Lawn tennis (indoor)	300 (500)	500 (750)	750 (1000)
Rodeo	(100)	(300)	(500)
Ski slopes (outdoor)	50 (10)	100	
Squash courts	300 (200)	400 (300)	750 (500)
Swimming pools (indoor)	200 (300)	300	1000 (500)
Table tennis	200 (200)	300 (300)	500 (500)
Volleyball (indoor)	300 (100)	500 (200)	750

* The unbracketed figures are UK recommendations for minimum levels from CIBSE (1990), the bracketed figures are target maintained values from the USA (IES, 1981, section 2). The values listed are the requirements for horizontal illuminance over the main playing area. There may be additional requirements, e.g. for vertical illuminances or illuminances over the spectator area. Higher levels may be required if a high proportion of participants are elderly (e.g. bowls, CIBSE, 1990).
† Figures from Sylvania Outdoor Lighting (1977).

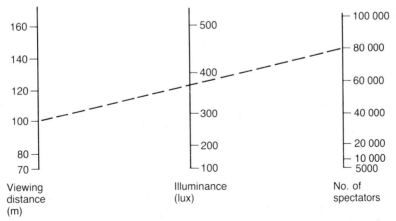

Figure 6.6   Nomogram showing the relationship between the number of spectators, the viewing distance to the centre of the pitch of the spectators who are furthest away and the recommended horizontal illuminance for sports stadia. (Reproduced from CIBSE, *Lighting Guide LG4: Sports* (1990), by permission of the Charted Institution of Building Services Engineers)

lights surrounding the playing area and mounted on masts at a height which ensures that the pools of illumination that they produce overlap satisfactorily. As noted earlier, a reasonable mounting height also minimizes glare problems. For indoor playing areas, rows of fluorescent lamps are often used. Figure 6.7 shows typical basic layouts for an outdoor national or international tennis court and for an indoor club or county court (IES, 1974). Note that, as in the case of other sports, when floodlights are used care must be taken to set the lighting poles far enough back from the playing area to minimize the risk of players colliding with them.

In some sports which are essentially unidirectional in nature it may be possible to direct floodlights so that negligible glare is experienced. In a target lane for archery, for example, floodlights can be mounted on a pole behind the shooting line and directed forward over the archer's head to illuminate the target, and a similar freedom from glare can be obtained on artificial ski slopes by directing the floodlighting down the slope in the direction in which the skiers are travelling (Figure 6.8).

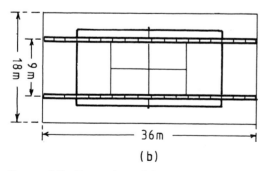

(a)

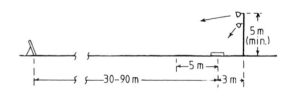

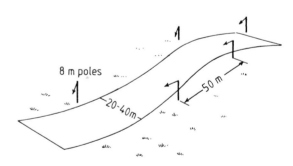

Figure 6.8 Examples of low-glare lighting for largely unidirectional sports. *a*, A single archery lane with a mast-mounted floodlight providing the main illumination. An intensity of about 300,000 cd is required to produce an illuminance of 100 lux on a target at 50 m: a second light may be used to provide additional illumination for the shooting zone if required. *b*, Lighting for an artificial ski slope to an illuminance of about 30 lux. (Reproduced from IES, *Lighting Guide: Sports* (1974, out of print) by permission of the Chartered Institution of Building Services Engineers)

(b)

Figure 6.7 Examples of lighting schemes for tennis courts. *a*, An outdoor court for use in major tournaments. It is lit to 500 lux by 1500 W tungsten halogen floodlights. *b*, An indoor court for club use lit to 300 lux by lines of trough reflectors, each housing two 1800 mm high-efficacy fluorescent lamps. (Reproduced from IES, *Lighting Guide: Sports* (1974, out of print) by permission of the Chartered Institution of Building Services Engineers)

Filters and other aspects

Although full-spectrum daylight or artificial light is desirable for most sporting purposes, there may be occasions when modification of the level, spectrum or polarization of the available light is beneficial. Table 6.3 (after Obstfeld, personal communication) summarizes the characteristics of filters which have been recommended by various authorities for particular sports. The filters may be made up in the form of spectacles, goggles or visors, depending upon the nature of the sport. In most cases it is desirable that the glazed appliance should provide impact protection to the appropriate national standard, as well as modifying the characteristics of the transmitted light. In general, too, all filters should have low transmittance to ultraviolet light which can be harmful to the eyes. Some of the basic types of filter will now be discussed in more detail.

Neutral density and photochromic spectacle lenses

Glare may be experienced when very high levels of daylight are available, particularly in highly reflecting environments such as sand or snow. Under such circumstances, light-absorbing spectacles, visors or goggles have obvious utility. In general, to avoid colour distortions, it is better that such devices have equal attenuation for all visible wavelengths, i.e, they should have neutral density (grey filters).

Table 6.3 Recommended filter characteristics for various sports

Sport	Filter characteristics
Clay pigeon shooting/skeet	Yellow filters may appear to improve contrast against blue sky. Green recommended for woodland. Red for orange clay shooting. All filters should be UV absorbing
Driving	UV and blue absorbing filters; photochromic plastics or toughened brown glass; neutral grey filter; single or double gradient mirror; anti-reflection coating (night driving)
Fishing	Polarizing: facilitates seeing into the water by absorbing reflected light or glare
Flying	UV and blue absorbing filter
Golf	Green–brown filter: improves visibility of the ball against grass and sky
Mountaineering	UV and blue absorbing filter; neutral grey filter; single or double gradient mirror
Shooting	Yellow filter: improves subjective appreciation of contrast
Skiing	Yellow filter: to improve contrast of irregularities on snow surfaces; UV and blue absorbing filter; orange–brown filter; photochromic plastics or toughened glass filter
Tennis	UV and blue absorbing filter
Water sports	UV and blue absorbing filter; photochromic plastics or toughened glass filter; single or double gradient mirror; brown filter; neutral grey filter; brown or grey polarizing filter

Source: After Obstfeld, personal communication, 1994

The only problem with conventional fixed filters of this type is that the wearer may omit to remove them when conditions change and they are no longer required. The sportsman's efficiency may then be impaired because too little light is reaching his eyes. The lenses of photochromic spectacles or sunglasses act as *active* filters, with transmission characteristics which change according to the ambient lighting levels. This is achieved by incorporating silver halide crystals in the glass or plastic of the lenses. The molecules partially dissociate under the action of high levels of shorter wavelength light to yield free silver, so that the lenses become dark and their transmittance is reduced: the process reverses when light levels fall, and the lenses clear again. The exact characteristics of photochromic lenses vary with the host material and its thickness, together with the mixture of silver halides and sensitizing dopants, such as copper, used by the manufacturer. Commonly, the basic tint is neutral or brown and the transmittance might change between about 20% in the fully darkened condition and 80% in the fully faded state. Transmittance changes roughly exponentially with time during both darkening and fading, each change being almost complete after about 5 minutes at 20 °C.

Lenses of this type have obvious attractions for use in various sporting situations when the weather is such that periods of bright sunlight are interspersed with duller periods. This is particularly the case for those who need to wear a prescription to correct their refractive error, since they do not need to change continually between prescription sunglasses and a conventional clear prescription. There are, however, two possible problems which must be borne in mind when considering the suitability of photochromic lenses for any particular sport: temperature effects and the wavelengths that induce the darkening. At lower temperatures, all photochromic materials tend to be darker at any light level, and to fade or darken more slowly as the light level changes. This may be significant in some 'cold weather' sports. Secondly, shorter solar wavelengths may be absorbed by window glass, so that certain types of photochromic lens may not respond adequately to changes in ambient lighting when, for example, worn by a saloon car driver.

Spectrally selective filters

In several sports, particularly shooting, skiing and night driving, it is often suggested that yellow or amber filters, which transmit only light of longer wavelengths and exclude the blue end of the spectrum, can improve performance. The yellow filters might be incorporated into gunsights or be in the form of spectacles or goggles. It is usually hypothesized (e.g. Miller, 1974) that an improvement in visual performance might be expected because blue light is likely to be scattered more in the ocular media than longer wavelengths: hence its exclusion will tend to improve retinal image contrast. A further supposed benefit is that restriction of the spectral band admitted to the eye will reduce the blurring effects associated with the longitudinal chromatic aberration of the eye, giving a crisper retinal image and increasing visual acuity. In night driving the chief claimed benefit is a reduction in glare from opposing headlights, again due to reduced intra-ocular scatter.

The bulk of the evidence fails to support the contention that yellow filters improve visual acuity (i.e. detection of high spatial frequency information) or reduce glare (Clark, 1969; Kelly *et al.*, 1984). Kinney *et al.* (1980, 1983) claimed, however, that the filters may enhance performance on tasks involving the detection of low contrast targets at intermediate spatial frequencies, a result supported by Yap (1984). This could justify the use of such filters by hunters, skiers, boaters and skeet shooters in low visibility conditions. In general it seems reasonable to conclude that although subjectively individuals might feel that objects look sharper when viewed through a yellow filter, there are considerable doubts as to whether visual performance is systematically improved. It remains possible that some individuals, perhaps in the older age group, might benefit more than others: filters passing only longer wavelengths have been shown to be beneficial for some low-vision patients with pre-retinal disease (Leat *et al.*, 1990).

Most of the debate on the use of yellow goggles as aids to skiers and others in improving visibility in overcast snowscapes centres on a slightly different argument, namely the enhancement of the contrast of irregularities in the snow when filters are worn, as a result of variations in the spectrum of the light reflected from different areas. It has been argued that the bottoms of holes, illuminated from the zenith sky, might appear bluer than the tops, illuminated by the horizon sky, so that a yellow filter by excluding the blue will enhance the contrast of the hole (Corth, 1985). Some experimental support for this general idea has been put forward by Troscianko (1986) who also suggested that light transmitted through the snow, which is preferentially absorbed at longer wavelengths, might contribute to the apparent blueness of the bottom of snow holes. Kinney (1985), citing arguments put forward by Wyszecki (1956), prefers a purely physiological explanation but all agree that there is a real improvement in ability to detect subtle variations in the contour of the snow when yellow goggles are worn.

There is no evidence to support the view that yellow or amber filters are helpful in night driving. Although the reduction in retinal illuminance that they produce may slightly diminish glare effects, it also degrades most aspects of visual performance (e.g. Lauer *et al.*, 1950; Haber, 1955; Phillips, 1967) and tends to negate the effects of improved vehicle and road lighting.

Polarizing filters

Light which is specularly reflected from smooth horizontal surfaces, such as water, tends to be predominantly polarized with its electric vector in the horizontal direction. Hence a linear polarizing filter which transmits only vertically polarized light will suppress these reflections (e.g. Freeman, 1990). This means that polarizing sunglasses are particularly helpful in environments where reflected glare from water or road surfaces is troublesome. They have particular advantages for anglers, as the specular reflections are removed, allowing objects located below the surface of the water to be seen more easily. They are also useful in a variety of water sports and for driving in wet conditions. Since only one plane of polarization is transmitted by a linear polarizer, such filters can only transmit a maximum of 50% of normal unpolarized light (a more usual figure in practice is 40%) and they effectively act as neutral filters as well reducing unwanted reflections.

Spectral transmission effects under water

It is interesting to note that even very clear water absorbs slightly at each end of the visible spectrum. Hence, in scuba diving in such water, as depth increases the available light becomes more and more dominated by blue–green wavelengths (Figure 6.9*a*). Thus full-spectrum flash is necessary in underwater photography if a full gamut of colours is to be recorded. (A useful discussion of techniques for underwater image recording is given in IES, 1981, section 18.) In waters with substantial concentrations of vegetable or mineral debris, which cause both absorption and scattering, such spectral effects may become even more pronounced with peak irradiance shifting more towards the green (Lythgoe, 1979). The diffuse attenuation coefficient, K, of irradiance (watts/unit area/unit wavelength interval) as a function of wavelength for some typical waters is shown in (Figure 6.9*b*) (the irradiance E_z at depth z is given by $E_z = E_o e^{-kz}$, where E_o is the irradiance at the surface). It can be seen that substantially different spectral distributions of underwater light may be expected in different locations

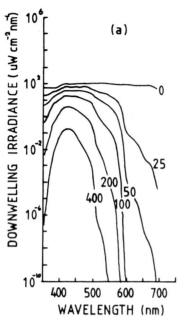
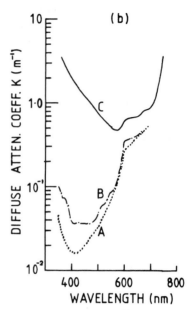

Figure 6.9 *a*, Spectral distribution of downwelling irradiance as a function of depth in metres for the very clear, pure, natural fresh water of Crater Lake in Oregon. Note that the spectral bandwidth of the available light becomes progressively narrower as the depth increases *b*, Spectral variation of the diffuse attenuation coefficient, *K*, in three types of natural water. A low attenuation coefficient corresponds to a high transmittance. **A**, Fresh water at Crater Lake; **B**, clear blue Gulf Stream sea water; **C**, green fresh water, rich in phytoplankton. (After Tyler and Smith, 1970)

(Kinney *et al.*, 1967; Tyler and Smith, 1970; Lythgoe, 1979; IES, 1981, section 18).

Navigation lights for aircraft and boats

Considerable theoretical interest attaches to the detection of what are essentially point stimuli under mesopic and scotopic conditions. Good discussions of the photometric problems involved will be found in Wright (1949) and IES (1984, 3–21 to 3–25). The lights of vessels, lighthouses and other beacons may be identified by different combinations of colour, temporal modulation and spatial arrangement (IES, 1981, section 16; Nautical Almanac, 1992). Aircraft visibility in recent years has been very substantially improved by the use of high intensity stroboscopic anti-collision flash beacons (IES, 1981, section 15).

Vehicle and traffic signals make similar use of colour, temporal modulation and shape.

One problem in the use of colour for signals is that, as noted earlier, about 8% of males (but less than 1% of females) have colour vision defects which may lead to errors in identifying the signals (e.g. Whillans and Allen, 1992). Errors may also occur when spectrally selective tinted lenses are worn (Hovis *et al.*, 1991).

At night, red light is frequently used to illuminate the navigation chart-plotting tables of yachts. Light levels must be high enough to give the navigator sufficient acuity to read the chart, so that illumination must necessarily be at least at the bottom of the photopic range. If red light of wavelength greater than about 600 nm is used, it is well within the spectral sensitivity of the essentially photopic cones but has relatively little effect on the visual pigment of the rods (see scotopic curve of Figure 6.1) which therefore remain in a near dark-adapted state (e.g. Miles, 1953; Le Grand, 1957; Optical Society of America, 1963). The navigator's night vision is therefore very little impaired when he returns from the chart table to the deck. Care must be taken that colour-coded features of charts are not mis-read when red illumination is used.

Summary

It is now possible to provide high quality, low glare lighting of good uniformity and colour for most sporting applications. For outdoor situations, adverse weather such as fog, rain or other precipitation is still a problem. It is not only uncomfortable for players and spectators alike but also reduces the contrast and visibility of features of the event, particularly for spectacle wearers. Perhaps the next phase of development, at least in larger stadia, will be the widespread adoption of moveable roof structures which can cover the entire stadium when conditions warrant. Such structures have already been pioneered in North America and elsewhere. Finally it should be remembered that the role of artificial lighting is not simply to optimize efficiency, safety and security: it can also have a powerful aesthetic impact. If properly designed, it can enhance the attractiveness of even the simplest of playing areas and, for major events, can accentuate the drama and spectacle of the sporting occasion. Lighting, then, deserves to be considered at all stages of the design of a sporting venue rather than, as all too often, being rather casually added on as an afterthought.

2. LIGHT DAMAGE AND THE EYE

Introduction

Light is around us every day and although necessary for us to see, its presence is taken very much for granted. This means that its potential for causing damage is probably the least considered of all mechanisms of eye injury during day-to-day life and sporting activities. Yet injuries due to light damage can, and do, occur, ranging from chronic insidious conditions (Taylor *et al.*, 1992) to acute severe sight-threatening damage (Jacobs *et al.*, 1985). Any outdoor sports or recreations, especially those taking place in bright conditions which are exaggerated by reflection from snow, sand or water, put the participants at risk from this form of eye injury. It is recognized that aircraft pilots, mountaineers and skiers are particularly susceptible, but recreational swimmers, sailors, anglers and windsurfers should be aware that they may also be at high risk.

Before proceeding to a detailed description of the specific effects of light on structures within the eye Figure 6.1 should be reviewed to remind the reader about the physical properties of light.

Absorption and transmittance of the ocular structures

By its very nature as a visual organ, the eye must be exposed to and process wavelengths within the visible spectrum. The refracting ocular media, comprising the cornea, aqueous, lens and vitreous body, need to transmit visible light freely to the retina in order to initiate the visual process. However, light is a form of energy, and as such may be harmful. So, in addition to allowing the light to pass through, the structures in the ocular media act as filters, absorbing certain wavelengths of light in order to protect the retina from the damaging effects of radiation. This is particularly important for shorter wavelength light, that is, the blue end of the visible spectrum and UV which have been implicated in causing retinal photodamage (Ham *et al.*, 1982).

The cornea is the most important filter. It is the main protector against infrared radiation and additionally is opaque to wavelengths of less than 300 nm which are either reflected or absorbed. The cornea does, however, allow the passage of wavelengths longer than this, which therefore include some UV-B and all of the UV-A part of the spectrum (Figure 6.10). The lens absorbs this UV-B and UV-A (i.e. the wavelengths between 300 nm and 400 nm) but little beyond this unless alteration in the lens properties due to ageing has taken place. The aqueous absorbs minimal amounts of UV and along with the vitreous has a small role as a heat (infrared) absorber.

The result of the filtering effects of these ocular structures is that the retina is exposed to radiation between 400 and 1400 nm. This range has been termed the 'retinal hazard region' (Marshall, 1984). Within this region the ocular media absorb only approximately 5% of the visible spectrum (400–760 nm) and 30% of the near infrared (IR-A 760–1400 nm) (Geeraets and Berry, 1968). Thus, because of these

effects, nearly all the visible and the majority of the infrared light reaches the retina. Some of this light is reflected back out of the eye but the remaining energy is absorbed.

There are five main systems for absorbing this light energy in the retina: the visual pigments, which convert the energy to neural transmission for vision, and four protective mechanisms to minimize any light damage. The protective mechanisms are the retinal pigment epithelium (RPE), haemoglobin, macular luteal pigment and the choroid. The RPE contains melanin which absorbs approximately 50% of the light entering the eye, predominantly at the blue end of the spectrum (Marshall, 1984). Some light damage may be caused by free radical generation, and in this situation melanin may act as a free radical scavenger (Lavail, 1980). Haemoglobin present in the retinal vessels also absorbs blue light but this has a minimal contribution because the retinal blood vessels are small and narrow. Macular luteal pigment is present maximally at the fovea and absorbs short wave blue light between 400 and 500 nm to protect this area of high acuity. Finally, the choroid absorbs light by both its melanin and haemoglobin content.

Mechanisms of damage

Light may damage susceptible tissues by either its thermal or photochemical effects (Lerman, 1985). Thermal damage occurs when sufficient radiant energy is absorbed by a structure to increase its temperature and thereby to increase the motion of its molecules. This type of burn requires a well-focused beam of high-energy light such as laser light. Such lesions are characterized by a central area of intense damage with surrounding sub-threshold damage. This is the mechanism of injury used beneficially in the treatment of diabetic retinopathy and is not really an area of concern for the sportsperson.

Photochemical damage to the eye by solar radiation is dependent on a number of factors,

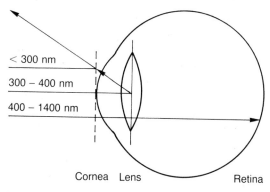

Figure 6.10 Wavelengths of light that are absorbed or reflected by the cornea and lens, and those that pass to the retina

including the compostion of the light to which the eye is exposed and any variation in absorption and transmittance characteristics of the different ocular structures. The power intensity required to produce photochemical damage is far lower than that needed to induce thermal damage. In this situation, absorption of light by the cell leads to an alteration in its molecular structure causing cell damage and tissue death. This process is highly wavelength-specific, depending on the absorption of light by specific macro-molecules and tending to occur maximally with the shorter wavelength visible and UV light. There is a latent period before the damage becomes evident and the affected area tends to be uniformly involved. Photochemical injury tends to be cumulative, with many sub-threshold exposures resulting in long-term injury to the ocular structures. Factors which might influence photochemical injury are pigmentation, pupil size, the effectiveness of protective lenses, if worn, and on-going regeneration and repair.

Reparative processes

Light plays a physiological role in maintaining the health of the outer segments of the retina, in that light reactions and any subsequent damage are followed by repair and regeneration of the photoreceptor membrane discs. This process is responsible for the maintenance of photoreceptor integrity and normal visual acuity. However, high levels of light energy or prolonged exposure may lead to receptor damage which outstrips the ability to regenerate, causing long-term cumulative cell loss (Lerman, 1980).

Specific examples of light damage to the eye

Lids

The skin, like the eye, contains elements which can absorb light and therefore can be damaged. Long-term exposure has been associated with the development of basal cell carcinoma of the eyelids, especially the lower lid.

Cornea

The cornea is the main protector against the effects of UV but is very susceptible to damage from a narrow band of wavelengths between 288 and 290 nm which is absorbed by chromophores in the DNA of the corneal epithelial cells (Lerman, 1980). This causes fragmentation of the nuclear proteins with resultant cell death. This process, recognized as 'snow blindness' or photokeratitis, was originally described in polar explorers. Clinically there is a latent period of between 6 and 12 hours after exposure to excessive UV light before the eyes become very painful and photophobic. These symptoms are due to exposure of the underlying corneal nerves which occurs when the devitalized epithelial cells slough off and are removed by the process of blinking. Photokeratitis is completely reversible after the epithelium has regenerated, although a recurrent corneal erosion may result in the long term.

Long-term effects of UV radiation on the external eye consist of pinguecualae, pterygia, exposure keratitis, Labrador keratitis and nodular shaped band keratopathy (Moran and Hollows, 1984; Lerman, 1985). In addition, herpes simplex keratitis and recurrent corneal erosions may be triggered by UV light (Taylor et al., 1992).

In contrast to the effect on the epithelium, the corneal stroma seems only to be affected by direct thermal damage. There is, however, experimental evidence which suggests that endothelial function may be damaged for a significant time following UV exposure (Cullen et al., 1984).

Lens

The cornea and aqueous transmit all wavelengths greater than 300 nm, therefore the lens is exposed to longer wavelengths and absorbs ambient UV from 300–400 nm. Epidemiological evidence suggests that this absorption throughout life may be associated with lenticular ageing changes, causing premature presbyopia (Miranda, 1979) and cataract formation (Heller *et al.*, 1977; Brilliant *et al.*, 1983; Taylor *et al.*, 1988). These chronic changes have been associated with both cortical and nuclear sclerotic lens opacities. The underlying mechanism is not clear, although a number of theories have been promoted. Iris pigment may absorb and convert light radiation into heat which is transferred to the underlying lens causing the development of cortical lens opacities (Miranda, 1980). Alternatively, direct photo-oxidative damage to the lens proteins, membrane lipids or epithelium may lead to an alteration in metabolism which prevents the maintenance of clarity (Pitts and Bergmanson, 1980). Secondary colour changes due to chromophore formation increase further absorption of UV and more chromophores are generated which cause further absorption and so on. This is manifest clinically as discoloration of the lens which changes from clear to yellow to brown with progressive reduction in the transmission of visible and UV light. These changes are, however, beneficial to the retina since they make the lens a more effective filter of UV and high energy blue visible light. Thus it protects the retina preferentially from photochemical damage, especially in the older age group when the reparative effects of the retina are becoming less efficient.

Vitreous

There are very few chromophores in the vitreous, however there are enough to absorb some infrared which may lead to shrinkage of the vitreous and to collagen denaturation causing premature syneresis, or degeneration of the vitreous gel.

As described above, UV light is filtered by the cornea and lens. In normal circumstances, therefore, the vitreous is not exposed to any UV. However, when the lens has been removed and either not replaced or replaced with an intra-ocular lens implant without UV absorption properties, the vitreous or retina may be more susceptible to light damage.

Retina

As everyone who comes inside on a bright sunny day knows, the normal dark adaptation response is delayed slightly after even short-term exposure to sunlight. With exposure to strong light for several hours overbleaching of the retinal pigments occurs with resultant significant changes in the dark adaptation curve with prolonged time to maximum sensitivity. This may be a chronic effect which can be present for many days (Clark *et al.*, 1946), as seen in climbers after long expeditions.

Only the retina is susceptible to damage by wavelengths in the visible spectrum, as the normal ocular media are transparent to such wavelengths (Lerman, 1985). Absorption of visible light by the retinal visual pigments is the basis of sight. It is also an integral part of the turnover of the outer discs of the photoreceptors. As long as the exposure to light is not excessive, the integrity of the disc membranes is maintained. However, if the loss of receptor discs is greater than the capacity for repair there will be damage (Marshall, 1984). With ageing, the retina becomes less capable of repair and, along with cumulative exposure to light over many years, there may be a reduction in the number of rods and cones with advancing age. The higher-energy, ultraviolet and blue end of the visible spectrum (320–450 nm) is especially damaging in this regard (Lerman, 1980). Prolonged exposure to high levels of blue and UV light may be related to the development of age-related macular degeneration in later life (Taylor *et al.*, 1992), and has been suggested to have a deleterious effect in certain retinal dystrophies (Adrian *et al.*, 1977).

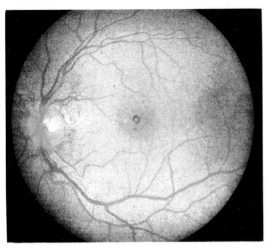

Figure 6.11   Solar retinopathy. (Courtesy of E.S. Rosen)

A particular type of acute retinal light damage has been recognized in the form of solar retinopathy, which occurs in patients who sungaze. This was originally thought to be a thermal burn to the retina, however, it is now considered to be a photochemical reaction caused by highly reactive free radicals. Solar retinopathy produces oedema at the macula with a surrounding pigmented halo and the foveal region may develop a lamellar hole (Figure 6.11). The clinical presentation is of reduced vision with a central scotoma, but the prognosis for visual recovery is good (Guerry *et al.*, 1985)

Factors that influence potentially hazardous radiation

The sun is essentially the only source of light intense enough to damage the eye under conditions in which sports are played. Fluorescent lighting does emit some UV-B, but protective filters should be built into the design of all such lamps.

There are a number of factors influencing the amount of radiation reaching the eye.

Ozone

One of the main concerns regarding the progressive loss of ozone is that this layer is responsible for filtering out the shortest wavelength UV-C and also selectively absorbing some of the UV-A and UV-B. Any decrease in the ozone layer leads to a disproportionate increase in the risk of photochemical retinal damage (Lerman, 1985).

Reflection

As one does not usually look directly at the sun because of discomfort and direct glare, it is not radiation which comes directly from the sun that tends to cause damage but rather that which is reflected from the earth's surface. As the reflected rays are from the sides and below, the forehead, eyebrows and headgear offer no protection. Earth and grass reflect 5% of incident light, sand reflects 17% and water 20%. Most dangerous of all is snow, which reflects a staggering 85% of incident light (Davis, 1987).

Local factors

Light cloud and haze may increase the amount of radiation reaching ground level from the sun, whereas dark clouds and pollutants reduce it.

Season and time of day

As one would expect, there is marked seasonal variation in the amount of light reaching sea level, with a seventeen-fold increase in the intensity of the solar radiation at midday from winter to summer (Blumthaler *et al.*, 1985).

When the sun is overhead at midday, the level of UV radiation reaching earth is ten times that at either three hours before or after that time.

Altitude

The filtering effects of the atmosphere decrease with increased height: for every 1000 metres of altitude there is an increase in radiation intensity of 16%. This is particularly concerning for activities carried out at high altitude on snow-covered terrain or aviation sports (Blumthaler *et al.*, 1985).

Body temperature

In experimental animals there is a relationship between body temperature and the amount of retinal damage caused by light. For a given level of exposure there is a marked increase in the amount of photic retinal damage if the body temperature is increased slightly (by 1–3°C above normal) (Noell *et al.*, 1966).

Drugs

A number of pharmacological preparations increase sensitivity to visible and UV light. Examples of such photosensitizing agents include some antibiotics, diuretics and oral contraceptives.

Protection and prevention

Like many sport-associated eye injuries the best way to manage light damage is to prevent it. There are basic reflexes which occur in response to strong light, such as turning the head away, blinking, screwing up the eyes and pupillary miosis. The direction of sunlight is obviously from above so there is the natural protection from the brows, forehead and hair. This can be augmented by wearing a large-brimmed hat or visor in bright sunlight. As mentioned above, however, a significant part of light coming into the eyes is reflected from the ground or surrounding structures. It is therefore important in some activities to have protection against UV from below and from the sides.

Sunglasses are potentially valuable protectors so long as they fulfil certain criteria. Unfortunately, the emphasis is often on whether or not they are fashionable rather than on their ability to absorb damaging wavelengths of light. The colour of tinted lenses cannot be regarded as a guide to their suitability as a protective filter. Appropriate information should be available about the properties of all sunglasses at the time and place of purchase. Guidelines such as BS 2724 (British Standards Institute, 1987) and ANSI Z-80.3 (American National Standards Institute, 1986) have been drawn up with the objective of establishing standards which should be met (Table 6.4). Sunglasses should absorb 100% of damaging UV, with a complete cut off below 400 nm. In addition, there should be low transmission at the blue end of the visible spectrum with a maximum of 10% of visible light being transmitted. Curved lenses which fit snugly around the face are useful in sports with a significant risk of peripheral UV exposure, and also will protect the eyes against strong winds which may be a problem for cyclists or riders. Any lenses, including sunglasses, which are to be worn during sporting activities should be made of polycarbonate as this will not fracture when struck (see Chapter 5).

All spectacles should fit comfortably over the nose and ears to prevent removal due to discomfort or loss due to a poor fit. In many instances, such as skiing or sailing, goggles which are securely attached to the face are required which also prevent light coming in from the sides and below. Contact lenses with UV absorbing properties are also available. These require to have complete corneal coverage in order to be effective and therefore a soft lens which extends to the limbus is necessary. All intra-ocular lens implants used nowadays should have UV absorbent properties.

In general there seems to be a lack of awareness that light is potentially damaging

Table 6.4 Classification and uses of sunglasses: extract from BS 2724

Classification	Use
Cosmetic spectacles	Lightly tinted spectacles not intended to give significant protection against sun glare and worn largely for their fashion properties
General purpose sunglasses	Sunglasses intended to reduce sun glare in bright circumstances, including the driving of motor vehicles in daylight
Special purpose sunglasses	Sunglasses intended to reduce sun glare in abnormal environmental conditions, e.g. near large expanses of water or in snow and mountain altitudes, or for persons who may be abnormally sensitive to glare as a result of medical treatment or otherwise
	Non-photochromic filters having a shade number of 4.1 are not considered suitable for use by persons when driving motor vehicles
Refraction class 1	Equivalent to prescription lens quality (see BS 2738) and recommended for continuous daytime wearing
Refraction class 2	Suitable for intermittent wearing
Break resistant sunglasses	Suitable for conditions where mechanical abuse is possible but will not be severe, e.g. driving, cycling, walking, camping or boating
Robust sunglasses	Suitable for conditions where mechanical abuse is possible and likely to be severe, e.g. soft ball sports and climbing
Impact resistant sunglasses	Recommended for more severe mechanical abuse hazards, e.g. hard ball sports and sports in which balls travel at velocities in excess of 10 m/s

Reproduced with the permission of British Standards Institution. Complete copies can be obtained by post from BSI Sales, Linford Wood, Milton Keynes MK14 6LE.

to the eye. This is partly because sunlight is taken for granted and is not thought to be harmful. However, health education is beginning to emphasize the message about the association between sunlamps, excess sunlight and the risk of skin cancer. Hopefully this will be extended to the effects on the eye and will lead to the introduction of eye protection.

The importance of light damage

While some studies have examined the occupational hazards of prolonged exposure of the eye to sunlight (Taylor *et al.*, 1992), none has yet clinically investigated the consequences of this for sporting activities. Numbers of winter sports enthusiasts, who are exposed to the particularly hazardous effects of UV, have more than doubled in recent times and overall there is more emphasis on the benefits of exercise and increased time available to pursue sporting activities both indoors and outdoors.

Some individuals are active in sport for prolonged periods during their youth, when the protective effect of the yellowing lens on the retina has not developed. This may be a vulnerable time when light damage could occur, particularly in sports such as sailing, windsurfing, skiing and climbing where there is a high amount of reflected light. The problem is that any effects may not be apparent for many years and it is therefore very difficult to prove a direct cause-and-effect relationship.

At the other end of the age spectrum, people of advanced age are also becoming more involved in sporting activities such as fishing, golf and water sports. This may cause particular problems in people who are aphakic or pseudophakic, particularly as the retinal reparative processes are less effective in older people.

From the above description of light damage and the factors which affect this, it is clear that any person who plays sport out of doors has an increased risk of light damage as there is increased exposure to solar radiation. This is a particular problem in sports which are carried out on snow or water and therefore have high levels of reflected radiation.

References and further reading

Adrian, W., Everson, R.W. and Schmidt, I. (1977) Protection against photic damage in retinitis pigmentosa. *Advances in Experimental Medical Biology,* **77,** 233–47

American National Standards Institute (1986) Z80.3 *Recommendations for Non-treatment Sunglasses and Fashion Eyewear,* ANSI, New York.

Blumthaler, M., Ambach, W. and Dexecker, F. (1985) Computation of radiation doses in changes of solar radiation with regard to photoelective keratitis. *Kliniks Monatsbl. Augenheilkd.* **4,** 275–8

Bradley, P.M. (1992) Sports hall lighting: Badminton players' attitudes. *Lighting Research and Technology,* **24,** 227–33

Brilliant, L.B., Grasset, N.C., Pokhrel, R.P. *et al.* (1983) Associations among cataract prevalence, sunlight hours and altitude in the Himalayas. *American Journal of Epidemiology,* **118,** 250–64

British Standards Institution (1968) BS667 *Specification for Portable Photoelectric Photometers,* BSI, London

British Standards Institution (1987) BSI 2724 *Sun Glare Eye Protectors for General Use,* BSI, London

Campbell, F.W., Rothwell, S.E. and Perry, M.J. (1987) Bad light stops play. *Ophthalmic and Physiological Optics,* **7,** 165–7

Cayless, M.A. and Marsden, A.M. (1983) *Lamps and Lighting,* 3rd edn, Arnold, London

CIBSE (1984) *Code for Interior Lighting,* Chartered Institution of Building Service Engineers, London

CIBSE (1990) *Lighting Guide: Sports.* Publication LG7, Chartered Institute of Building Service Engineers, London

CIE (1978) CIE 42 *Lighting for Tennis,* Commission Internationale de l'Eclairage, Vienna

CIE (1979) CIE 45 *Lighting for Ice Sports,* Commission Internationale de l'Eclairage, Vienna

CIE (1983a) CIE 57 *Lighting for Football,* Commission Internationale de l'Eclairage, Vienna

CIE (1983b) CIE 58 *Lighting for Sports Halls,* Commission Internationale de l'Eclairage, Vienna

CIE (1984) CIE 62 *Lighting for Swimming Pools,* Commission Internationale de l'Eclairage, Vienna

CIE (1989) CIE 83 *Lighting of Sports Events for Colour TV Broadcasting,* Commission Internationale de l'Eclairage, Vienna

Clark, B.A.J. (1969) Color in sunglass lenses. *American Journal of Optometry and Archives of the American Academy of Optometry,* **46,** 825–40

Clark, B., Johnson, M.L. and Dreher, R. (1946) The effect of sunlight on dark adaptation. *American Journal of Ophthalmology,* **29,** 826–36

Corth, R. (1985) The perception of depth contours with yellow goggles: an alternative explanation. *Perception,* **14,** 377–8

Cronly-Dillon, J., Rosen, E.S. and Marshall, J. (eds) (1985) *Hazards of Light,* Pergamon Press, Oxford

Cullen, A.P., Chou, B.R. and Glover, R.F. (1984) Corneal endothelial recovery following irradiation with UV-B. *Investigative Ophthalmology and Visual Science,* **25** (Suppl.), 331

Davies, L.F., Jackson, M.G.A and Rogers, B.C. (1972) Lighting techniques and associated equipment for outdoor colour television with particular reference to football stadium lighting. *Lighting Research and Technology,* **4,** 181–201

Davis, J.K. (1987) Lenses for sports vision. In *Sports Ophthalmology* (eds L.D. Pizzarello and B.G. Haik), Charles C. Thomas, Springfield, Ill., ch. 2

Freeman, M.H. (1990) *Optics,* 10th edn, Butterworths, London, p. 375

Geeraets, W.J. and Berry, E.R. (1968) Ocular spectral characteristics as related to hazards from lasers and other light sources. *American Journal of Ophthalmology,* **6,** 15–20

Guerry, R.K., Ham, W.T. and Mueller, H.A. (1985) Light toxicity in the posterior segment. In *Clinical Ophthalmology* (ed. T. D. Duane), Harper and Row, Philadelphia, vol. 3, ch. 37.

Haber, H. (1955) Safety hazards of tinted automobile windshields at night. *Journal of the Optical Society of America,* **45,** 413–19

Ham, W.T., Muller, H.A. Ruffolo, J.J., Guerry, D. and Guerry, R.K. (1982) Action spectrum for retinal injury from near ultra-violet radiation in the aphakic monkey.

American Journal of Ophthalmology, **93**, 229–306

Hargroves, R.A., Henry, I.C. and Trezzi, M. (1986) Glare evaluation of tennis court lighting. *Lighting Research and Technology,* **18**, 157–60

Heller, R., Giacometti, L. and Yuen, K. (1977) Sunlight and cataract: an epidemiologic investigation. *American Journal of Epidemiology,* **105**, 450–9

Hovis, J.K., Cranton, D. and Chou, B.R. (1991) Tinted lenses and the ANSI standards for traffic signal transmittances. *Optometry and Vision Science,* **68**, 750–5

IES (1974) *Lighting Guide: Sports,* Illumination Engineering Society, London

IES (1981) *IES Lighting Handbook: 1981 Application Volume* (ed. J.E. Kaufman, and H. Haynes, Illumination Engineering Society of North America, New York

IES (1984) *IES Lighting Handbook: 1984 Reference Volume* (ed. J.E. Kaufman and J.F. Christensen), Illumination Engineering Society of North America, New York

Jacobs, N.A., Headon, M. and Rosen, E.S. (1985) Solar retinopathy in the Manchester area. *Transactions of the Ophthalmology Societies of the United Kingdom,* **6**, 625–8

Kelly, S.A., Goldberg, S.E. and Banton, T.A. (1984) Effect of yellow-tinted lenses on contrast sensitivity. *American Journal of Physiological Optics,* **61**, 657–62

Kinney, J.S., Luria, S.M. and Weitzmann, D.O. (1967) Visibility of colors underwater. *Journal of the Optical Society of America,* **57**, 802–9

Kinney, J.A. (1985) The perception of depth contours with yellow goggles: comments on letter by Richard Korth. *Perception,* **14**, 378–9

Kinney, J.S., Schlichting, C.L., Neri, D. and Kindness, S.W. (1980) Various measures of the effectiveness of yellow goggles. Naval Submarine Medical Research Laboratory, Report No. 941. Naval Medical Research and Development Command, RWU-MF58.524.0.13–1039. Naval Submarine Medical Research Laboratory, Groton

Kinney, J.S., Schlichting, C.L., Neri, D.F. and Kindness, S.W. (1983) Reaction time to spatial frequencies using yellow and luminance-matched neutral goggles. *American Journal of Optometry and Physiological Optics,* **60**, 132–8

Lauer, A.P., Fletcher, F.K., Winston, P. and Takahashi, E.S. (1950) Effect of nightglasses and colored windshields. *Optometry Weekly,* **41**, 951

Lavail, M.M. (1980) Circidian nature of rod outer segment disc shedding in the rat. *Investigative Ophthalmology and Visual Science,* **19**, 407–11

Leat, S.J., North, R.V. and Bryson, H. (1990) Do long wavelength filters improve low vision performance? *Ophthalmic and Physiological Optics,* **10**, 219–24

Le Grand, Y. (1957) *Light, Colour and Vision* (trans. R.W.G., Hunt, J.W.T. Walsh and F.R.W. Hunt), Chapman and Hall, London, pp. 252–3

Lerman, S. (1985) Ocular phototoxicity. In *Recent Advances in Ophthalmology 7* (eds S.I. Davidson and F.T. Fraunfelder), Churchill Livingstone, Edinburgh, ch. 7

Lerman, S. (1980) *Radiant Energy and the Eye,* MacMillan, New York, chs 2, 3

Long, W.F. and Woo, G.C.S. (1980) Measuring light levels with photographic meters. *American Journal of Optometry and Physiological Optics,* **57**, 51–5

Lumsden, W.K., Aldworth, R.C. and Tate, R.L.C. (1974) *Outdoor Lighting Handbook,* Gower, Epping

Lynes, J.A. (1968) *Principles of Natural Lighting,* Applied Science Publishers, London

Lyons, S. (1992) *Lighting for Industry and Security,* Butterworth-Heinemann, Oxford

Lythgoe, J.N. (1979) *The Ecology of Vision,* Clarendon, Oxford

Marshall, J. (1984) Light damage and the practice of ophthalmology. In: *Intra-ocular Lens Implantation* (eds E.S. Rosen, W.M. Haining and E.J. Arnott), Mosby, St Louis, ch. 19

Miles, W.R. (1953) Effectiveness of red light on dark adaptation. *Journal of the Optical Society of America,* **43**, 435–41

Miller, D. (1974) The effect of sunglasses on the visual mechanism. *Survey of Ophthalmology,* **19**, 38–44

Miranda, M.N. (1980) Environmental temperature and senile cataract. *Transactions of the American Ophthalmological Society,* **78**, 255–64

Miranda, M.N. (1979) The geographic factor in the onset of presbyopia. *Transactions of the American Ophthalmological Society,* **77**, 603–21

Moran, D.J. and Hollows, F.C. (1984) Pterygium and ultra violet radiation: a positive correlation. *British Journal of Ophthalmology,* **68**, 343–6

Murdoch, J.B. (1985) *Illumination Engineering – From Edison's Lamp to the Laser,* Collier Macmillan, London

Nautical Almanac (1992) *The Macmillan and Silk Cut Nautical Almanac 1992* (eds B. D'Oliveira and I.J. Lees-Spalding), Macmillan, London

Noell, W.K., Walker, V.S., Kang, B.S. and Berman, S. (1966) Retinal damage by light in rats. *Investigative Ophthalmology,* **5**, 450–73

Optical Society of America (1963) *The Science of Color,* Optical Society of America, Washington, p. 111

Perry, M.J., Campbell, F.W. and Rothwell, S.E. (1987) A physiological phenomenon and its implications for lighting design. *Lighting Research and Technology,* **19**, 1–5

Phillips, A.J. (1967) Amber night driving spectacles. *British Journal of Physiological Optics,* **24**, 161–205

Pitts, D.G. and Bergmanson, J.P.G. (1980) The UV problem: have the rules changed? *Journal of the American Optometric Association,* **60**, 420–3

Pritchard, D.C. (1990) *Lighting,* 4th edn, Longmans, London.

Rothwell, S.E. and Campbell, F.W. (1987) The physiological basis for the sensation of gloom: quantitive and qualitative aspects. *Ophthalmic and Physiological Optics,* **7**, 161–3

Schiler, M. (1992) *Simplified Design of Building Interiors,*

Wiley, Chichester

Sliney, D. and Wolbarsht, M. (1980) *Safety with Lasers and Other Optical Sources*, Plenum, New York, p. 20

Smith, G. (1982) Measurement of luminance and illuminance using photographic (luminance) light meters. *Australian Journal of Optometry*, **65**, 144–146.

Steward, J.M. and Cole, B.L. (1989) What do color defectives say about everyday tasks? *Optometry and Vision Science*, **66**, 288–95

Sylvania Outdoor Lighting (1977) *Sports Lighting Made Easy*, GTE Sylvania, Fall River, Mass

Taylor, H.R., West, S.K., Rosenthal F.S. *et al.* (1988) Effect of ultra-violet radiation on cataract formation. *New England Journal of Medicine*, **319**, 1429–33

Taylor, H.R., West, S.K., Munoz, B. *et al.* (1992). Long term effects of visible light on the eye. *Archives of Ophthalmology*, **110**, 99–104

Tekelenburg, J., Fischer, D. and Van Bommel, W.J.M. (1982) Evaluation of discomfort glare in outdoor sports lighting. *Procedings CIBS National Lighting Conference Proceedings*, p. 168

Troscianko, T. (1986) Snowhole blues: comments on Kinney and Corth. *Perception*, **15**, 219–21

Tyler, J.E. and Smith, R.C. (1970) *Measurements of Spectral Irradiance Under Water*, Gordon and Breach, New York

Van Bommel, W.J.M., Tekelenburg, J. and Fischer, D.A. (1983) Glare evaluation system for outdoor sports lighting and its consequences for design practice. *Proceedings CIE 20th Session*, Amsterdam, p. D505/1

Whillans, M.G. and Allen, M.J. (1992) Color defective drivers and safety. *Optometry and Vision Science*, **69**, 463–6

Wyszecki, G. (1956) Theoretical investigation of colored lenses for snow goggles. *Journal of the Optical Society of America*, **46**, 1071–4

Wright, W.D. (1949) *Photometry and the Eye*, Hatton Press, London, ch. 5

Yap, M. (1984) The effect of a yellow filter on contrast sensitivity. *Ophthalmic and Physiological Optics*, **4**, 227–32

Sports vision correction

Henri Obstfeld, Roger Pope, Nathan Efron and Emanuel Rosen

This chapter is divided into 3 main sections, each dealing with methods of correcting ametropia for the sports person. The first part by Henri Obstfeld and Roger Pope deals with methods of correcting vision using spectacles. Nathan Efron then gives a comprehensive review of different forms of contact lenses and the advantages and disadvantages of each type for different forms of sports activity. In the last section, Emanuel Rosen explores the most recent advances in refractive surgery. The opening section is by all three contributors and brought together as an introduction to the concept of sports vision correction.

1. INTRODUCTION

Each sport carries its own specific visual demands, and in order to select the best method of correction for the ametropic sportsperson it is important to understand these demands. The choice of correction should be based not only on optimizing vision, but also on the environment in which any particular sport is performed and on the inherent risk of eye injury. Task analysis and hazard evaluation of each sport requires the practitioner to be knowledgeable about the sport in question (see Figure 7.1). Since there are hundreds of sports, it is not possible to have expert knowledge about each one. Apart from relying on the information obtained from the sportspeople who seek a consultation, there are some reference works on the visual and protective requirements of sports such as the *Sports Vision Guidebooks* (Carlson 1984, 1985, 1991). Sports vision consultants should obtain and be familiar with such a reference book.

What to correct

Refractive errors are not uncommon, affecting approximately 25% of the white Caucasian population. Overall 11% are myopic and 15% are hypermetropic (Stromberg, 1993) (Table 7.1 and Figure 7.2). With increasing age presbyopia becomes common, making the ability to focus on near objects difficult.

When to correct

In general, practitioners avoid prescribing contact lenses or spectacles to correct small refractive errors. However, when correcting the sportsperson's vision, such relatively small visual dysfunctions may make a considerable difference, especially where critical distance visual acuity is required. Hyper-

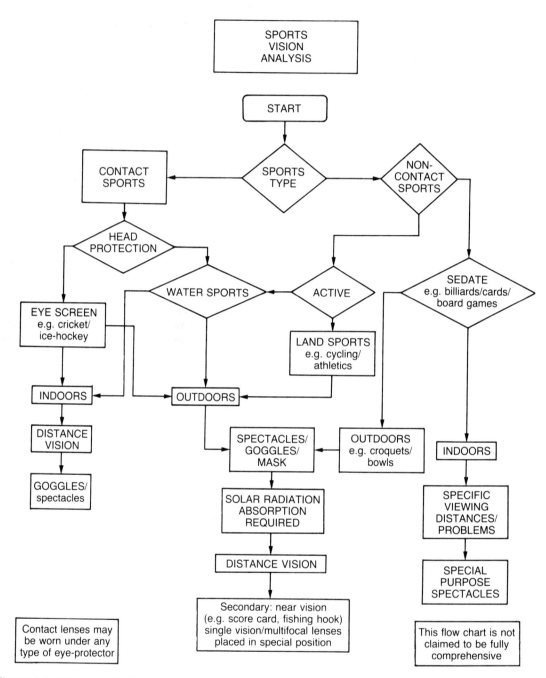

Figure 7.1   Flow chart of how to analyse tasks and hazards in each sport with a view to considering the optimum type of optical correction (flow chart contributed by H. Obstfeld)

Table 7.1   Classification of refractive errors

Astigmatism: a condition of refraction in which the image of a point object is not a point (stigma = point, astigmatism = no point focus)

Emmetropia: the refractive state of the eye in which with accommodation relaxed the conjugate focus of the eye is at infinity. In this condition the vision is normally clear without spectacles or contact lenses

Hypermetropia: a refractive condition in which distance objects are focused behind the retina when accommodation is relaxed. (Syn: far sight, long sight, hyperopia)

Myopia: a refractive condition in which images of distant objects are focused in front of the retina when the accommodation is relaxed. (Syn: short sight, near sight).

Presbyopia: a refractive condition which is a normal ageing process in which the accommodative ability of the eye becomes insufficient for satisfactory near vision without the use of corrective convex or plus lenses

---

After Millodot, 1993

metropic people can muddle through life and sport more easily than myopes who, if they have as little as 1.00 dioptre of myopia, cannot see clearly beyond one metre. All myopic refractive errors (even 0.25 dioptres) should be considered for correction in sport. Correction of anisometropia of 0.50 dioptres or more should also be contemplated, especially if accurate depth perception is required. Correcting hypermetropia over 1.00 dioptre can alleviate fatigue, particularly in sports requiring sustained visual attention at middle distance targets. Astigmatism of more than 0.50 dioptres may reduce sharp focus and therefore should be corrected.

For the young sportsperson a slight over minus correction will afford maximum distance visual acuity. One should bear in mind that, in a typical consulting room with a test distance of 6 metres, the distance correction actually represents a fog of 0.17 dioptres. Thus, by adding at least 0.25 dioptres of minus to the final refraction, as determined in a standard 6 metre consulting room, this will ensure that the sportsperson has maximum acuity for observing true far distance targets, albeit at the expense of having to exert a minor accommodative effort.

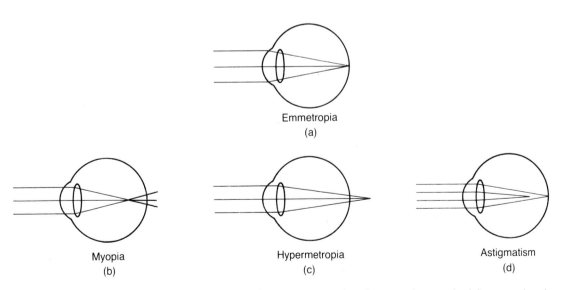

Emmetropia
(a)

Myopia
(b)

Hypermetropia
(c)

Astigmatism
(d)

Figure 7.2   Diagrammatic representation of light rays coming from an image in (a) emmetropic, (b) myopic, (c) hypermetropic and (d) astigmatic eyes

Table 7.2 Sports and vision requirements

1. Requirement for sharp vision
   (a) Distance vision
       Ball sports
       Stick, racquet and bat sports
       Target sports
       Motor sports
       Fishing
   (b) Near vision
       Fishing

2. No requirement for very sharp vision
       Contact sports
       Track and field
       Gymnasium
       Water sports
       Cerebral sports.

3. Glasses (or rigid corneal contact lenses) an
   impediment to sports performance
       Contact sports
       Ball sports
       Water sports

It is, however, important to remember the precise requirements for sharp vision vary tremendously according to the nature and form of each sport, and in some cases any corrective lenses may in fact impede performance (Table 7.2).

How to correct

Spectacles were invented about 1275 and have been the traditional method of correcting refractive errors (Figure 7.3).

The first human trials of lenses placed directly on the surface of the eye, or contact lenses (Figure 7.3) were undertaken by Fick in 1888. Since then, contact lens technology has come a long way. The modern contact lens era really began in the 1970s with the development of the soft contact lens which has allowed many athletes to be successfully fitted with contact lenses. Since 1975 surgical methods for reducing myopia by radial corneal incisions or radial keratotomy (RK) (Lynn *et al.*, 1987) and astigmatic errors by transverse or arcuate incision (TK or AK) have been applied and intensively studied. Since 1983 experimental, and latterly clinical, investigations into a new modality of effecting a permanent alteration of the optical status of the eye has emerged using laser treatment in the form of photorefractive keratectomy (PRK). Myopic individuals may be potentially treated by RK or PRK in order to reduce their myopia to a level which would make them, at least, less dependent on optical aids.

Each of these methods of correction have their place in providing optimum visual acuity for the sportsperson, while also taking different environmental conditions and requirements of maximum safety into account. Each will now be considered.

References

Carlson, N.J. (ed.) *Sports Vision Guidebook*, vol. I (1984), vol. II (1985), vol. III (1991), American Optometric Association, St Louis, Mo

Lynn, M., Arentsen, J. and Asbell, P. (1987) Factors affecting outcome and predictability of radial keratotomy in the PERK study. *Archives of Ophthalmology*, **105**, 42–51

Stromberg, (1993) In *Refractive Eye Surgery* (ed. C.D. Bores), Oxford, Blackwell

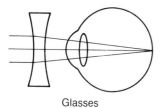

Glasses

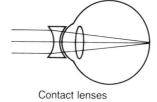

Contact lenses

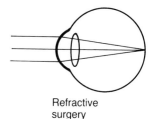

Refractive surgery

Figure 7.3 Diagrammatic representation of how spectacles, contact lenses and surgery can correct a myopic refractive error

2. SPORTS VISION CORRECTION WITH SPECTACLES

Introduction

This section is concerned with the design and selection of spectacles for the sportsperson, and for descriptive purposes the frame (or a derivative such as goggles) and the lenses will be considered as separate entities. Sporting activities may be classified as those that require eye (and possibly also face, neck and head) protection and those that do not. Where eye protection only is necessary, for a sportsperson with good vision, prescription lenses are not required. Where eye protection is not required, as in card games or target sports, then spectacles will be prescribed to improve vision only.

Davey (1984) has pointed out that most protective eye wear is not specifically designed for, and may be unsuitable for many sports, where a greater amount of protection is frequently required. For instance, impact resistant lenses usually conform to industrial standards BS 2092 (to be replaced by BS EN 166, 167 and 168, British Standards Institution, 1987a; BS 7028, British Standards Institution, 1981; ANSI Z80.1, American National Standards Institute, 1987; ANSI Z87.1, American National Standards Institute, 1989). However, standards developed for racquet sports (ASTM F803.3, American Society for Testing and Materials, 1983; CSA P400-M1, Canadian Standards Association, 1982; CSA Z262.2-M90, Canadian Standards Association, 1990; AS/NZS 4066, Standards Association of Australia, 1992) ensure that adequate physical protection is afforded by them. It is important to be aware that standards are reviewed and updated regularly and may be modified as a result of regional and international cooperation.

Although sunglasses should be designed with large-sized and possibly wraparound frames, no useful purpose is achieved if the field of view through the lenses exceeds the limits of the wearer's visual fields (Bouman, 1955). Sunglasses should be comfortable, well fitting, of high quality, provide adequate spectral transmittance, not cause colour distortion and meet published standards (BS 2724, British Standards Institution, 1987b; ANSI Z80.3, American National Standards Institute, 1986; prEN 172, European Committee for Standardization, 1989; draft DIN 58 217, Deutsches Institut für Normung, 1989).

Spectacle frames

Spectacles are the desired method of correction by many athletes and the advantages and disadvantages of spectacles, goggles and eye screens over contact lenses depend on the refractive error and the type of sport being played. Possible advantages are that they provide a large choice of special purpose appliances that can often be adapted for other purposes. They are easily stored as no special facilities, other than a hard case, are required, although because of its bulk this may take up some space. The protection provided against a variety of physical and radiation hazards is unrivalled by contact lenses and refractive surgery. They are easily removed and may be adjusted periodically as and when required to provide the most comfortable fit.

Spectacles are, however, prone to problems due to external factors, e.g. they may perform badly in wet and muddy situations and may also attract dust. This can be avoided by a special coating. Sometimes spectacles are dislodged, although this can be avoided by using a head strap. Frames made of unsuitable materials may lead to skin sensitivity and metal frames may corrode with time, making replacement of parts a necessity. Most importantly, however, spectacle wear has its limitations in a number of sports, especially the contact sports, because the appliance may cause injury, either to the players themselves or to their opponents. Because of this, some sports (such as soccer) do not allow spectacles of any type to be worn during play. If spectacles are to be worn, they should be made of plastics frames and the frame rim should be wider on the side towards the player to ensure that the lenses fall outwards if struck. Polycarbonate lenses should always be used and the athlete should be advised about the possibility of injury and the availability of appropriate protectors where indicated (e.g. in the racquet sports, hockey).

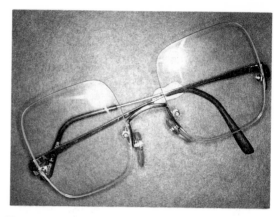

Figure 7.4   A pair of rimless billiards spectacles. Note the large vertical dimension of the lenses: horizontally 53 mm × vertically 57 mm. The optical centre of the lenses must be decentred upwards. The joint has been engineered to provide an angle of side subtending 10° above the perpendicular to the back plane of the front. (Courtesy of Norville Optical Co., Gloucester, UK)

Spectacle frames for specific sports

Although the following is not an exhaustive list of optical appliances specially designed for specific sports purposes, it highlights some major sports in which spectacle frames are used. If they include padding and an eye screen, they are described as goggles.

Billiards frames

Billiards frames are spectacles incorporating joints which enable the wearer to adjust the angle of the side (BS 3521, British Standards Institution, 1991). Billiards, pool and snooker players frequently assume a semi-prone position and, in general, the best foveal image is assured when the visual axis of the eye and the optical axis of the spectacle lens coincide. For this to occur, the spectacle front needs to be tilted away from the face and the optical centres of the lenses should be decentred upwards. The upper rim of the frame then protrudes above the wearer's eyebrows and the bridge appears to be very low. Some billiards frames incorporate a joint with a 'negative' angle while others have a normal

joint, but include a second joint which allows the front to be tilted upward. The second joint is usually positioned along the side and a short distance behind the front (Figure 7.4).

Cycling goggles

Cycling goggles may incorporate an eyescreen or separate lenses made from polycarbonate material. They are designed to give protection against small stones thrown up by passing vehicles, adverse weather conditions such as wind and rain, and radiation. Some styles may be fitted with prescription lenses placed in a separate holder (Figure 7.5).

Diving face masks

These are designed for the wearer to see clearly underwater (Obstfeld, 1982) and to prevent water from being breathed inadvertently up the nose (BS 4532, British Standards Institution, 1969). There are several styles available, but all have one transparent eyescreen and the mask makes a watertight

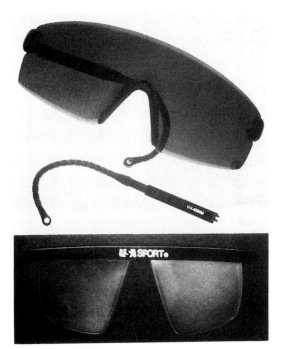

Figure 7.5 A sports frame. A click-stop mechanism is provided so that the length of the sides can be altered. The shape of the curl is adjustable. A strap may be attached to the side, to secure the frame on the wearer's head. An insert (shown below) can be fitted with correcting lenses. It fits behind the front which carries absorbing lenses

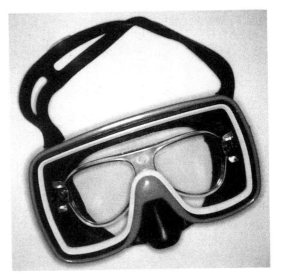

Figure 7.6 A diving mask fitted with an insert for spectacle lenses

seal with the wearer's face while the area surrounding both eyes is covered by the eyescreen (Figure 7.6). BS 4532 states that the eyescreen shall be made of toughened glass or plastics conforming for general robustness, optical qualities and light transmission to the requirements of BS 2092, and that laminated glass shall not be used. It is advisable for the seal and fit of the mask to be tested by the wearer prior to purchase. The wearer should try on a mask and, without using a headstrap, breath in forcibly though the nose. If the mask stays in position for as long as the breath is held, the fit is considered to be satisfactory. The standard also specifies that a label shall be attached to the eyescreen stating 'For safety and greater enjoyment learn to use this equipment correctly. Before entering the water read

the enclosed instructions.' The wording of the instructions is clear. The standard additionally includes a test for watertightness of the mask. Face masks should also be suitable for contact lens wearers.

Flip-up frames

These provide a wide field of view for a combination of any two viewing distances (distance, intermediate, near) and/or radiation absorbing lenses (Figure 7.7) and either or both fronts may be fitted with multifocal lenses. It is better to supply toughened glass rather than plastic lenses since the former are

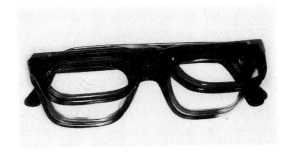

Figure 7.7 A flip-up frame consisting of two fronts. Other forms are available

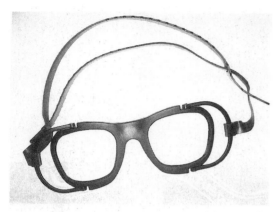

Figure 7.8 This pair of flying goggles consists of a stiff, polyamide front which fits very closely to the eyes. It is held on to the head by means of an adjustable head strap. Designed to be worn under a face mask or helmet.

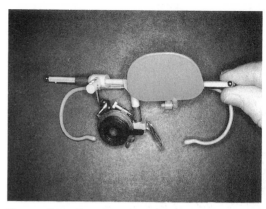

Figure 7.9 The 'Champion' shooting frame shown here fitted with an adjustable iris diaphragm and flip-up occluder. It is universally adjustable, and has curl sides

less likely to mark each other. If the fronts are held together with two joints, it is imperative that the screws or dowels have a common axis, otherwise torsion will cause breakage. This type of appliance may be useful where, for example, a driver requires temporary tinted lenses or a presbyopic pilot needs to view overhead instruments.

Flying goggles

Flying goggles are intended for aircraft pilots in open cockpits who require eye protection and prescription lenses (Figure 7.8). These fit closely to the eyes, and are kept in place by means of a strap which passes behind the head. Flying goggles are also suitable for use with helmets and masks used for other purposes.

Shooting frames

These may be used for archery, clay pigeon/skeet shooting, pistol and rifle shooting and are also suitable for billiards, pool and snooker. Modern designs (Figure 7.9) consist of a bar instead of a front, a nose rest and, in some cases, side shields. A lens holder is suspended from, and can be moved laterally

along the bar allowing accurate horizontal centration. Because sportspeople aim with one eye, often directing that eye to the contralateral side of the body, the lens holder can also be rotated around a vertical axis so that visual and optical axes coincide to provide the best foveal image. The lens holder may also include an aperture, a filter or a tint. The non-aiming eye may be placed behind a second lens holder into which a lens or occluder is fitted. The former serves either to correct or to suppress vision, whilst the occluder, which may be opaque (black or grey) or a matt glass, inhibits vision.

Ski goggles

These are similar to face masks, but do not fit as tightly and incorporate ultraviolet (UV) and visible radiation absorbing screens which are replaceable. (Figure 7.10). They also include anti-misting devices or vents. Prescription lenses can be fitted in a holder, or contact lenses can be worn underneath. This type of goggle may also be used for hang-gliding and various water sports, when the eyescreen may be polarized in order to reduce glare. A draft European Standard (on downhill skiing goggles) has been published for

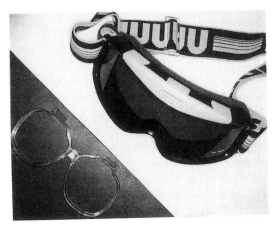

Figure 7.10 A pair of ski goggles incorporating wrap-round, impact resistant, tinted lenses. Insert for correction lenses shown below.

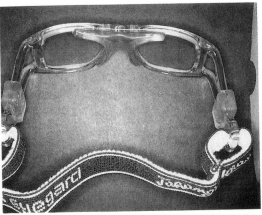

Figure 7.11 A pair of sports goggles without joints. Note the padded bridge and the head strap

public comment (prEN 174, European Committee for Standardization, 1993).

Sports goggles

Specifications for sports goggles have been published by several organizations including ASTM Standard F803–3, CSA P400–M, AS/NZS 4066 and prEN 967 (American Society for Testing and Materials, 1983; Canadian Standards Association, 1986; Standards Association of Australia, 1992; European Committee for Standardization, 1992, respectively). They provide protection for racquet sports such as squash or badminton, for baseball, hockey and war games. A draft British Standard for eye protectors for squash and other racquet sports and a draft International Standard for face protectors and visors for use in ice-hockey have been circulated for comment and approval (British Standards Institution, 1993; International Organization for Standardization, 1994). The goggles and lenses are made of polycarbonate material without joints (Figure 7.11). The disadvantage, however, is that the sides cannot be folded. Jointless frames made of polyamide of which the sides can be folded are also available (Figure 7.12). Frames may be fitted with curl sides, or with a strap from side end to end, to retain the frame on

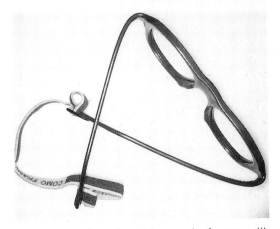

Figure 7.12 A polyamide sports frame with jointless sides and head strap. (Courtesy of W.T. Rees Ltd, Harrow, UK)

the wearer's head. Attachments are also available which convert a drop-end into a type of curl side (Figure 7.13). A 'military' frame with a very thin polyamide side can be worn under a helmet (Figure 7.14) and one-piece polycarbonate goggles are recommended as protective eyewear over contact lenses. Goggles with open apertures should never be recommended for sports. Such designs are positively dangerous as they admit, and even direct, projectiles to the eye thus facilitating injury (see Chapter 5).

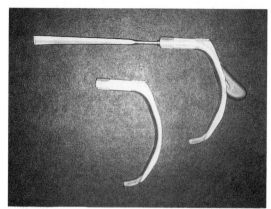

Figure 7.13 An auxiliary curl (*below*) which can turn a drop-end side into a curl side (*above*)

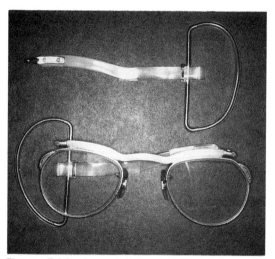

Figure 7.14 A metal front with joints, polyamide sides and semi-circular loops which fit around the ear. The side length can be adjusted. The frame fits under masks and helmets

Surface swimming goggles

Specifications are given in BS 5883 (British Standards Institution, 1980). The goggles have individual cup-type lenses and to form a seal between the goggles and the face, expanded rubber or plastics foam cushioning, at least 4.5 mm thick, should be affixed to the flange of the lens. The seal material must cover the lens flange and overlap the outside periphery by at least 1 mm. The lenses should transmit more than 69% of the energy within the visible spectrum and withstand the impact of a steel ball travelling at a speed of 45.7 m/s. The headstrap should also include elasticated material and connect the outer edges of each cup-type lens and be adjustable in length so as to provide a minimum goggle assembly circumference of 430 mm. Methods to test the adhesion of the eye seal to the lens, the slippage resistance of the headstrap and the tensile strength of the bridge strap are also described in the standard. The goggles should come with a specified safety warning. There are several goggles, not necessarily according to BS 5883, that can be fitted with pairs of spherical correcting lenses and, in at least one, separate spherical prescription cup-type lenses can be fitted.

Vehicle users

Eye-protectors are designed for the use of car and motor cycle drivers. The grades of impact resistance, optical quality and abrasion resistance of these visors, goggles and spectacles are specified in BS 4110 (British Standards Institution, 1979) (Figure 7.15).

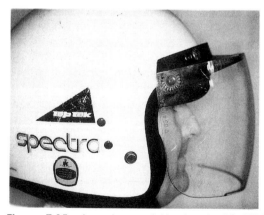

Figure 7.15 A motor cyclist's visor to BS 4110 fitted on a helmet to BS 6658

Table 7.3 Comparison of soft lenses versus rigid lenses versus spectacle lenses for the sportsperson (table constructed by Professor N. Efron)

Characteristic	Soft lenses	Rigid lenses	Spectacles lenses
Field of view	Full	Full	Restricted
Stability of vision (post-blink)	Excellent	Good	Excellent
Glare	None	In low light	None
Glare protection tint possible	Cosmetic only	No	Yes
UV protection tint possible	Yes	Yes	Yes
Initial comfort	Good	Poor	Good
Long-term comfort	Good	Good	Good
Adaptation required	Very little	Yes	Sometimes
Suitability for intermittent use	Yes	Not usually	Yes
Disposability viable	Yes	No	No
Risk of loss	Low	Moderate	Low
Risk of dislodgement during wear	Low	Moderate	High
Risk of damage during wear	Low	Low	High
Risk of damage with handling	High	Low	Low
Ease of care	Multiple-step	Fewer steps	Simple
Initial cost	Moderate	High	High
Ongoing costs	High	Moderate	None
Cost to correct astigmatism	High	Low	Low
Bifocal correction possible	Compromise	Very difficult	Yes
Use in rain	Good	Good	Poor
Susceptibility to fog-up	No	No	Yes
Susceptibility to dirt-up	No	No	Yes
Risk of complication	Low	Negligible	None

Lenses

The advantages and disadvantages of spectacle lenses and contact lenses for the sportsperson are outlined in Table 7.3. **Polycarbonate** is the lens material of choice, where physical protection of the eyes is the prime consideration. The advantages and disadvantages of polycarbonate, as summarized by North (1993) and modified by the present author, are as follows.

Advantages

1. A much greater impact resistance than heat-toughened glass; if the material fractures on impact, it will crack but does not break into particles.
2. Does not warp, chip or discolour with age.
3. A very low density: 1.2g/cm^3.
4. Its refractive index of 1.586 is relatively high compared to other suitable materials.
5. It absorbs UV radiation (completely below 380 mm).

Disadvantages

1. The surface quality is poorer than that of other ophthalmic lens materials although this is being improved.
2. Polycarbonate lenses are usually tinted by a vacuum coating process, to about 50% absorption. Greater absorption is about to be introduced. A solid tinted material with a greater absorption but a limited range of lens powers may also be obtained.
3. Under certain circumstances chromatic aberration may produce colour fringes around objects.
4. Abrasion resistance coatings can decrease impact resistance.

Another complication is the need for special lens edging equipment which may increase the cost of glazing. Eyescreens, afocal eye protectors and fronts can be made in one piece by injection moulding.

CR39 is another plastics material suitable for limited eye protection. It can withstand an impact of 45 m/s, specified in BS 2092 as Grade 2, can easily be tinted and made to absorb UV radiation. CR39 may break into sharp, jagged and, therefore, dangerous fragments. Polymethyl methacrylate, also known as PMMA, 'perspex' or 'plexiglass', has almost completely been replaced by CR39 as a plastics lens material. Photochromic lenses are available in CR39 but not polycarbonate and may be considered in recreations and sports with a low risk of eye trauma such as bowls, croquet and snooker.

It is recommended that **glass** lenses should be 'toughened', either thermally or chemically, for protective purposes in sports. Since the density of spectacle crown glass is about twice that of plastics, glass spectacle lenses are heavier than plastics. So-called mid-refractive-index and high-index glass lens materials are usually as heavy as the equivalent power spectacle crown glass lenses. In addition, they tend to show colour fringes and scratch more easily than crown glass. Nowadays, protective glass lenses are usually avoided. Mid-index and high-index lenses should be provided with an anti-reflection coating. This will not only reduce reflections thus avoiding irritation and, possibly, confusion caused by multiple images of the same object, but also help to admit more light to the eye thus improving vision, particularly in the presence of glare at low light levels.

Prescribing

The following sections deal with some aspects of vision that may be encountered in sports and may be important when prescribing lenses. The list is presented in alphabetical order, and is not meant to be exhaustive.

Colour vision

Sports people with colour defects may be handicapped as they are unable to distinguish different colours, for example, a coloured ball may not be noticed against another colour. Whether or not the person will be able to see the ball will depend on the type and severity of the colour vision defect. In the general population, about 8% of males and 0.5% of females are red/green colour defective. Amongst sportspeople these percentages are lower (Heere, 1985), and one may speculate that this is the result of self-selection. Filter lenses may either aggravate or improve the problem, depending on the colour combination(s), type of filter used and/or colour vision defect present (see p. 140).

Lens powers

Spectacle lenses over six dioptres are unsuitable for sports. Convex lenses to correct hypermetropia have fields of view with a blind area in the shape of the rim which varies with the power of the lens. The greater the power, the larger the blind area. On the other hand, myopic corrections have an overlap of the fields of vision seen through the lenses and the one seen outside the frame. This may cause confusion when the same object is seen twice, but occupying different positions in space.

Multifocal lenses also have drawbacks for certain types of sport. For example, bifocals which provide clear vision in the distance and (usually) for reading, are unsuitable for card players who require clear vision at an intermediate distance. On the other hand, older golfers may like to have a near vision segment added to their distance glasses so that they can see their score card clearly.

Misting

Spectacle lenses can be provided with a permanent anti-mist coating, or a temporary coating may be applied from a bottle, lens cleaning tissue or stick. This problem does not arise with contact lenses. One should consider prescribing contact lenses for those involved in water and other sports where atmospheric conditions between the lens and the player's skin give rise to droplet formation on the lens surface.

Night vision

Some individuals tend to become more short-sighted under low levels of illumination compared with normal light levels. To compensate for this 'night myopia', a small amount of extra negative sphere power should be added to the distance spectacle prescription for night vision. Undercorrected, short-sighted people are particularly affected. At night human vision is reduced to the recognition of white, black and shades of grey, as central foveal vision is suspended. Hence, in order to see a small object, the observer must look to the side of that object. In Germany, car drivers must not use filter lenses that transmit less than 80% visible light at night (DIN 58 216, Deutsches Institute für Normung, 1980). The British Highway Code (Department of Transport, 1993) states that the windscreen and windows of a motor vehicle should be 'clean and clear', that spray-on or other tinting materials should not be used on them, nor should tinted glasses, lenses or visors be used at night (see Twilight vision).

Soiled lens surfaces

Anti-static lens coatings are designed to prevent dust from being attracted to the lens surface. Removable thin layers of cellophane or similar substances that cover the front surface of the lens provide a clean surface after removal of a soiled layer.

Twilight vision

Human colour vision deteriorates steadily over 'twilight' until colour can no longer be perceived (Millodot, 1986). Short wavelength radiation (such as blue) is then perceived as brighter than long red wavelengths (Schober, 1970). This change in sensitivity is known as the Purkinje shift (see Glossary).

Multi-purpose spectacles

Most sports participants are likely to require distance vision correction only. However, some, for instance card game players, require a correction suitable for intermediate distance, such as arm's length vision and those who need to mark a score card will require a near correction if they are presbyopic. The reading segment in conventional bifocal glasses is placed such that it may interfere with the game; for example in golf, while addressing the ball, the player looks through the reading segment so that the ball cannot be seen clearly and may also appear too close. One solution is to fit 'golf glasses' with one distance single vision lens and one small diameter near segment, bifocal lens. The reading segment of the bifocal lens should then be placed well out of the lens area normally used to observe the ball: instead of placing the segment on the lower nasal side, it should be positioned on the temporal side (right temporal displacement for a right-handed person and visa versa for left-handed). For pilots, Backman and Smith (1975) suggest half-eye frames for presbyopes who only require a reading correction, and wide-segment bifocals for presbyopes who require a distance and near correction. For pilots flying aircraft where the flight chart viewing distance is nearer than the forward instrument panel distance, they suggest custom-made solid bifocal lenses with an additional cemented segment so that the lens looks like an E-type trifocal.

Summary

Spectacles are a convenient, versatile and efficient modality to both correct vision and protect the eyes of sports participants. To provide a comprehensive sports vision service, practitioners need to be familiar with the available appliances and also to understand the sports or recreations of their patients. In order that the most appropriate optical appliance may be supplied each consultation requires a detailed sports visual task analysis as outlined in Figure 7.1. Additionally the visual sports requirements and spectacles of sports people must be evaluated on a regular and continuing basis.

References

American National Standards Institute (1986) ANSI Z80.3 *American National Standard for Ophthalmics: Nonprescription Sunglasses and Fashion Eyewear – Requirements*, ANSI, New York

American National Standards Institute (1987) ANSI Z80.1 *American National Standard Recommendations for Prescription Ophthalmic Lenses*, ANSI, New York.

American National Standards Institute (1989) ANSI Z87.1 *American National Standard Practice for Occupational and Educational Eye and Face Protection*, ANSI, New York

American Society for the Testing of Materials (1983) ASTM Standard F803–3. *Standard Specification for Eye Protectors for Use by Players of Racquet Sports*, ASTM, Philadelphia

Backman, H.A. and Smith, F.D. (1975) The design and prescription of multifocal lenses for civil pilots. *American Journal of Optometry and Physiological Optics*, **52**, 591–9

Bouman, M.A. (1955) *Memorandum over zonnebrillen*, Rapport WW 1955–11 RVO–TNO, Soesterberg

British Standards Institution (1969) BS 4532 *Snorkels and Face Masks*, BSI London

British Standards Institution (1979) BS 4110 *Eye Protectors for Vehicle Users*, BSI, London

British Standards Institution (1980) BS 5883 *Surface Swimming Goggles*, BSI, London

British Standards Institution (1985a) BS 2495 *Protective Helmets for Vehicle Users (High Protection)*, BSI, London

British Standards Institution (1985b) BS 5361 *Protective Helmets for Vehicle Users*, BSI, London

British Standards Institution (1985c) BS 6658 *Protective Helmets for Vehicle Users*, BSI, London

British Standards Institution (1987a) BS 2092 *Eye-Protectors for Industrial and Non-Industrial Uses*, BSI, London

British Standards Institution (1987b) BS 2724 *Sun Glare Eye Protectors for General Use*, BSI, London

British Standards Institution (1988) BS 7028 *Guide to Selection, Care, Maintenance of Eye-protectors for Industrial and Other Uses*, BSI, London.

British Standards Institution (1991) BS 3521: Part 2 *Glossary of Terms Relating to Spectacle Frames*, BSI, London

British Standards Institution (1994) Draft: PSM/129 *Specification for Eye Protectors for Squash and Other Racquet Sports*, BSI, London

Canadian Standards Association (1982) CSA P400–M1 *Racquet Sports Eye Protection*, CSA, Ontario

Canadian Standards Association (1990) CSA Z262.2 M90 *Face Protectors and Visors for Ice-Hockey Players*, CSA, Ontario

Davey, J.B. (1984) Incompatibility and eye protection. *Optician*, **187**, 16–23

Davey, J. (1990) Tints in a fix. *Optician*, **200**, 12–15

Department of Transport (1993) *Highway Code*, HMSO, London

Deutsches Institut für Normung (1980) DIN 58 216 *Brillen für Fahrzeugführer; Teil 1*, DIN, Berlin

Deutsches Institut für Normung (1989) Draft: DIN 58 217 *Persönlicher Augenschutz: Sonnenschutzfilter für den allgemeinen und gewerblichen Gebrauch*, DIN, Berlin

European Committee for Standardization (1989) prEN 172 *Personal Eye Protection: Sunglare Eye Protectors for Industrial Use*, European Committee for Standardization (CEN), Brussels

European Committee for Standardization (1992) prEN 967 *Head Protectors for Ice Hockey Players*, European Committee for Standardization (CEN), Brussells

European Committee for Standardization (1993) prEN 174 *Personal Eye Protection for Downhill Skiing*, European Committee for Standardization (CEN), Brussels

Heere, L.P. (1985) Het gezichtvermogen van topsporters. In *Sport en zien: beter zien is beter sporten*, De Vrieseborch, Haarlem, pp. 9–13

International Organization for Standardization (1994) Draft: ISO/DIS 10257.3 *Face Protectors and Visors for Ice Hockey Players*, ISO

Keeney, A.H., and Reynaldo, D.P. (1975) Impact resistance of ophthalmic lenses of various strengths and influence of frame design. *Canadian Journal of Ophthalmology*, **10**, 367–76

Lean, A.E. (1994) A study into the misting characteristics of spectacle lenses and their effect on contrast levels. Final Year Project, City University, London

Millodot, M. (1986) *Dictionary of Optometry*, Butterworths, London

North, R.V. (1993) *Work and the Eye*, Oxford University Press, Oxford, p. 100

Obstfeld, H. (1982) *Optics in Vision*, 2nd edn, Butterworths, London, pp. 366–72

Obstfeld, H., Constantinides, M. and Needham, C.M. (1991) An objective determination of the abrasion resistance of coated CR 39 lenses. *Optical World*, **20**, 142, 18–20

Schober, H. (1970) *Das Sehen*, vol. I, Fachbuchverlag, Leipzig p. 201

Standards Association of Australia (1992) AS / NZS 4066 *Eye Protection in Racquet Sports*, Standards Association of Australia, Sydney

Taylor, S. (1994) Lenses for drivers. *Dispensing Optics*, **9**, 6–7

3. SPORTS VISION CORRECTION WITH CONTACT LENSES

Introduction

With modern contact lens technology, there is no reason why an ametropic sportsperson cannot compete with a normally sighted opponent on an equal basis from the standpoint of visual function. Paradoxically, the fully corrected contact lens wearing ametropic sportsperson may have a visual advantage over an apparently emmetropic counterpart who, in fact, may have a slight refractive error that has hitherto been undiagnosed. The extensive array of contact lens materials and designs, the variety of lens maintenance solutions, and the different forms of lens wearing modality and lens replacement frequencies available today allow the sports vision specialist ample choice from which to develop the optimum contact lens system for any given sportsperson.

This section presents an overview of factors that should be considered when prescribing contact lenses for those participating in sports and leisure pursuits. A brief introduction to the current 'state of the art' is provided for the non-specialist. Consideration is given to environmental factors, as well as likely physical forces acting on the eye and body, since these can influence the choice of lens type. Special attention is given to the visual and ocular demands imposed by endurance sports and combination sports. Activities involving critical visual acuity are discussed, and con-sideration is given to the specific visual needs of presbyopic sportspersons and referees. Guidelines for the fitting of various lens types are provided, as well as some useful hints for coaching staff.

Lens types

There are essentially three types of contact lenses – soft lenses, rigid lenses and scleral lenses. Certain lens types are more suited to particular sports, and a central theme of this section will be to discuss the visual demands of the various sports and to present arguments and evidence as to which lens is best in given circumstances. Thus, it is important to understand the key characteristics of the three categories of contact lens.

Soft lenses are manufactured mainly from materials known as hydrogels – jelly-like plastics that for contact lens usage are made with water contents ranging from 35% to 80% (Figure 7.16). Higher water content lenses are more oxygen-permeable but suffer the disadvantage of being more fragile and susceptible to environmental influence. Soft lenses are typically larger than the diameter of the cornea, and they move around much less on the eye compared to rigid lenses. Although soft lenses impinge upon the sclera, they are not classified as true scleral lenses.

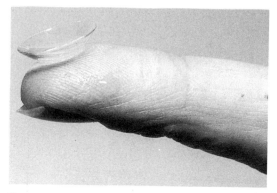

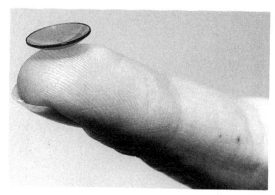

Figure 7.16 Soft contact lens. (From N. Efron, (1991). Contact lens correction. In *Vision and Visual Dysfunction*, vol. 1 (ed. J.R. Cronly-Dillon), Macmillan, London, with permission)

Figure 7.17 Rigid contact lens. (From N. Efron, (1991). Contact lens correction. In *Vision and Visual Dysfunction*, vol. 1 (ed. J.R. Cronly-Dillon), Macmillan, London, with permission)

Rigid lenses (also known as rigid gas permeable lenses) are made of solid but flexible plastic materials (Figure 7.17). They were originally made from perspex (PMMA; polymethylmethacrylate). Such lenses, which are also known as hard lenses, are very stable and long-lasting. However, hard lenses are impermeable to oxygen and cause adverse long-term and short-term complications. As a consequence of this, the hard lens is now virtually obsolete. All modern rigid lenses are made of materials such as fluoro-acrylates and fluoro-silicone-acrylates, and are permeable to oxygen. Rigid lenses are smaller in diameter than the cornea; they glide over the tear film and adhere loosely to the cornea via capillary attraction.

Scleral lenses are made of rigid materials and are larger in size. They must be custom-made and are only available from hospitals and a small number of speciality clinics. In some respects, scleral lenses could be used for virtually all sports. They are almost impossible to dislodge accidentally and offer maximum protection to the eye from the harsh elements such as wind, rain, snow, dust and dirt. However, these lenses are expensive and difficult to fit, and require many days or weeks for proper adaptation. In view of these drawbacks, and the general lack of availability of scleral lenses, discussion throughout the rest of the chapter will be confined primarily to the use of rigid and soft lenses.

A comparison of typical dimensions of the three types of contact lenses is presented in Figure 7.18. When considering the linear dimensions given in this figure, it should be noted that the human cornea is approximately 12 mm in diameter.

Lens care systems

As with other medical devices which come into frequent contact with the human body, contact lenses must be routinely cleaned and disinfected so that they cannot act as vectors for contaminating the eye with micro-organisms during lens insertion. The essential components of contact lens care systems are as follows: surfactant clean, saline rinse, disinfection, protein removal and in-eye lubrication.

Certain sports are played intermittently, due to a variety of factors such as long scheduled periods between ongoing sporting fixtures, seasonal breaks, being 'sidelined' because of suspension or injury, or merely the inclination of the sportsperson. Even if prepared correctly, virtually all contact lens storage solutions permit microbial growth, especially fungi, given sufficient time. If lenses

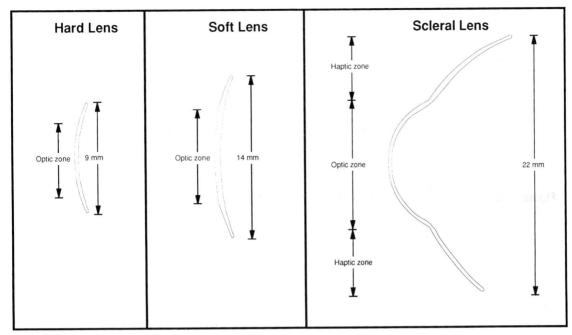

Figure 7.18   Typical contact lens dimensions (not drawn to scale). (From N. Efron, (1991). Contact lens correction. In *Vision and Visual Dysfunction*, vol. 1 (ed. J.R. Cronly-Dillon), Macmillan, London, with permission)

have not been worn for a prolonged period, they should be cleaned and disinfected prior to use (Lowe, 1993).

Lens wear modalities and frequency of lens replacement

Theoretically, contact lenses may be broadly categorized into five modalities of wear: continuous wear, extended wear, casual wear, daily wear and intermittent wear. The first two in this list involve sleeping in lenses, which should generally be avoided.

It is now generally accepted that no soft lenses should be used for more than one year (some say 6 months), except perhaps when special custom lenses (e.g. very high power toric) have been prescribed, or when lenses are worn only occasionally; in both such cases, regular replacement is uneconomic. Soft lens disposability is a concept that is particularly

suited to the sportsperson (Davis, 1990). Optimum vision and comfort are maintained. Torn or lost lenses are inconsequential, since the sportsperson will have a large supply of replacement lenses. A fresh supply is guaranteed.

The key choice: soft lenses, rigid lenses or spectacles?

The three primary correction options are: soft contact lenses, rigid contact lenses or spectacles. Scleral lenses are sometimes prescribed, but usually only in the most extenuating circumstances; they will therefore not be considered in detail in this section. A comparison of the key features of the three primary options is presented in Table 7.3. Refractive surgery of course represents a more radical alternative and is considered in the final part of this chapter.

In a small number of cases, a specific form of refractive correction will be indicated on medical grounds. For example, a sportsperson with advanced keratoconus or marked corneal distortion often must wear rigid lenses; a sportsperson with epithelial surface disease may need soft lenses; and a psychological aversion to touching the eye may necessitate spectacles. Such circumstances are fortunately rare, and the vast majority of sportspersons can be prescribed a form of visual correction that best suits their specific visual needs. Unique solutions to specific problems – such as the soft–rigid combination system described by McKinnon (1989) for an athlete with keratoconus – are always possible.

The major advantages of soft lenses are their instant comfort, security in the eye (difficult to dislodge), full field of view and sound visual acuity. They are certainly the first lens of choice for many sports vision specialists (Lieblein, 1986; Del Pizzo, 1993; Spinell, 1993), although others (Andrasko, 1993; Bennett, 1992) argue that rigid lenses are satisfactory for a vast majority of sports. Visual acuity is perhaps slightly better with rigid lenses, although this marginal consideration rarely outweighs the disadvantages of rigid lenses with respect to the greater possibility of accidental dislodgement, reduced comfort, the requirement for an adaptation period, and the occurrence of glare and flare in low illumination.

The question of adaptation is particularly relevant to the sportsperson who wears lenses intermittently (e.g. only when participating in the sport). Adaptation is a poorly understood phenomenon whereby, to avoid extreme discomfort, wearing time must be substantially reduced following a period of cessation of lens wear. Thus, unless a lens is worn for a significant length of time every day, adaptation will be required. Because this phenomenon occurs with rigid lenses and is virtually non-existent with soft lenses, soft lenses are the lens of choice for the intermittent wearer, which category includes a significant proportion of sportspersons.

It is often the case that lenses specifically designed and prescribed for certain sports may be unsuitable for general purpose wear. For example, large diameter, thick, low water content lenses may be perfectly suitable for certain water sports, but they may only be worn comfortably for a few hours because of their poor oxygen performance. Thus, practitioners should be aware that in many cases a sportsperson may need different lenses for sporting activities versus leisure or vocational pursuits. This section will consider only the most appropriate form of correction for a given sport *without regard* to the lens type that the sportsperson would wish to wear at other times.

There are often compelling ergonomic and functional reasons why contact lenses are preferred to spectacles. In certain sports such as American football and ice-hockey it is mandatory to wear protective helmets. Although specially strengthened safety spectacles can be worn beneath such protective headgear, contact lenses are generally more comfortable and convenient. Furthermore, in poor weather conditions it is particularly difficult to attend to dislodged or soiled spectacles, often necessitating removal of the mask.

Some clinicians have offered the anecdotal opinion that, compared to spectacles, contact lenses enhance visual skills of the ametropic sportsperson; however, properly controlled clinical trials do not support these claims. Schnider et al. (1993) applied a battery of tests (including measurement of high and low contrast visual acuity, assessment of lens fit and subjective assessment of visual performance) to ametropic athletes wearing their spectacle correction versus low water content soft contact lenses. The authors found that, although contact lenses did *not* offer a measurable advantage over spectacles in terms of visual performance under these testing conditions, the psychological advantages were significant, and in this way contact lenses may enhance overall sports-orientated visual performance.

Choosing an appropriate type of contact lens

The choice of contact lens for use in a given sport must be made with reference to the length of time that it takes to play the sport, the environment in which it is played and the general physical demands of the sport. A comprehensive (but not necessarily complete) list of sporting pursuits, together with an indication of the environmental and physical demands that generally pertain to each, is presented in Table 7.4.

In many cases the best lens design for a given sport will *not* necessarily afford an optimum physiological ocular response. For example, a thick soft lens may be essential for in-eye stability, but this will have poor oxygen transmissibility which could induce corneal oedema. Such a compromise is inconsequential as long as the lens is worn for a limited period of time; thus, the time taken to play various sports is an important consideration. An analysis of the sports listed in Table 7.4 reveals that the majority of sports are completed within 2 hours (Figure 7.19), which equates to a total period of lens wear of 4 hours, allowing for pre- and post-match activity during which lens insertion and removal would be impractical and/or undesirable.

The environmental and physical demands of the sports listed in Table 7.4 are discussed in some detail below. Even when these factors are understood, the lens of first choice may not be obvious. The most appropriate lens is sometimes only determined by trial and error.

Environmental conditions

Sports are played in almost every environment. Perhaps the only environment that is *not* sought for the playing of sport is extreme heat. The environmental conditions considered below will directly affect the choice of lens for the sportsperson.

Cold

It is evident from Table 7.4 that 19% of sports take place in cold environments, typically in close proximity to ice and snow. Although the question of a cold environment will be

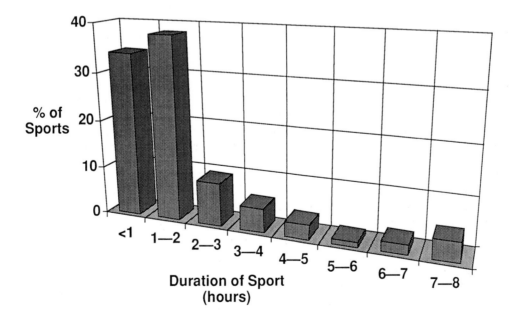

Table 7.4 Environmental and physical demands of different sports

Sport	Critical static vision	Cold	Altitude	Dirt and dust	Aquatic	Sub-aquatic	UV light	Body contact	Extreme body movement	Air flow	G forces
Aerobatic flying		*	*				*				*
Aerobics									*		
Archery	*						*				
Athletics (field)				*			*		*		
Athletics (track)							*		*		
Badminton									*		
Baseball				*			*		*		
Basketball								*	*		
Bobsleigh		*	*	*			*			*	*
Bowling (indoor)											
Bowling (outdoor)							*				
Boxing								*	*		
Bungee-jumping										*	*
Canoeing					*		*		*		
Cricket				*			*		*		
Croquet											
Curling		*					*				
Cycling				*			*		*	*	
Darts	*										
Diving (high)				*				*	*		
Diving (scuba)		*				*			*		
Equestrian (dressage)				*							
Equestrian (jumping)				*					*	*	
Equestrian (speed)				*					*	*	
Fencing								*	*		
Fishing		*		*	*		*				
Football (American)				*				*	*		
Football (Australian)				*				*	*		
Football (Gaelic)				*				*	*		
Football (soccer)				*				*	*		
Gliding		*	*				*				*
Golf				*			*		*		
Gymnastics									*		
Handball									*		
Hang gliding		*	*				*			*	
Harness racing				*						*	
Hockey (field)				*				*	*		
Hockey (ice)		*		*				*	*		
Horse racing				*					*	*	
Hurling				*				*	*		
Iron man				*	*		*		*		
Judo								*	*		
Karate								*	*		
Kayaking					*		*		*		
Lacrosse				*				*	*		
Luge		*	*	*			*			*	*

Table 7.4 Continued

Sport	Critical static vision	Cold	Altitude	Dirt and dust	Aquatic	Sub-aquatic	UV light	Body contact	Extreme body movement	Air flow	G forces
Motor cycling				*					*	*	
Motor racing											*
Mountaineering		*	*	*			*				
Netball								*	*		
Orienteering				*					*		
Parachuting		*	*				*		*	*	*
Polo (horse)				*					*	*	
Polo (water)					*			*	*		
Powerboat racing					*		*			*	*
Power lifting									*		
Racquetball									*		
Rodeo				*					*		
Rowing					*		*		*	*	
Royal (real) tennis									*		
Rugby league				*				*	*		
Rugby union				*				*	*		
Sailing		*			*		*			*	
Shooting (clay)	*						*				
Shooting (pistol)	*						*				
Shooting (rifle)	*						*				
Skateboarding									*	*	
Skating (ice; dance)		*							*		
Skating (ice; race)		*							*	*	
Skating (roller)								*	*	*	
Skiing (alpine)		*	*	*			*		*	*	
Skiing (freestyle)		*	*	*			*		*	*	
Skiing (jet)					*		*			*	
Skiing (nordic)		*	*	*			*			*	
Snooker (billiards)	*										
Softball									*		
Squash								*	*		
Surf lifesaving					*		*		*		
Surfing					*		*		*		
Swimming					*				*		
Swimming (synchro)					*				*		
Table tennis									*		
Tennis							*		*		
Trampolining									*		*
Volleyball									*		
Water polo					*			*	*		
Weight lifting									*		
Wheelchair sport									*	*	
Wind surfing		*			*		*		*		
Wood chopping				*			*		*		
Wrestling (Olympic)								*	*		
Wrestling (sumo)								*	*		

considered here in isolation, it is important to note that many other environmental factors will affect the choice of vision correction. For example, the eyes of a downhill skier will be exposed (in addition to low temperatures) to rapid air flow, altitude hypoxia, ultraviolet light, snow and rain, and the skier will typically experience extreme body movements and falls. These other factors are considered elsewhere in this section.

Because of the intrinsic temperature of the eye and tear film (33 °C), contact lenses cannot freeze up in the eye. In an extensive survey of 105 contact lens wearers who were frequently engaged in cold weather sports, Socks (1983) found no evidence of eye injury or disease. 'Eye redness' was the most common complaint of rigid lens wearers; soft lens wearers most frequently complained of slightly reduced vision. Socks (1982) found that the eyes of rabbits fitted with hard (polymethyl methacrylate, PMMA) contact lenses and exposed simultaneously to temperatures of –28.9 °C and winds of 125 km/h (wind chill factor –67.8 °C) were largely unaffected; only 15% of eyes suffered minor irritation which recovered a few hours after exposure.

Kolstad and Opsahl (1969) examined the corneas of 29 skiers (one of whom wore contact lenses) who had just completed a 15 km cross-country race in an average of 50 min with ambient temperatures of –15 °C without wearing protective goggles. Three skiers suffered a slight loss of vision. All displayed mild epithelial trauma to the inferior cornea, except for the contact lens wearer who showed no signs or symptoms of ocular distress. Kolstad and Opsahl (1969) suggested that contact lenses can protect the eyes of skiers in cold weather.

Large diameter, low water content soft lenses may provide the best results in cold conditions. Such environments are often associated with low humidity, which in turn tends to induce lens dehydration; low water content lenses will afford maximum resistance to lens dehydration. Thick, low water content lenses will provide suboptimal *physiological* perform-

ance, which may necessitate a reduction in wearing time.

Altitude

The ability of oxygen to reach the cornea through a contact lens, which is a key prerequisite to sustain good ocular health during lens wear, is a function of the oxygen transmissibility of the contact lens and the partial pressure of oxygen in the atmosphere. This argument is particularly relevant to the 11% of sports which are carried out at altitude (Table 7.4). Practitioners have some control over the oxygen performance of the contact lens; lenses made of materials of higher water content have a higher oxygen performance, and reducing lens thickness will have a similar effect. However, the partial pressure of oxygen in the atmosphere decreases with altitude, which effectively means that the tolerance of the eye to a lens of given oxygen performance will decrease with increasing altitude. In addition, temperature falls about 10 °C per 1500 m increase in altitude to a minimum of –50 °C; the effects of extreme cold on the cornea were discussed above.

A paradox faced by the sports vision specialist is that lower water content lenses, which perform best in cold, low humidity environments, will reduce corneal oxygen availability. Large, thick lenses, which provide greater in-eye stability, will have the same deleterious effect on oxygen performance. As a result, such lenses can only be tolerated for relatively short periods of time. This does not often pose a problem since most high altitude events are of a relatively short duration – typically a matter of minutes. Nevertheless, a sportsperson may wish to wear contact lenses on the snow fields for most of the day for convenience. Marathon Nordic skiing events can last up to 3 hours and the lenses may need to be worn for up to 5 hours. Marathon downhill skiing expeditions, where skiers are dropped at remote sites by helicopter, can also involve many hours at very high altitude. In such cases, medium to high water content lenses may need to be considered.

The prolonged high altitude conditions experienced by mountain climbers wearing contact lenses demand the wearing of lenses of maximum oxygen performance – that is, either highly gas permeable, large diameter rigid lenses or soft lenses of at least 70% water content. This is because prolonged hypoxia is the greatest threat to ocular integrity; in-eye stability is a less critical factor compared with more active snow sports. During the 1975 British assault on Mount Everest, two climbers wore high water content extended wear soft lenses for 50 continuous days on the mountain up to an altitude of 7925 m (26 000 ft), with no observed corneal problems (Clarke, 1975).

Simple multi-purpose maintenance solutions, which are available for rigid and soft lenses, are best suited to such harsh conditions in which there is also a limit to the amount of supplies that can be carried.

Dirt and dust

Rigid contact lenses are prone to trap debris beneath the lens and are clearly contraindicated in dirty and dusty environments, in which some 37% of sports are played (Table 7.4). These sporting environments are typically associated with intense physical activity and a greater risk of lens dislodgement, which are further factors contraindicating the use of rigid lenses. Large diameter soft lenses are therefore the lens of first choice. Lens water content is a less critical factor.

Aquatic environments

Aquatic sports are defined here as those that take place immediately above or in water, but generally not deeper that 2 m; these constitute 16% of the sports listed in Table 7.4. Contact lenses can be worn safely for such sports as long as a few basic rules are observed. Certainly, the fear of lens loss while engaged in water sports is well founded, with low but significant rates of loss of up to 12% being reported, depending on the sport (Stein, 1976; Solomon, 1977; Galkin and Semes, 1983; Peterson, 1989). Although Peterson (1989) reported an average of one lens lost for every 500 hours of surfing, there was considerable individual variation; some lost a lens every 50 hours of surfing whereas others surfed for many thousands of hours without lens loss. With disposable or frequent replacement lens systems, occasional lens loss is a relatively minor inconvenience.

Edmunds (1992) has suggested that sportspersons engaged in aquatic activities be advised of the following strategies for avoiding lens loss and preserving eye health.

- Close eyes on impact with water.
- Do not open eyes fully when under water; instead, squint and maintain a head position in the direction of gaze.
- Upon surfacing, gently wipe water from closed lids before opening eyes.
- Irrigate eyes with fresh saline upon leaving the water.
- Remove and disinfect lenses shortly thereafter.

Contact lens wear is known to slightly increase the risk of infection, and the use of lenses in aquatic environments must be considered as an additional risk factor. Despite this, the absolute risk is still very small – approximately four contact lens wearers per 10 000 wearers per year have serious infections of any type with soft lenses (Schein et al., 1989). With respect to activity in aquatic environments, the risks are different depending on whether the environment is salt water or fresh water. In fresh water (which would include chlorinated swimming pools), the main risk is of infection from Acanthamoeba – an amoebic micro-organism that can ultimately lead to painful corneal ulceration and visual loss. Halophilic (salt-loving) organisms pose the greatest threat of infection in marine or salt water environments; specifically, these include Vibrio alginolyticus and Vibrio parahaemolyticus. Fortunately, all of the above forms of infection are rare, and the risk of lens-related eye disease can be reduced to almost zero if lenses are removed, cleaned and disinfected in the prescribed manner soon after leaving the water.

Some general guidelines are to be observed when prescribing contact lenses for water sports. The prescription of rigid lenses should generally be avoided in view of the greater risk of loss with this type of lens. Larger, thicker, low water content lenses provide the greatest stability, which is of particular benefit when engaged in dynamic water sports (Banks and Edwards, 1987). Such a lens design may provide sub-optimal *physiological* performance and is therefore only suitable for short duration events (less than 3 hours). Higher water content lenses, and in particular disposable lenses, may afford better tolerance for longer duration sports.

Practitioners should be aware that soft lenses perform differently in the eye depending on whether the lenses are used in fresh water (hypotonic) or salt water (hypertonic). Theoretically, one would expect soft lenses to swell when worn in a hypotonic environment such as swimming pool water, and to deswell when worn in a hypertonic environment such as sea water, leading to differences in lens tightness and in-eye movement. However, in both of these environments, lenses tend to cling to the cornea (Diefenbach *et al.*, 1988). Examination of the sportsperson at the site of their activity will allow such variances to be detected, and compensated for, if deemed to be clinically necessary. High water content lenses may be contraindicated for use in salt water environments due to excessive burning and stinging.

Contact lenses are generally considered to be beneficial for those engaged in water sports in that they provide protection against tonicity differences, water flow trauma, particulate matter in the water and chlorine and other disinfection agents in various aquatic environments (Josephson and Caffery, 1991). Nevertheless, if the eyes of a contact lens wearing sportsperson are still compromised, then goggles may be of benefit. These are worn over contact lenses in the same way as worn by a non-lens wearer, and will ensure both good vision and preservation of ocular health in that individual. The wearing of goggles may also help to reduce lens loss.

Sub-aquatic environments

Various authors advocate the use of both rigid lenses (Holland, 1993) and soft lenses (Bennett, 1985) for scuba diving. All seem to agree that the use of contact lenses with a standard face mask is preferred to the use of prescription face masks. The former option results in better image quality and a wider field of view since vision is not restricted by the perimeter of the optical correction fixed to the mask. Furthermore, vision is preserved in situations where the mask must be removed either under water or out of the water.

There has been much confused discussion in the literature over the years concerning the appearance of gas bubbles beneath contact lenses during scuba diving, and the relevance of this phenomenon to lens fitting (Holland, 1993). As a result of the increased pressure experienced during deep dives, inert atmospheric gases, in particular nitrogen, dissolve in body tissues. As the diver returns to the surface slowly, these gases are released and, in the case of rigid contact lens wearers in particular, can be seen as minute bubbles beneath the lens.

The degree of bubble formation and subsequent corneal insult is less with soft lenses (Molinari and Socks, 1986) compared with rigid lenses (Socks *et al.*, 1988). A key consideration in lens fitting for scuba diving is to ensure that a good degree of tear exchange is possible so that any bubbles that do form beneath the lens during controlled decompression are readily flushed out. If the bubbles are not flushed out, minute dry spots form on the cornea resulting in slight 'dimple veiling'; this can cause mild discomfort and slight fogging of vision but is transient in nature (lasting only 20 minutes after lens removal) and not sight-threatening. Calculation of the maximum amount of gas that can dissolve in the cornea demonstrates that gas bubbles are not capable of enlarging to a size whereby the lens is forced off the cornea (Holland, 1993).

Strategies for enhancing tear exchange beneath rigid lenses include the prescription of lenses of reduced diameter, greater edge lift and looser or flatter fit. Lens diameter should not be reduced too much so as to reduce the risk of lens dislodgement during a dive. Adequate wetting is important, and high permeability materials will further facilitate the efflux of gasses trapped beneath the lens (Holland, 1993).

Tear exchange beneath soft lenses can be enhanced by the prescription of lenses of reduced diameter and looser or flatter fit. In addition, thicker, low water content lenses will tend to display greater movement with each blink. The disadvantage of lower water lenses is their inferior oxygen transmissibility compared to higher water content materials.

Scuba divers tend to blink less during a dive because the high humidity (approaching 100%) within the mask prevents ocular surface drying, which is normally a powerful stimulus to blink. Intense concentration can also result in less blinking. This is potentially a problem since blinking, apart from other benefits to the eye, is the driving force for tear exchange beneath the lens. Thus, the sports vision specialist must reinforce good blinking behaviour among scuba divers – especially during the decompression phase of the dive, where full rapid blinking will prevent the entrapment of bubbles.

Ultraviolet light

Sporting activities conducted on water, sand or snow (30% of sports listed in Table 7.4) will result in the sportsperson being exposed to excessive ultraviolet (UV) radiation. In addition to potentially causing sunburn, excessive UV radiation can cause a very painful form of keratitis, which is temporarily blinding (see Chapter 6). Snow skiers at altitude are at greatest risk of developing this condition.

Long-term exposure to excessive UV has been implicated in the aetiology of cataracts (Taylor *et al.*, 1988) and pterygia (Hill and Maske, 1989). Thus, it is in both the short-term and long-term interests of contact lens wearing sportspersons exposed to such environments to explore the possibility of incorporating some form of UV protection into their contact lenses.

Although contact lenses can be ordered with tints that specifically absorb excessive ultraviolet light (Cullen *et al.*, 1989), they will not prevent excessive and potentially damaging ultraviolet light from reaching those parts of the external eye that are not covered by the lens – such as the exposed cornea in rigid lens wearers and the bulbar conjunctiva in rigid and soft lens wearers. The use of goggles with UV absorbing tints, to be worn over UV absorbing contact lenses (as an extra precaution for periods when the mask is removed), is therefore essential on the snow fields. (Skiers should be reminded also to apply UV protection creams to the remaining exposed skin on the face and neck.)

Physical extremes

Special consideration needs to be given to ametropic sportspersons to facilitate their full participation in sports characterized by extreme body movement, body contact, air flow and gravitational forces. In many such cases, eye, head or even general body protection is mandatory for the sportsperson subjected to such physical extremes.

Extreme body movements

Stability of a contact lens in the eye is essential for the sportsperson participating in activities that involve extreme body movements (73% of sports listed in Table 7.4). Spectacles and sunglasses may be unsuitable or even banned in many of these sports. Rigid lenses are contraindicated in view of the high risk of dislodgement during the sports action.

The body and eye may be subjected to vibrational stress, particularly in sports involving vehicular movement (motor car or motor cycle racing, bicycle racing, luge, bobsleigh). Vibration of 10–25 Hz is considered to be most detrimental to visual performance (Hornick, 1973). Brennan and Girvin (1985) subjected individuals wearing spectacles and soft contact lenses to sinusoidal vibrations of between 2 and 32 Hz. Visual acuity was impaired between 6–8 Hz with both types of correction. No contact lenses became dislodged when individuals were subjected to excessive vibration. Cullen (1992) suggests that contact lenses are to be preferred to spectacles in situations where excessive vibration is a problem.

Large diameter soft lenses provide the greatest stability when excessive eye, head and body movements are involved. The lens should centre well and display minimal movement. Slightly thicker, lower water content lenses resist folding up in the eye, although long-term comfort is reduced with such a lens design.

Body contact

The same considerations as above apply here, along with the additional factor of physical contact (25% of sports listed in Table 7.4). Those participating in full body contact sports can be subjected to excessive body shock and jarring, and there is also the possibility of direct physical insult to the face and eyes. The obvious extreme example is boxing; most authorities governing this sport (such as the British Boxing Board of Control) ban the use of contact lenses.

The governing bodies of many body contact sports encourage the wearing of eye and face protection via the use of helmets and masks. In sports where this is optional, the contact lens wearing sportsperson is advised to wear such protection to preclude accidental dislodgement of the lens through direct physical contact to the eyes by an opponent. In such situations, large diameter soft lenses offer greatest stability, with rigid lenses being contraindicated.

Air flow

Twenty-five percent of sports listed in Table 7.4 involve significant air flow over the eyes. This typically occurs in the course of speed sports, such as luge or motor cycle racing, while the most extreme conditions of air flow over the eyes are experienced by parachutists during freefall, which can last up to 60 seconds. Air flow over the eyes in these circumstances can reach up to 290 km/h. Although contact lenses afford some mechanical protection for the eyes during freefall, they will not provide complete relief from the rapid and constant air flow or from flying debris and particles in the air (Gauvreau, 1976).

In a series of experiments involving 93 parachute jumps, Gauvreau (1976) observed that 39% of soft lenses were lost when protective goggles were not worn, versus a loss of 2% with goggles. Clearly, it is preferable for ametropic parachutists to wear contact lenses beneath protective goggles. This arrangement is preferable to not wearing contact lenses (and having an optical correction built into the goggles), to afford full functionality when the goggles are not being worn immediately before or after the action.

The rapid action and intense concentration required when participating in such sports leads to infrequent and incomplete blinking. To avoid consequent lens dehydration, sportspersons should be counselled in good blinking behaviour and should be fitted with large diameter, low water content lenses. These considerations also apply to sports where the air flow is less severe and goggles are not necessarily worn.

Gravitational forces

Aerobatic pilots can be subjected to gravitational forces between +6G and −3G. Participants in luge, bobsleigh, motor car and motor cycle racing are generally subjected to lower G forces – typically less than +2G. Brennan and Girvin (1985) fitted volunteer pilots with 50% and 75% water content soft lenses and subjected them to +4G and +6G (in the downward or 'z' direction). Lenses displaced 1.50 mm downwards in response to +4G and 1.75 mm downwards in response to +6G; tightly fitted lenses remained central regardless of G forces. Dennis *et al.* (1989) observed that positive forces of up to +9G caused rigid lenses to decentre downwards with a maximum of 2–3 mm, without adversely affecting vision. There is no evidence that prism-balasted toric contact lenses will mislocate as a result of excessive G forces.

In view of the evidence described above, a sportsperson who is likely to be subjected to significant G forces may find that a large, tight fitting soft lens provides maximum stability with minimum interference to visual performance. Of the sports listed in Table 7.4, it is estimated that 10% involve the body being subjected to intermittent G forces greater than +1.

Endurance sports

Participants in endurance events such as rally car driving, ocean racing and mountaineering, which are typically spread over weeks and months, are faced with numerous visual as well as physical and emotional demands. The need for physical effort will vary considerably and often unpredictably over the course of such events. Ocean yachting is one example. Due to the possibility of unpredictable adverse weather, the resting crew are constantly 'on call' and will be in no position to pause and insert lenses in turbulent conditions (in itself dangerous) when urgent assistance is required on deck.

Extended wear contact lenses (either rigid or soft) may be the best option in many of these sports. Rigid lenses in particular have the following advantages for endurance sports: they require relatively low mainte-

nance; they can deliver very high levels of oxygen to the cornea to sustain good comfort and ocular health; and vision is excellent. Rigid lenses should not be worn if the consequences of lens dislodgement are critical to performance. Simple, multiple purpose care systems should be used to lighten the supply pack of mountaineers; these systems cause minimal interference to the normal schedule of activity (ocean racing and rally car driving).

Sports requiring critical static visual acuity

A disadvantage of contact lenses generally is the transient instability of vision following a blink. Although measured in milliseconds (ms), this is a phenomenon that may impinge on the performance of an athlete when critical static visual acuity is required in a particular phase of a sporting pursuit. Certainly, the transient fluctuation in vision following a blink is one reason why patients complain that vision with soft lenses is more variable and of poorer quality compared with spectacles. Ridder and Tomlinson (1991) found that vision with soft lenses was considerably degraded when a target was presented less than 100 ms after the blink. They explained their finding in terms of blink suppression and prismatic shift of the retinal image induced by the movement of the contact lens produced by the blink. This explanation was reinforced by their observation that loose-fitting contact lenses caused an even greater decrement in immediate post-blink vision.

In view of the above considerations, spectacles are preferred to contact lenses when critical static visual acuity is the fundamental requisite for optimum sports performance. The four general sporting pursuits that are of relevance here are archery, static shooting, darts and snooker (and billiards, 8-ball etc.). The stability and acuity of vision afforded by precision ophthalmic lenses cannot be matched by rigid or soft contact lenses.

Contact lenses to correct deficient colour vision

The use of a red tinted contact lens (the other being clear) to compensate for deficiencies in colour perception has been advocated, although the efficacy of this procedure has not been proved (Weisbarth, 1994). Since very few sports require critical colour discrimination, this option will generally not be needed. Nevertheless, if it is thought that a colour defective sportsperson may benefit from such a strategy, a brief trial while participating in the sport (in addition to standard colour vision testing in the consulting room) will provide the answer. Interference with normal stereo-acuity as a result of the Pulfrich phenomenon may interfere with critical depth perception when a tinted lens is worn in one eye only, and this may affect performance in certain sporting pursuits.

Combination sports

In terms of vision correction, and especially contact lens correction, combination sports such as biathlon, triathlon, heptathlon, decathlon, Nordic biathlon, Nordic combined and modern pentathlon pose perhaps the greatest challenge to ametropic athletes and their practitioners. Many of these sports combinations are wildly diverse and the individual events impose very different specific visual demands. The final choice of correction may involve considerable compromise if there is no pause between component events (e.g. triathlon, Nordic biathlon and Nordic combined); when the competition is spread out over many days, various forms of correction may be used (e.g. decathlon and modern pentathlon).

A good example of a combination sport with diverse visual demands, during which there is time to change the form of optical correction, is the modern pentathlon. As an Olympic event, the component events are contested in the following sequence – day 1:

fencing; day 2: swimming and shooting; day 3: running; and day 4: horse riding (show jumping). The pentathlete may find that large diameter soft lenses are suitable for fencing (with face mask), swimming (with goggles), horse riding (with helmet) and running, but a spectacle correction is best for shooting.

Prescribing contact lenses

As a general rule, sports vision practitioners should be familiar with details of the particular sport or sports in which their patients are participating. The rules and objectives of the specific activity should be understood, as well as the visual demands likely to be encountered. Consideration should be given to any specific difficulties or ergonomic constraints that could be a mitigating factor with respect to contact lens wear – for example, in constraining attempts to insert, remove or manipulate the lens during pauses in the activity. Rapport with the sportsperson will be strengthened if the practitioner becomes familiar with, and uses, the terminology and slang that is part of the culture of that sport.

Most sports have seasonal cycles, which can be of relevance to prescribing and fitting contact lenses to a sportsperson. Mid-seasonal contact lens fitting or alteration should be avoided as this could provide an unnecessary distraction. Of course, in certain circumstances, a mid-seasonal adjustment may be essential, and could improve performance. However, for routine care, the best time is immediately following the conclusion of the season, so that the sportsperson has time to become familiar with their new vision correction during the off-season.

Although general contact lens fitting techniques are also applicable to fitting the sportsperson, there are certain technical aspects of lens fitting that are of particular relevance to sport.

Soft lens fitting

Soft lenses are typically manufactured with a total diameter of between 13.50 mm and 14.50 mm. Such diameters are suitable for most sportspersons, although those who are susceptible to lens loss as a result of individual anatomical characteristics or involvement in particularly rigorous sports should be fitted with the largest possible diameter for maximum stability. Katz and Malin (1990) report successful application of soft lenses of 15.50 mm diameter which were specifically designed for sporting activities. Although such large diameter lenses may not be readily available in all countries, they can be ordered from custom laboratories for a moderate additional cost.

The physical fit of a soft lens is not a critical consideration (as distinct from rigid lens fitting) because hydrogel materials 'drape' over the cornea; accordingly, most manufacturers of stock lenses operate a 'one lens fits all' philosophy. If more than one lens back central optic radius (lens back surface shape) is available, the steeper fit should be selected as the lens of first choice with a view to achieving greater lens stability. The choice of soft lens water content is often governed by the prevailing environmental conditions (see Environmental extremes above).

Rigid lens fitting

If a rigid lens is to be fitted, an important design consideration is to minimize the risk of the lens dislodging; this can be achieved by fitting a lens of larger total diameter than usual – say, 10.00–10.50 mm, instead of a typical rigid lens size of 9.20 mm. A slightly tight central alignment fit will improve in-eye stability. A large optic zone size will reduce flare (a form of glare due to light reflections from the lens edge).

Maximum tolerance is usually achieved with a highly oxygen permeable material, especially since the extent of tear exchange will be reduced with such a lens. However, there is a 'trade off' here in that higher oxygen performance materials are more susceptible to warpage and may not provide optimal vision in an astigmatic athlete. Warpage can be avoided by manufacturing the lens with a greater thickness, but again this will offset the oxygen advantage. High oxygen performance materials are also less wettable (which means that they may develop surface deposits more readily) and are more easily scratched with handling. Often the best material for a given individual can only be arrived at after a period of systematic trial and error.

Another consideration in rigid lens fitting is the 'fitting philosophy', which defines the relationship between the back surface of the lens and the shape of the cornea. Corneal shape is a unique personal trait, like a fingerprint, which means that an ideal lens form for one person may be unsuitable for another. A variety of lens shapes are available, such as tricurve, multicurve and aspheric. The best lens form for a sportsperson is one that affords minimal movement (bearing in mind that *some* movement is essential). This could be achieved with an aspheric design, which tends to conform more closely with the corneal contours. Again, only systematic trial and error can reveal the best lens for an individual. Additional stability can be achieved with a slightly steeper fit and reduced edge lift.

Scleral lens fitting

Lens dislocation or loss is virtually impossible with scleral lenses because of their very large diameter. Some people involved in dynamic water sports such as water polo or surfing therefore wear such lenses. The main disadvantages of scleral lenses are that they are expensive, they take a long time to fit, they are initially very uncomfortable and wearing time is limited. It is impossible to replace a lost or broken lens with an identical copy as each lens is custom made; however, there is the possibility of making a good reproduction if the original stone cast of the eye is retained. Scleral lenses should be made of materials of the highest possible oxygen permeability, and sealed lenses (that is, without holes or fenestrations) must be prescribed for water sports.

Compliance

The normal rules of good hygiene that apply to the general population also apply to the sportsperson. It is axiomatic that the sportsperson should adhere to the instructions issued by their practitioner; however, with so many other factors demanding their attention in a competitive sporting environment, the level of compliance necessary for safety and efficacy may be compromised.

Athletes often come in to contact with grip rosin, grease, tape dressings or ointments which are toxic to the eye and highly irritative. The hands of the sportsperson may also become covered with dirt, soil or general contaminants from their particular sporting environment (track, sand, grass, water or other synthetic surface). It is therefore imperative that hands are washed thoroughly before handling, inserting or removing contact lenses, or manipulating a lens in the eye.

Lee (1993) has drawn attention to certain psychological and personality traits that may influence the level of compliance among elite sportspersons. Often eye care is provided without charge, so less value may be attributed to the lenses and care systems. The normal practice for a contact lens wearer is to remove an uncomfortable lens. A sportsperson, however, may be inadvertently conditioned to persist with a troublesome lens due to the general competitive culture to press on in the face of adversity – a concept encapsulated by the adage 'no gain without pain'. Failure to remove an uncomfortable lens at the earliest possible opportunity can lead to an adverse ocular response.

Hints for coaching staff

The coach of a contact lens wearer should have full knowledge of the type of lenses being worn, the limitations of the particular lens type, the care system used, and any special constraints on lens wear. With this information, the coach can provide encouragement and reinforcement of information relating to lens wear and care. In many instances it is also important that the coach has been trained in lens handling – in particular, lens insertion, in-eye recentration and removal. Such skills could be invaluable in providing assistance during a brief pause in the action, or in an emergency where it is essential that lenses be removed from an unconscious sportsperson.

In team sports, one member of the coaching/management team should be assigned the responsibility of maintaining a register of contact lens wearers in the team, with full documentation of the lens type and prescription, the care system being used, and contact details of the eye care practitioner of each team member. This staff member should be skilled in lens handling and emergency procedures. It is essential that periodic checks are made to ensure that the documentation and supply kits are current. All contact lens wearers should be encouraged by the coach to visit their practitioner for regular aftercare examinations.

Another responsibility of this staff member should be the maintenance of a central supply kit of lenses and solutions that pertain to each team member, even if it duplicates their own personal supply. Apart from specific care products, the following general items should be included in such a kit: large quantities of saline solution, re-wetting drops for rigid and soft lenses (some are suitable for both), general purpose rigid and soft contact lens cases, special miniature suction cup for rigid lens removal, hand cleaning towels, mirror, tissues and a penlight.

Supplementary eye protection

The topic of eye protection was dealt with in Chapter 5; nevertheless, it is worth providing a few specific guidelines concerning protection of the contact lens wearing eye. From a survey of twenty-five eye injuries to sportspersons wearing hard PMMA contact lenses, Rengstorff and Black (1974) concluded that the lenses afforded some protection to the eyes and rarely contributed to ocular damage. On the other hand, Loran (1992) surveyed the ocular injuries suffered by twenty-eight contact lens wearing squash players and formed the opinion that those wearing rigid lenses were more prone to eye injury. Notwithstanding this conflicting evidence, it is important to follow this basic 'rule of thumb': the contact lens wearing eye should be treated the same as a non-lens wearing eye. Since contact lenses will not protect the eye against potential trauma, the usual protective eyewear or headgear used in a given sport should also be used by the sportsperson who wears contact lenses.

Supplementary protection for contact lens wearers, in particular for outdoor sports, must also be considered in order to provide maximum comfort. In particular, sunshades and/or supplementary sunglasses may be of benefit in reducing glare when participating in outdoor events. Although ultraviolet absorbing tints may be incorporated into contact lenses to prevent long-term damage to the eyes, it is important to note that tinting for relief of glare is relatively ineffective with contact lenses. (In general, the only benefits obtained from tinting contact lenses are cosmesis – that is to change the appearance of the eyes by altering the apparent iris colour or to entrance visibility and handling). For effective glare relief, sunglasses (to be worn in addition to the contact lenses) and sunshades or visors are the only option. In exceptional cases where the wearing of sunglasses is contraindicated, such as water sports, very dark tinted lenses (70% absorption) can provide some relief (Edmunds, 1992).

Contact lens wearing sportspersons who have a tendency to perspire profusely, or who typically play their sports in warm environments, may be troubled by sweat from the forehead entering the eyes. This can result in intense stinging and lens discomfort, due to the high salinity of sweat. Many athletes (including contact lens wearers) will therefore choose to wear an absorbent head band to prevent perspiration from entering the eyes.

Contact lenses for the presbyopic sportsperson

Virtually all persons over the age of 45 require an optical correction for clear vision at close distance due to presbyopia (see Glossary).

In the case of the ametropic sportsperson, this means that separate distance and near vision optical corrections are required. In general, presbyopic sportspersons are less often engaged in sports that are physically demanding such as rugby or football, and may be more prominent in sports like golf that require attention to near tasks such as score cards and strategy notes (Carlson, 1990).

For sports in which there is virtually no need for near visual tasks – such as bowling – a distance correction in the form of spectacles or contact lenses will suffice, even for presbyopes. If contact lenses are worn, presbyopic sportspersons should always carry with them a pair of spectacles with a near vision overcorrection as there is always the possibility of exceptional circumstances where a reading correction is required (e.g. consulting the rule book).

The two basic types of bifocal contact lens – simultaneous vision and alternating vision – result in sub-optimal distance and near vision compared with separate single vision lenses. Because of this, bifocal contact lenses are contraindicated for sport. Thus, if both a distance and near correction is required for participating in a certain sport, then either separate single-vision and near-vision spectacles, or bifocal *spectacles*, are indicated. If contact lenses are the only option, the best form of correction may be monovision, whereby the non-dominant eye is given the minimum necessary additional power to conduct vital near tasks. Alternatively, a distance correction in one eye and simultaneous vision correction in the other eye may be prescribed. Bifocal contact lenses and monovision correction interfere with stereopsis; thus, such lenses should not be prescribed if critical depth perception is an important requisite for optimum performance in a given sport.

Similar considerations will apply to the emmetropic sportsperson who has become presbyopic. For action sports in which a spectacle correction is contraindicated, a soft lens with minimum sufficient plus power in one eye could suffice. In such circumstances, this may be the first time that the contact lenses have been worn, so additional time must be invested by the sports vision specialist in providing advice and encouragement.

Contact lenses for referees, umpires and judges

Every sport requires some form of adjudication, so referees, umpires and judges are an integral part of the sporting culture (the term 'referee' will be used in this section to cover all active sports officials). Such referees are coming under increased scrutiny in the modern television and video age with action replays in slow motion and high resolution. Certain sports have incorporated television replays to facilitate adjudication with respect to 'line decisions' (as distinct from decisions requiring interpretation or opinion).

The ametropic referee is subject to the same environmental extremes and visual demands as the athletes; therefore, many of the factors considered above regarding the choice of appropriate contact lens or spectacle correction apply equally well here. For example, a starting official at an alpine downhill ski event will be subjected to sub-zero temperatures; a football referee may well be in a windy and dusty environment; a swimming official could experience a humid environment complete with fumes derived from pool chlorination and ample water being splashed about.

Three main factors will govern the choice of vision correction for the ametropic referee: (a) age (in particular, whether or not the referee is presbyopic); (b) orientation (whether the referee is seated or moving with the action); and (c) field of vision (whether or not there is a need for considerable head and eye movement). These will be considered in turn.

Age

In many cases, the key prerequisite for a sports official is experience and wisdom, which means that such people are more senior than the athletes and they often will be over 45 years of age. This places many referees in the presbyopic age group, whereby a separate correction is required for distance versus near vision. Although participation in virtually all sports necessitates good distance vision, in some circumstances the referee must conduct intermittent near tasks such as recording a result on a score sheet, viewing a timekeeping device or referring to a computer terminal. The topic of presbyopic correction for sport is considered earlier in this chapter; some additional specific issues relevant to presbyopic sports officials who wear contact lenses are discussed below.

For the adjudication of indoor events with stable environments, such as gymnastics, a spectacle correction may be preferred to afford maximum critical vision and avoid transient post lens-movement vision loss with contact lenses (Ridder and Tomlinson, 1991). If contact lenses are worn, a pair of spectacles with a near vision over-correction should always be at hand in case of need.

As is the case with presbyopic sports-persons, all forms of bifocal contact lens correction are contraindicated for presbyopic referees in view of the significant reduction of visual function. Thus, if both distance and near corrections are required for refereeing a certain sport, then either separate distance-vision and near-vision spectacles, or bifocal spectacles, are indicated. An important exception is in the case of an active presbyopic referee who must 'run with the action', as in hockey or soccer. Such officials must conduct near tasks such as checking the time on a wrist watch and recording fouls in a notebook. Since spectacles are clearly contraindicated for such referees, monovision contact lens correction is the preferred option.

Orientation

The orientation, position and perspective that officials adopt with respect to the action that they are adjudicating are important considerations when choosing the most appropriate form of vision correction. Depending on the particular sport, the referee may be seated (e.g. tennis, canoeing gate official), standing essentially in one position (e.g. volleyball, starting official for swimming or track and field), running with the action (e.g. football, hockey), or even intermittently lying down (e.g. wrestling referee attempting to decide if shoulders are pinned to the floor). As a general rule, a spectacle correction may be more suited to a 'static' official and a contact lens correction to a 'dynamic' official. Obviously, there will be a greater risk of dislodgement of spectacles in dynamic situations, and adverse environmental conditions such as rain may render spectacles a hindrance to optimal decision making.

Field of vision

The decision as to whether spectacles or contact lenses are preferred will also be governed by the typical field of view of the action. A static referee of a sport that is played out over a wide field of view relative to the viewing position may prefer contact lenses. A typical example here is the tennis umpire, who must monitor rapid action over a field of approximately 200°. Although a spectacle-wearing tennis umpire will retain sharp vision within the field of view of the spectacles (of the largest possible eye size), there is always the possibility of extreme action or a critical line call falling outside this field of view. Line judges are present to assist in the adjudication, but the risk of missing such incidents would be reduced with contact lenses. An exception here is the ametropic referee who is also presbyopic, who may prefer bifocal spectacles.

If the referee is static and the required field of view is relatively narrow (say, less than 70°) – as in the case of adjudicating gymnastics or diving – then spectacles are clearly indicated to afford maximum critical vision and avoid transient post lens-movement vision loss with contact lenses (Ridder and Tomlinson, 1991).

Conclusions

When so many factors govern the choice of optical correction of the ametropic sports-person, it is difficult to make general conclusions. Nevertheless, some consistent themes have emerged that are worth highlighting. Both soft and rigid contact lenses are capable of affording optimal visual function for any given sport; however, for certain specific activities where visual acuity is critical, such as shooting, archery and darts, spectacles may be the best option.

For most sports, soft lenses appear to be the preferred option. Relatively tight, large diameter, medium thickness, low water content lenses will provide the greatest in-eye stability, which appears to be an important prerequisite for the majority of sports. Although such lenses will suffer from poor oxygen performance, which may limit wearing time to a few hours, this will not represent an inconvenience for most sports. Notwithstanding the above arguments, a significant proportion of elite athletes wear rigid lenses for sport. Of the 35 contact lens wearing Olympic athletes who accepted an open invitation to visit a vision screening centre at the 1992 Winter Olympic Games in Albertville, France, 30 (86%) wore soft lenses during competition and 5 (14%) wore rigid lenses. Similarly, of 64 contact lens wearing Olympic athletes screened at the 1992 Summer Olympic Games in Barcelona, Spain, 55 (86%) wore soft lenses and 9 (14%) wore rigid lenses (Roncagli, 1992).

It is interesting to observe that a typical soft lens for cosmetic use would be smaller and thinner than the 'sports lens' described above, and be made from a low to medium water content material. Therefore, when such 'sports lenses' are prescribed, an alternative form of lens for general wear may be required, especially by the sportsperson with a medium to high refractive error who needs a correction at all times.

Successful contact lens correction for sporting activities requires patience, perseverance and understanding. By employing modern contact lens technologies, the keen sports vision specialist will be able to meet the challenge. The reward is the knowledge that the sportsperson in their care is not hampered by their ametropia and is capable of performing to his or her maximum visual capabilities.

References

Andrasko, G. (1993) Guest editorial: another contact lens myth bites the dust. SportsVision, 9, 4

Banks, L.D. and Edwards, G.L. (1987) To swim or not to swim. A remedy for patients prone to losing lenses while taking a dip. Contact Lens Spectrum, 6, 46–8

Bennett, E.S. (1992) Rigid gas permeable contact lenses for the athlete. SportsVision, 8, 30–4

Bennett, Q.M. (1985) Contact lenses for diving. Australian Journal of Optometry, 68, 25–6

Brennan, D.H. and Girvin, J.K. (1985) The flight acceptability of soft contact lenses: an environmental trial. Aviation and Space Environmental Medicine, 56, 43–8

Carlson, N.J. (1990) Contacts and golf: more presbyopic options. Contact Lens Forum, 14, 16

Clarke, C. (1975) Contact lenses at high altitude: experience on Everest south-west face. British Journal of Ophthalmology, 60, 479–80

Cullen, A.P. (1992) The environment. In Clinical Contact Lens Practice, 2nd edn (eds E.S. Bennett and B.A. Weissman), J.B. Lippincott, Philadelphia, pp. 1–29

Cullen, A.P., Dumbleton, K.A. and Chou, B.R. (1989) Contact lenses and acute exposure to ultraviolet radiation. Optometry and Vision Science, 66, 407–11

Davis, R.A. (1990) Disposable contact lenses and the athlete. Contact Lens Forum, 15, 24

Del Pizzo, N. (1993) Fitting hard or fitting soft. SportsVision, 9, 6–8

Dennis, R.J., Woessner, W.M., Miller, R.E. et al. (1989) The effect of fluctuating +Gz exposure on rigid gas permeable contact lenses Optometry and Vision Science Supplement, 66, 167

Diefenbach, C.B., Soni, P.S., Gillespie, B.J. and Pence, N. (1988) Extended wear contact lens movement under swimming rule conditions. American Journal of Optometry and Physiological Optics, 65, 710–16

Edmunds, F.R. (1992) Contact lenses and sports. In Sportsvision Program, Bausch & Lomb Inc., New York, pp. 1–33

Galkin, K.A. and Semes, L. (1983) Risk of loss of Soflens during water skiing. Journal of the American Optometrical Association, 54, 267–9

Gauvreau, D.K. (1976) Effects of wearing Bausch & Lomb Soflens while skydiving. American Journal of Optometry and Physiological Optics, 53, 236–40

Hill, J.C. and Maske, R. (1989) Pathogenesis of pterygium. Eye, 3, 218–26

Holden, B.A., Sweeney, D.F., Vannas, A. et al. (1985) Effects of long-term extended contact lens wear on the human cornea. Investigative Ophthalmology and Visual Science, 26, 1489–501

Holland, R. (1993) Rigid contact lenses for scuba diving. SportsVision, 9, 13–21

Hornick, R.J. (1973) Vibration. In Bioastronautics Data Book, 2nd edn (eds J.F. Parker and V.R. West), NASA, Washington, DC, p. 312

Josephson, J.E. and Caffery, B.E. (1991) Contact lens considerations in surface and subsurface aqueous environments. Optometry and Vision Science, 68, 2–11

Katz, H.D. and Malin, A.H. (1990) A new lens for sports proves an excellent troubleshooter. Contact Lens Spectrum, 5, 27–37

Kolstad, A. and Opsahl, R. (1969) Cold injury to corneal epithelium. A cause of blurred vision in cross-country skiers. Acta Ophthalmologica, 47, 656–9

Lee, P.N. (1993) Contact lens compliance and the athlete.

SportsVision, **9**, 29

Lieblein, J.S. (1986) The athlete's choice: contact lenses. *Contact Lens Spectrum,* **1**, 55–8

Loran, D.F.C. (1992) Eye injuries in squash. *Optician,* **203**, 18–26

Lowe, R. (1993) The role of disinfection in contact lens care – current perspectives. *Optician,* **205**, 19–29

McKinnon, T.J. (1989) Case report: contact lens correction of keratoconus for contact sports. *Clinical and Experimental Optometry,* **72**, 179–80

Molinari, J.F. and Socks, J.F. (1986) Effects of hyperbaric conditions on cornea physiology with hydrogel contact lenses. *Journal of the British Contact Lens Association,* **9**, 3–7

Peterson, W.L. (1989) Contact lenses and surfing. *Contact Lens Spectrum,* **4**, 59–60

Rengstorff, R.H. and Black C.J. (1974) Eye protection from contact lenses. *Journal of the American Optometric Association,* **45**, 270–6

Roncagli, V. (1992) Contact lenses of the olympians. Paper presented at the European Symposium on Contact Lenses, Bordeaux, France, 16–19 October

Ridder, W.H. and Tomlinson, A. (1991) Blink-induced, temporal variations in contrast sensitivity. *International Contact Lens Clinic,* **18**, 231–7

Schein, O.D., Glynn, R.J., Poggio, E.C., Seddon, J.M. and Kenyon, K.R. (1989) The relative risk of ulcerative keratitis among users of daily-wear and extended-wear soft contact lenses: a case control study. *New England Journal of Medicine,* **321**, 773–8

Schnider, C.M., Coffey, B.M. and Reichow, A.R. (1993) Comparison of contact lenses versus spectacles for sports oriented vision performance. *Investigative Ophthalmology and Visual Science* (Suppl.), **34**, 1005

Socks, J.F. (1982) Contact lenses in extreme cold environments: Response of rabbit corneas. *American Journal of Optometry and Physiological Optics,* **59**, 297–300

Socks, J.F. (1983) Use of contact lenses for cold weather activities. Results of a survey. *International Contact Lens Clinic,* **10**, 82–91

Socks, J.F., Molinari, J.F. and Rowey, J.L. (1988) Rigid gas permeable contact lenses in hyperbaric environments. *American Journal of Optometry and Physiological Optics,* **65**, 942–5

Solomon, J. (1977) Swimming with soft lenses. *Contact Lens Forum,* **2**, 13–15

Spinell, M.R. (1993) Soft hydrophilic lenses. The visual correction of choice for athletes. *SportsVision,* **9**, 5

Stein, H. (1976) Swimming with soft lenses. *Contact Lens Journal,* **5**, 10–12

Taylor, H.R., West, S.K., Rosenthal, F.S. *et al.* (1988) Effect of ultraviolet radiation on cataract formation. *New England Journal of Medicine,* **319**, 1429–33

Weisbarth, R.E. (1994) Tinted hydrogel contact lenses. In *Contact Lens Practice* (eds M. Ruben and M. Guillon), Chapman & Hall, London, ch. 30

4. REFRACTIVE SURGERY AND SPORT

The need

Breaking free from three would-be tacklers, the 250 lb rugby prop forward surged towards the line. Triumphantly he dived over for the winning try – or so he thought. He had grounded the ball over the 22 metre line, such was the degree of his myopia! Rugby is not a game to be played in glasses or, arguably, contact lenses. Britain's best known heavyweight boxer was not allowed a professional licence until his uncorrected visual standard had been achieved through refractive surgery. These are just two examples of how refractive errors can have an impact on sport at the highest level. Extrapolate these examples to sport at all levels, bearing in mind that 25% of all participants are potentially visually disadvantaged either by having to, or not being able to, wear an optical aid. Sporting activities are very common motivating factors amongst patients enquiring about the potential of refractive surgery.

Blurred vision is generally a negative factor for those participating in sport. Essentially sportsmen and sportswomen with refractive errors delight in the visual freedom afforded them by a successful surgical intervention to neutralize their refractive error. This is the case for emmetropia for sport participants, whatever the nature of their sport.

The concept

The concept of refractive surgery for eyes with a refractive error but no coincident pathology is relatively new and still accepted by some professionals with misgivings or caution. New 'treatments' for nature's endowment of individuals are typically resisted. For example, the invention of spectacles was not without controversy: 'The newly invented optick glasses are immoral as they pervert the natural sight and make things appear in an unnatural and false light' (Mr Cross, Vicar of Chew Magna, Somersetshire, 13th century).

The cornea is the main refracting element of the eye, or more correctly, the air/tear film interface provides the most abrupt change in the refractive index of the visual system, and the cornea provides the proper curvature for the tear film. In the majority of eyes, the refracting power of this interface is about plus 45 dioptres. Approximately 75% of the overall refractive power of the normal adult eye is, therefore, provided by this air/tear film interface on the cornea. The remaining 20–25% of the eye's focusing power, which is provided by the lens, is primarily needed for near vision focusing or accommodation of the eye. The corneal curvature provided to the anterior tear film is therefore effectively the 'lens' of the eye. Thus, the cornea is the most accessible and effective target for surgical intervention. It is not, however, the only facet of the eye which may be modified or added to by refractive elements. The corneal refraction may be modified by surface additions, e.g. contact lenses as discussed above, to provide a temporary solution; but permanence requires surgical intervention. Surgery aims at emmetropization of an eye at best, or reduced reliance on optical aids at least. These objectives can be attained by following the natural principles of surgery, namely: understanding the problem, effecting the treatment and studying the consequences by serial clinical observation and analysis of the pathological processes of healing.

Understanding corneal refraction

The central cornea is rarely spherical; indeed the cornea is designed as an aspheric system, so as to minimize any spherical aberrations. In recent years there has been increased research and interest in the field of corneal topography, i.e. measuring and mapping the curvature of the anterior corneal surface (Bogan et al., 1994). Today's computer assisted corneal topography systems are based on a concept developed in 1880 by Antonio Placido. He placed a planar concentric ring target with alternating black and white rings in front of a patient's eye and then observed the shape of the rings in the virtual image of the target created from the reflection off the patient's cornea. If the cornea is spherical the rings appear circular and concentric. Deviations of the corneal shape appear as either distortions in shape or concentricity of the rings. This method provides the observer with qualitative information about the patient's corneal curvature.

Computerized corneal topography is the logical advance from the basic principles of keratometry and photokeratoscopy developed over the twentieth century. Photokeratoscopy (photographing the reflections of concentric rings in a 'Placido disc') provided qualitative information about the curvature of the cornea and changes that accompany surgery, contact lens wear and progressive corneal pathologies, but its uses were limited because only a small area of the central cornea was studied. In contrast, computerized video keratographic systems measure corneal refractive power at thousands of points on the corneal surface from inside the 1 mm optic zone to outside the 9 mm optic zone. With the capabilities of modern computers and software technology it is therefore now possible to analyse the radius of curvature (mm) and corresponding refractive power (dioptres) across the whole corneal surface. This information can be presented as a complete colour coded representation of the corneal shape and can therefore monitor corneal curvature chan-

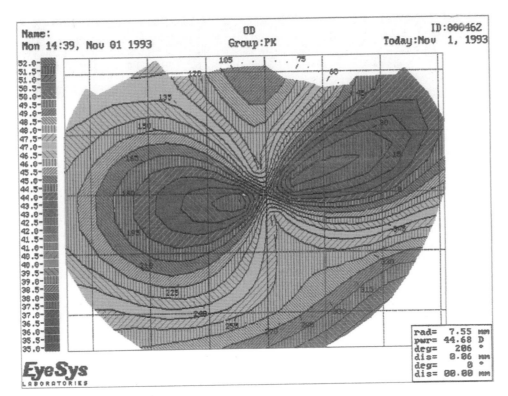

Plate 18 Corneal topography

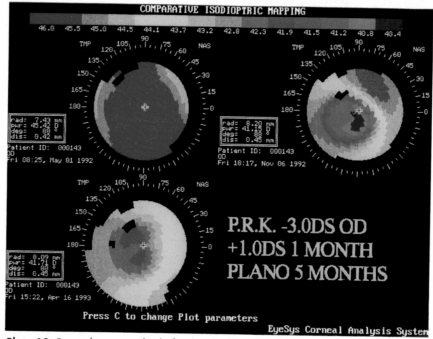

Plate 19 Corneal topography before and after PRK. Top left: cornea before treatment. Top right: postoperative hyperopia. Bottom: regression to emmetropia at 5 months.

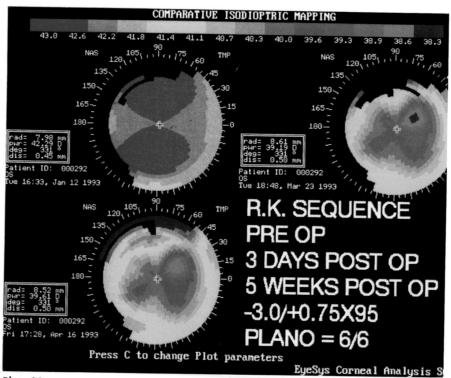

Plate 20

ges from the apex to the periphery. Having the ability to measure refractive power across the corneal surface and to follow corneal shaped changes induced by corneal pathology and surgery has provided us with a much greater understanding of refractive complaints.

Computerized corneal topography systems utilize personal computers to quantify the data obtained from reflected Placido disc images. The topography information must be displayed in a clinically relevant manner such as the isodioptric colour coded display (Plate 18). For most systems, the scaled colour range is normalized, i.e. the central value of the range of colours and/or the step size of the individual colours is scaled to the examination under consideration. Caution must be used when viewing these colour coded maps to be certain of the step size. In order to minimize the risk of misreading these colour coded maps, one system (EyeSys Tm, EyeSys Company Houston, Texas) provides a high resolution absolute scale covering a range of 35 dioptres to 52 dioptres in clinically significant 0.5 dioptre steps to provide a true colour coded representation of the cornea. The colours and patterns assigned to each dioptric range remain fixed for all examinations and do not scale to the examination under consideration. By use of this dynamic scale for printing or reviewing patient records, it is quite simple to observe changes from one examination to the next.

Measurement of refractive errors and examination

Comprehension of refractive errors when surgical treatment is to be considered requires a deeper analysis of eye measurement than usually required for spectacle or contact lens correction. Accurate measurement of the axial length of the eye using ultrasound is necessary. Pre- and postoperative corneal topography is carried out. Ophthalmic examination should include uncorrected and corrected visual acuity, refraction, including cycloplegic refraction (see Glossary) in younger patients, intra-ocular pressure measurements and a complete routine eye examination. Accurate corneal thickness mapping (pachymetry) is essential before incisional surgery. This ensures maximum incision depth without perforation, as incisions need to penetrate almost to Descemet's membrane to create their effect. Rigid contact lens wearers should be advised to remove their lenses two weeks prior to treatment.

Criteria for refractive surgery and patient characteristics

Refractive surgery is relatively new in the ophthalmic surgeon's armamentarium and needs to be subject to certain criteria before it is practised on a wide scale. Refractive surgery must not only be effective and safe but its effect should be stable and above all predictable (Rowsey et al., 1994).

Sporting activities, with the associated requirement of freedom from optical aids, are a major indication for refractive surgery. Patients must be both well informed and well motivated as to the rationale for treatment and its predictability. Contraindications include: personality problems, particularly obsessive, compulsive or perfectionist types; young patients (generally under 21 years) who may not yet have stable myopia; and ophthalmic abnormalities which include monocularity, coincidental ocular disease such as keratoconus, irregular astigmatism and known herpes simplex virus keratopathy.

The majority of patients are in their third or fourth decade of life, nevertheless they must be aware of the problems of incipient presbyopia. They should be advised that near vision glasses will be a consequence of emmetropia when they become presbyopic in their 40s or early 50s. It is possible, however, that multifocal effects may be achieved serendipitously in those undergoing photorefractive keratectomy (PRK). Whatever the modality of treatment applied, they should be aware that their best acuity may still require the use of a spectacle correction fine tuning.

Corneal aspects of refractive surgery

There are two main modalities in current practice for the modification of corneal refraction, with other processes undergoing evaluation for early clinical application. These present techniques are:

1. Laser refractive surgery to ablate the corneal surface, or photorefractive keratectomy (PRK).
2. Incisional methods, radial and astigmatic keratotomy (RK and AK).

The essential difference between laser ablative and surgical incisional methods is the location of application. Laser PRK treats the optical zone of the cornea whereas RK/AK achieve their effect on the optical zone indirectly by application to the corneal mid-zone.

Excimer laser photorefractive keratectomy (PRK)

Lamellar keratectomy is a corneal refractive surgical process utilizing removal of a lamella of corneal tissue. Both automated and laser enhanced methods are being developed currently with limited application, but with immense prospects for addressing a wide range of refractive errors. Excimer laser PRK is effected by argon/fluoride excimer lasers which emit ultraviolet light (193 nm) with high photon energy capable of breaking intermolecular bonds within proteins and other macromolecules without causing thermal damage to adjacent tissues (Trokel et al., 1983). Excimer lasers, used in industry since 1971,

were introduced to ophthalmic surgery in 1983 (McDonald et al., 1991). Experimental application confirmed the possibility of executing precise and smooth changes to the corneal surface allowing progress to large scale human clinical trials. These lasers can remove sub-micrometre (μm) portions of tissue from the anterior corneal surface, altering the anterior radius of curvature and yielding a very precise refractive change (Trokel et al., 1983). Tissue ablation is actuated at a rate of 0.25 μm per pulse by a beam which is shaped to conform to the requirement of tissue removal. A graduation of the edges of the shaped cornea is required to avoid epithelial filling which would result in a subsequent reduction of the optical effect. Sub-epithelial deposition of new extra-cellular matrix occurs after all excimer laser procedures. This may cause thickening of the ablated area and thereby reduce the refractive element. The healing response is also responsible for a sub-epithelial haze which is always present in varying degrees of severity.

Indications for PRK

Indications for this technique are currently based on the limited period of clinical study which predicts that treatment to within 1.00 dioptre of expectation may be achieved in eyes with a spherical myopic refraction of 2.00–6.00 dioptres and with no more than 1.00 dioptre of astigmatism (Seiler and Wollensak, 1991; Gartry, 1992; Salz et al., 1992). Intermediate myopia of 7.00–12.00 dioptres may be treated with less predictable results (Figure 7.20), i.e. there is a greater chance of regression, increased corneal opacification, consequent upon the greater depth of corneal penetration, and a danger of lasting corneal scarring. Treatment of astigmatism remains experimental with insufficient evidence for predictable and stable treatment yet realized, while the methods of laser application are continuing to be developed. Similarly claims for treatment of hypermetropia are not yet substantiated.

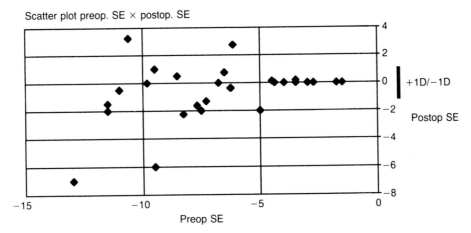

Scatter plot preop. SE × postop. SE

Figure 7.20   Scatter plot to show results of PRK at 90–140 days in 26 eyes: range myopia 3 to 13D; SE = spherical equivalent. (From Rosen, 1993, with permission)

The procedure

Treatment is performed on an outpatient basis under topical anaesthesia. Following operation, pain may be severe in the first 12–36 hours, but can be moderated by the immediate application of lubricant ointment, cycloplegic eye drops and systemic analgesics. Thereafter vision may be blurred for the first few days or even weeks as the healing process invariably produces an over-correction which is followed by a period of regression. A period of 2–4 days off work is necessary. Anisometropia will result after treating the first eye and early PRK on the second eye is contingent upon the status of the fellow eye. Patients undergoing photorefractive keratectomy, therefore, must be aware there may be an interim period of some months between each eye being treated with associated ocular dissociation, however this may be ameliorated by contact lens wear in the unoperated eye.

Postoperative effects

Outpatient follow-up visits for medical supervision are required on a frequent and regular basis in order to monitor the eye for any complications and to appraise the refractive result. A constant feature following treatment is a variable corneal haze in the treated zone, which generally does not disrupt visual function and largely disappears within 6–12 months. Steroids are widely used in an attempt to reduce haze and modify the refractive effect, although evidence for their influence is disputed (Hann *et al.*, 1992). If deeper treatments are effected for higher degrees of myopia in too small an optical zone, denser degrees of opacification may occur and persist. Patients may, therefore, note moderate glare in the first 2–3 months after treatment and a longer lasting flare effect, especially if the treatment zone is decentred. A similar halo effect may be noted, particularly at night, if the treatment zone is smaller than the pupil diameter. In 80% of cases healing is predictable with a modest over-correction followed by regression towards the target refraction, and PRK for myopia invariably results in the desired refraction after a period varying from a few weeks to several months (Plate 19). During this period a progressive improvement in visual acuity is to be expected. In 15% of cases, however, corneal haze associated with persistent hypermetropia may occur and in 5% regression towards the original myopia may be significant (Seiler and Wollensak, 1991). The recurrent corneal abrasion syndrome does not occur after PRK as the epithelium becomes especially adherent.

Diurnal fluctuation of vision which has been reported after radial keratotomy does not appear to be a problem following PRK, and evidence to date suggests that all eyes are stable by 12 months. The psychological effects are generally favourable. Salz *et al.* (1992) reported that 75% of those treated with PRK felt that their lifestyle had improved and 84% were completely satisfied with the result. Seventy-four per cent of his cases did not require a spectacle correction 1 year after PRK and no patient felt that their vision was worse after the procedure.

Reported results

Clinical results of PRK indicate that relatively low degrees of uncomplicated myopia (2.00–6.00 dioptres) can be predictably neutralized with up to 90% of treated eyes being within 1.00 dioptres of the intended refraction after one year and none of the eyes treated losing or gaining more than one line of spectacle corrected acuity (McDonald *et al.*, 1991; Salz *et al.*, 1992).

Incisional corneal surgery for myopia and astigmatism (AK/RK)

Simple myopia can be addressed by radial incisions or radial keratotomy (RK) wherein a central optical zone of 3.00–4.50 mm is affected by radial incisions through the corneal mid-periphery. The effect is varied by the number, depth and length of the incisions. The longer the incisions, the smaller the optical zone (OZ). Other variables with minor effects on central corneal flattening in order of importance are: age, gender, corneal curvature (steep respond better than flat corneas) and intra-ocular pressure (IOP) (more effect with higher IOP than lower IOP within normal range). Surgical technique can also influence the effect, with two-way incisions more effective than single-direction incisions. Mixed

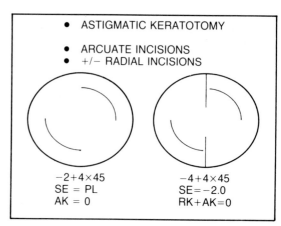

Figure 7.21 Example of radial and arcuate keratotomy for neutralization of mixed astigmatism. *Left*, refraction –2.0 /+4.0 × 45, spherical equivalent (SE) = plano, 2 × 45° arcuate incisions at 7 mm OZ; postoperative refraction = plano, coupling ratio 1/1. *Right*, preoperative refraction –4.0 / +4.0 × 45, spherical equivalent (SE) = –2.0D, 2 × 45° arcuate incisions at 7 mm OZ, + two radial incisions, coupling ratio 1/1; postoperative refraction = plano

astigmatism therapy is effected by arcuate or transverse incisions in the corneal mid-periphery coupled if necessary with non-intersecting radial incisions for the residual myopic component (Figure 7.21).

As the procedure is not reversible, overcorrection must be avoided at all costs. Accordingly, a staged approach to higher corrections is advocated. The sensible expectation for correction is no more than 6.00 dioptres. A limit of eight incisions is generally practised, though in the early application of the technique up to 64 incisions were reported which should be categorized as mutilation of the cornea!

Postoperative effects

Outpatient follow-up is required to monitor the results in a similar manner to those undergoing PRK. However, there is not the period of over-correction in PRK (Plate 20), which means that the second eye can be treated within days to weeks of treating the first. There may be fluctuation of the vision for a prolonged period, with alterations in the refraction throughout the day. Patients may be bothered by glare, due to the peripheral wounds, which is particularly troublesome at night when the pupil dilates. In addition, some long-term complications have been identified in a few patients, such as deep corneal vascularization around the cuts, fluffy white corneal scars, persistent corneal oedema, epithelial microcysts, central corneal erosions, bacterial endophthalmitis and endothelial cell loss.

Clinical results

Figure 7.22 illustrates the author's 1993 PRK results on 45 eyes with a spherical equivalent refraction at 60 days, an optical zone of 3–4 mm and a myopia range of 1.50–7.00 dioptres. The PERK study group published their results of prospective evaluation of radial keratotomy study after 5 years of surgery (Waring *et al.*, 1991). This long-term study achieved close follow-up of a large group of patients (Table 7.5), demonstrating the overall safety, predictability and efficacy of the technique, if practised without too great an ambition to correct higher degrees of myopia. In the USA today, PRK is performed

Table 7.5   PERK study: 5-year review

793 eyes of 435 patients
2.00–8.00 D myopia
Eight incisions 100% paracentral depth
OZ 3 mm–4.5 mm
97 eyes (12%) additional eight incisions
757 eyes (95%) follow-up 3–6.3 years
Uncorrected acuity > 20/40 = 88%
± 1DS in 64% eyes
19% > 1D myopic
17% > 1D hyperopic
6 months – 5 years 22% hyperopic shift > 1D
25 eyes (3%) loss two or more lines acuity

on a large scale, driven by patient requirement, professional enthusiasm and limited access to laser photorefractive keratectomy by Federal regulatory control.

The clinical applications for each technique

Incisional methods are more effective the older the patient, but have limited effect (approximately 6.00 dioptres) to reduce myopia. Laser PRK is equally effective at any age and is capable of treating higher ranges of myopia (Gimbel *et al.*, 1993). However, the

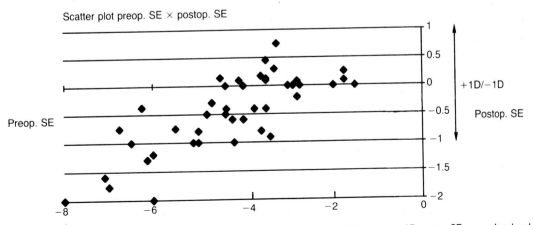

Figure 7.22   Scatter plot to show results of retinal keratotomy at 60 days in 45 eyes; SE = spherical equivalent. (From Rosen, 1993, with permission)

Table 7.6 PRK results: psychosocial study in 26 patients

Motivation = improve vision
  cosmetic reason minor importance
74% no glasses after PRK at 1 year
72% felt visual acuity improved
28% felt visual acuity no change, i.e. none worse
75% improved lifestyle
84% completely satisfied

Source: Salz *et al.,* 1992

higher the degree of myopia, the less predictable the outcome. Laser PRK causes central corneal scarring which may be unpredictable and the time scale of healing is several weeks or months, especially when greater degrees of ablation are effected. On the other hand, incisional methods give almost instant results, allowing early rehabilitation by completion of bilateral treatment in a matter of days, or a week or two compared with several months for PRK. In essence the two techniques are most effective in the lower ranges of myopia but incisional surgery achieves an almost immediate effect compared with a variable time delay of weeks or months before satisfaction is achieved with the laser method.

Early sports experience with radial keratotomy for myopia

A survey of recreational athletes who had undergone radial keratotomy showed that an overwhelming majority felt that the procedure had improved their sports performance and they would undergo the surgery again. The survey was carried out on 1500 patients who had undergone radial keratotomy across the USA. The objectives of the study were to discover not only how patients felt about RK, but how it affected their sports performance.

There was an overwhelming response indicating that performance in sports was significantly improved after RK (Seiller, 1992).

The survey was distributed throughout eight RK centres across the USA. All patients had undergone RK at least six months prior to responding to the survey. Of 1500 questionnaires despatched 554 responses were analysed in three postoperative groups: 6–12 months, 12–24 months and more than 24 months.

Questions ranging from patient satisfaction to the level of sports participation were answered. One fact to emerge was that the mean age of the survey group was 40 years (range 16–86 years) indicating that RK can improve the quality of life for sports people of all ages. Ninety per cent of the patients indicated that they would undergo RK again in both eyes or would recommend surgery to a family member or friend. Another 5% said they would find the need to have it undertaken on one eye. Despite the strong endorsement of RK in the survey, 70% reported visual phenomena relating to the procedure which included star bursts and diurnal variation, though this did not sway the athletes' belief in the procedure or affect their overall satisfaction.

While this survey documents certain benefits of refractive surgery for athletes, RK is not commonplace at higher levels of athletic competition. At the time of writing there are no data available on the prevalence of RK amongst professional athletes in the USA or elsewhere.

Intrastromal devices

Intrastromal surgical devices, such as corneal PMMA ring technology (Keravision Co., California, USA) are presently undergoing clinical evaluation. This concept embraces the insertion of 7 mm PMMA rings of varying thickness into the corneal mid stroma. The thicker the ring, the greater the central corneal flattening and the greater the correction factor for myopic eyes. Preliminary studies with a ring designed to correct 3.00–4.00 D of myopia are very promising (Schanzlin *et al.* 1993). The most attractive aspect of this approach to refractive surgery is its reversibility; removal of the ring allows the cornea to revert to its former refractive status, a unique feature, so far, in the evolution of refractive surgery.

Hypermetropia

Surgical treatments for hypermetropic eyes are currently not as predictable as surgical methods for addressing myopic refractive errors. The methods available include incisional, lamellar and thermal methods. Their common basis is the steepening of the central (optic axis) corneal radius of curvature (refractive power) in order to bend light rays sufficiently to focus on the fovea in eyes which are generally shorter than their emmetropic counterparts.

Incisional method

This is based on a hexagonal pattern of peripheral corneal incisions, the purpose of which is the induction of tissue shrinkage through healing processes. The pattern of the incisions determines the central corneal steepening. The predictability of the process has been so poor and the instability of the process so common, that this form of surgery has not been widely used (Waring, 1992).

Lamellar method

Micro-engineering technical advances have made lamellar corneal surgical methods a practical reality. The principal of treatment in hypermetropic eyes is to remove an anterior lamella of 6 mm diameter by 300–400 μm thickness and then simply replace it. In reality the dissected lamella is hinged and replaced. The effect is to cause the residual posterior corneal stroma to be fractionally weakened, allowing the intra-ocular pressure to cause a slight forward bowing and hence steepening with greater refractive power. The device utilized is the corneal micro-keratome or corneal shaper (Chiron-intra-optics Co., California, USA).

Thermal methods

There are two methods available. Placing a hot needle (**cautery**) into corneal stroma causes collagen shrinkage and corneal steepening. The effect is unpredictable; it was suggested by Fyodorov in the USSR but without supporting data to confirm its efficacy and stability. The second technique employs **laser thermal methods**. The holmium (infrared) laser has been developed in various forms for the treatment of hypermetropia. Technology changes rapidly and obsolescence is ever present. One system uses an add-on facility to the (myopic) excimer laser (Summit technology), utilizing an adaptation of the probe developed for holmium laser sclerostomy for the surgical management of glaucoma. The holmium laser probe is placed onto the corneal periphery and the applied energy causes heating of the collagen fibres in the corneal stroma inducing fibre bundle shrinkage and modulation of the corneal curvature. Healing of the cornea involves collagen shrinkage, damage to Bowman's layer, repair of epithelial defects, collagenase with corneal necrosis or melting. The overall outcome is stromal scarring which alters the corneal shape.

Lenticular aspects of refractive surgery

Discussion of cataract surgery is generally beyond the scope of this section but it is worthy of note that cataract and lens implant surgery is the major form of refractive surgery practised today. This may take the form of lens extraction with lens implantation or may simply involve the supplementary implantation of an intra-ocular lens in the anterior or posterior chamber. We are now in an era of small incision cataract surgery with the whole process of cataract removal and lens implantation taking place through incisions as small as 2.7 mm. This is the obvious method of choice, especially for younger patients with cataracts who have a sports interest. Cataract surgery aims generally at emmetropization of the patient's refraction whatever the prior condition.

Supplementary intra-ocular lenses may be incorporated into phakic eyes, thus retaining the combination of the younger eye which otherwise would be sacrificed by lens extraction and implantation. Supplementary anterior chamber lens implants for the refractive correction of high myopia are being introduced on a small scale, particularly in France and Germany (Fechner and Wichmann, 1992). In Russia, Fyodorov and his group are placing type IV collagen lenticules onto the crystalline lens in young ametropic patients, both myopic and hypermetropic, but hard data on their efficacy and safety are not available.

Trauma and the eye after refractive surgery

Refractive surgery involving radial or transverse corneal incisions will create marginal weakness of the cornea in relation to direct trauma. The same comment applies to standard larger incision cataract surgery. The force of the direct blow is all important, but it is generally accepted that an incised cornea will be intrinsically weaker than a virgin one. In day-to-day life the chances of a direct blow to the eye are more remote than in certain sports, e.g. small ball sports such as squash or equivalent sports such as badminton where the diameter of the ball or shuttlecock is smaller than the protective orbital rim. Similarly, any contact sport wherein a finger might inadvertently hit an eye, e.g. wrestling or rugby, may be regarded as a contra-indication to incisional methods of refractive surgery, where proactive and appropriate polycarbonate eye protectors should be worn for sports participants who have undergone refractive surgery.

Age and vision

Finally, it must be remembered that ocular anatomy and physiology change with age, especially with reference to the crystalline lens and cornea from the refractive perspective. Loss of accommodation, yellowing of the crystalline lens and to a lesser extent the cornea each alter the visual process. Presbyopia, essentially due to the crystalline lens increasing in thickness and hardness with age, with reduction or loss of accommodation, may alter the requirement for visual aids. Eventually, surgical processes may find a complete answer to all these problems, but meanwhile the decade of the 1990s is realizing the first major steps in refractive surgery on an ever-widening scale.

References

Bogan, S.J., Maloney, R.K., Drews, C and Waring, G.O. (1994) Computer assisted videokeratography of corneal topography after radial keratotomy. *Archives of Ophthalmology*, in press

Fechner, P.U. and Wichmann, W. (1992) Correction of myopia by implantation of a concave lens into the anterior chamber of phakic eyes. *European Journal of Implant and Refractive Surgery*, **5** (1), 55–60, September

Gartry, D.S. (1992) Excimer laser photorefractive keratectomy: 18 month follow up. *Ophthalmology*, August, 1209–20

Gimbel, H.V., Van Westenbrugge, J.A. and Johnson, W.H. (1993) Visual, refractive and patient satisfaction results following bilateral photorefractive keratectomy for myopia. *Refractive and Corneal Surgery*, 9, 5–11

Hann, K.D., Puliquen Y., Waring, G.O. III, *et al.* (1989) Corneal stromal healing in rabbits after 193 nm excimer laser surface ablation. *Archives of Ophthalmology*, **107**, 895–901

McDonald, M.B., Liu, J.C., Byrd, T.J. *et al.*, (1991) Central photorefractive keratectomy for myopia. Partially sighted and normally sighted eyes. *Ophthalmology*, **98**, 1327–37

Millodot, M. (1993) Dictionary of Optometry, 3rd edn, Butterworth Heinemann, Oxford

Rowsey, J.J., Waring, G.O. and Monlux, R.D. *et al.* (1994) Results of the prospective evaluation of radial keratotomy (PERK) study after 10 years of surgery. *Archives of Ophthalmology (USA)*, **112** (10), 1298–1308

Salz, J.J., Maguen, E., Macy, J.I. *et al.* (1992) One year follow up of excimer laser photorefractive keratectomy for myopia. *Refractive and Corneal Surgery*, **8**, 269–73

Schanzlin, D.J. and Waring, G.O. (1993) Intrasomal corneal ring, one year results of first implants in humans: a preliminary non-functional study in refractive corneal surgery. *Refract. Corneal. Surg.*, **9** (6), 452–58

Seiler, T. and Wollensak, J. (1991) Myopic photorefractive keratectomy with the excimer laser. One year follow up. *Ophthalmology*, **98**, 56–63

Seiller, B.L. (1992) Ninth annual meeting of the International Academy of Sports Vision, 1992. Visual Fitness Institute of Vernon Hills, Keratorefractive Study Group

Trokel, S.L., Strinivasan, R. and Braren, B. (1983) Excimer laser surgery of the cornea. *American Journal of Ophthalmology*, **96**, 710–15

Waring, G.O. III. (1992) *Refractive Keratotomy for Myopia and Astigmatism*, Mosby Year Book, St Louis

Waring, G., Lynn, M.J., Nizam, M.K. *et al.* (1991) Results of prospective evaluation of radial keratotomy study after 5 years of surgery. The PERK study group. *Ophthalmology*, **98**, 1164–76

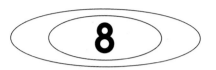

Visual performance enhancement in sports optometry

Bradley Coffey and Alan W. Reichow

Introduction

This chapter presents a practical and logical approach to the enhancement of sport-related visual skills beyond the provision of optimum refractive compensation and protective eye wear. General and specific methodologies are suggested for each area based upon research findings and clinical observations. Emphasis is placed upon procedures designed for the individual athlete rather than procedures which might be used with groups or teams. As the public's awareness of sports vision enhancement training grows, it becomes increasingly important that practitioners utilize a shared core of knowledge for both evaluation and enhancement services. It is hoped that the information presented here will facilitate greater standardization in the discipline and enhance communication between practitioners.

Sports visual enhancement training: introduction and scope

Visual enhancement training provided by sports vision specialists is based upon a logical approach to the multi-tasking sensory motor environment in which the athlete competes. Training procedures may be conceptually divided into three categories:

1. Enhancement of inefficient or inconsistent visual abilities.
2. Enhancement of visually dependent motor functions that are not as fast, quick, accurate or automatic as desired.
3. Enhancement of visual cognitive functions that are critical for visual decision making during competition.

Training in each of these areas requires different procedures and approaches for best efficacy to be attained.

Inefficient or inconsistent visual abilities

Inefficient visual abilities may limit competitive potential or may be responsible for inconsistencies in performance under certain circumstances or at specific times, such as when fatigued or when competitive pressure is extreme. Our current understanding of complex information processing tasks suggests that humans have limited pools of attention available at any moment in time

(Broadbent, 1982). Breakdowns, errors or inconsistencies in performance arise when the demands on the limited attention pool exceed its capacity. If any necessary task-related sensory or motor ability is inefficient, it draws an enlarged share from the limited attention pool. The excessive draw reduces the amount of attentional energy available for control of other critical processes and presents the potential for a reduction in quality of the overall performance output (Navon, 1985).

Consider the alpine slalom skier. If the skier has a tendency to suppress intermittently in association with a decompensating esophoria, momentary losses of stereopsis may be experienced. If noticed, attention may be shifted to the reduction in visual spatial information and the skier may blink rapidly or make a rapid eye movement to disrupt the sensory suppression. If the blinking, eye movement, or attentional shift required to produce these motor actions occurs at the moment of a critical balance shift necessary to complete the slalom course, the skier may lose balance or necessary momentum to achieve a peak performance. If the suppression is not noticed, overall performance is likely to be affected because available visual spatial information will be compromised, and timing of turns through the gates and over irregular terrain will be less than optimal.

Similar compromises in overall performance may occur for the trapshooter who has reduced accommodative or vergence facility. If the shooter has been concentrating on the sighting bead or other relatively near target prior to calling for the target, there is a potential slowness in identifying and localizing the target. If the shooter has a vague awareness that the visual process is 'slow', greater attention may be paid to shifting visual focus when the target appears. This greater-than-normal attentional allocation reduces the amount of attention available for control of the other components of the shooting task and creates the potential for reduced or inconsistent performance. If the shooter does not notice the effects of reduced accommodative or vergence facility, less precise target acquisition and localization may occur and therefore the competitive potential is never reached. Similar examples can easily be conceived to involve any of the visual skills typically considered by the sports vision specialist.

Motor functions

Given the absence of inefficiencies in visual input processes such as visual sensitivity (visual acuity and contrast sensitivity), binocularity, spatial perception, colour vision, visual fields and other primarily sensory functions, the sports vision specialist must consider the primarily motor components involved in sport-related visual function. In sports where speed is critical, sports which are largely dynamic and reactive in nature such as ice-hockey, soccer or basketball, sports vision enhancement training may include techniques designed to increase the speed, quickness, accuracy or automaticity of visually dependent motor functions. The player defending a legendary offensive player in the National Basketball Association has a significant demand placed upon eye–hand reaction and response speeds and upon automaticity of those functions. The visual system of the defender may function very efficiently, but if the specific eye–hand reaction ability is inefficient or compromised, the legendary offensive player will have little trouble avoiding the defender's attempts to steal the basketball. Similar parallels can be drawn for the ice-hockey player controlling the hockey stick or the racing car driver piloting the car. In a sport such as soccer, the demands for eye–hand reaction and response speeds are replaced by eye–foot demands, and the soccer player must have excellent eye–foot automaticity to achieve and maintain peak performance.

Cognitive functions

The enhancement of visual cognitive functions that are critical for visual decision making during competition is the area of training that is by far the most ambiguous for the sports vision specialist. Although it is easy to conceptualize the nature of these skills, it is very difficult to isolate them for measurement in order to assess or improve efficacy of training. Indeed, of the published protocols for sports vision assessment (Reichow *et al.*, 1985; Coffey and Reichow, 1987; Christenson and Winkelstein, 1988; Coffey and Reichow, 1990; Berman, 1993), none include procedures for sport-related visual cognitive skills. These skills tend to be rather complex and involve the whole of the visual system in the process of visual thinking. Perhaps the most discussed of the skills in this area is that of visual imagery or visualization as described in Chapter 2. Much has been written on the importance of this skill in several different aspects of sport (Harris and Harris, 1984; Heil, 1984; Suinn, 1984; Finke, 1986), yet there are no visualization evaluation procedures with demonstrated validity that are specifically sport-related. Despite the lack of measurement procedures, sport psychologists and some sports vision specialists use methods designed to improve visual imagery ability, often with good success based upon subjective feedback from the athlete.

Another visual cognitive skill that is obviously critical in sport is the control of visual attentional focus and facility. This skill area has been emphasized primarily in 'closed' (Poulton, 1957; McLeod, 1985) sports such as diving, rifle and pistol shooting and gymnastics in which there is an internal locus of control and performance is relatively independent of environmental factors. Visual attention variables have been the subject of much scrutiny in Olympic training programmes, particularly in the former Soviet bloc countries (Raiport, 1988). Visual attentional skills such as breadth of attentional focus and speed of movement of attentional focus can be measured using several different procedures in the laboratory setting (Posner, 1980; Downing and Pinker, 1985), but there are no published standardized methods for clinical assessment of these skills. Some practitioners derive subjective information in this area by observing the athlete in a controlled multi-tasking environment (sometimes called 'loading' or 'cognitive loading', and usually involving variables such as simultaneous visual, auditory, motor, cognitive and vestibular stimulation), or by observing the athlete when confronted with tasks which require the simultaneous integration of information presented to central and peripheral vision. An example of the latter task is a quantitative procedure developed at Pacific University which requires the athlete to perform an eye–hand task using peripheral vision while simultaneously identifying visual stimuli presented to central vision.

When contemplating an approach to sports optometry enhancement training for a specific athlete, the authors recommend that the three areas of enhancement training introduced above be provided in hierarchical fashion. Evaluation and enhancement of basic visual input skills should precede any higher-level enhancement training that is dependent upon those skills (Coffey and Reichow, 1990). It is inappropriate, for example, to begin enhancement of spatial localization ability when the athlete has unstable binocularity or compromised visual sensitivity. Any type of enhancement training programme should be preceded by the provision of appropriate protective eye wear and ophthalmic lenses to compensate any refractive condition that may have a negative impact upon contrast sensitivity. The fact that reduced visual sensitivity creates negative ramifications for higher-order visual skills is intuitively obvious, yet many practitioners continue to provide to athletes contact lenses which do not optimize visual sensitivity. In this regard, the practitioner should have available many types and designs of contact lenses including toric and bitoric designs to assure the best possible fit and lens performance for the athlete. The fitting process must include an evaluation of the lens performance in non-primary positions of gaze, particularly those positions that are common in the athlete's sport. The practitioner should anticipate possible contact lens problems associated with the sport environment, and should provide the athlete with appropriate solutions and a minimum of one spare pair of lenses. Also, the practitioner or a trusted colleague should have available many different types of protective eye wear and should select this in the context of the visual task demands of the specific sport.

Although the authors recommend well-fitting contact lenses as the first choice option for refractive compensation, there are instances where the use of protective eye wear that incorporates the athlete's refractive prescription is desirable. This option should be considered in sports that do not have significant demands for non-primary positions of gaze nor peripheral vision, for athletes who have a prior corneal condition that precludes the use of contact lenses, or in the rare cases where adequate refractive compensation cannot be attained with contact lenses. In cases of extreme refractive prescriptions (especially those involving astigmatism) it may be desirable to compensate a portion of the condition with contact lenses and to compensate the residual amount using the protective eyewear lenses. High refractive prescriptions in polycarbonate lenses should be avoided due to the higher degree of peripheral optical aberrations associated with this material.

Developing the enhancement programme

There are three primary components to the development of an enhancement training programme.

1. The sport visual task analysis.
2. The profile of the athlete's visual performance skills.
3. The athlete.

The sport visual task analysis

The sport visual task analysis is an examination of the sport to determine which visual skills are most critical to meet the demands of the sport. A sport such as tennis is dynamic and reactive in nature and visual skills such as eye movement ability, accommodative vergence facility, eye–hand coordination, eye–hand reaction speed, peripheral vision and balance are critical. In contrast, golf is primarily non-dynamic in nature and requires different visual skills. The golfer requires excellent visual sensitivity, stable visual spatial perception, precise depth perception and facile visual imagery ability. The visual evaluation of the tennis player and golfer should therefore emphasize different assessment procedures and the interpretation of the test results should reflect the different relative importance of the visual skills in the two sports. Slower eye–hand reaction time for the golfer, for example, may not present a barrier to achieving consistent peak performance in that sport. The same finding for the tennis player may represent a barrier to achieving competitive potential. When preparing the enhancement training programme, techniques and procedures should be utilized that offer the best cost/benefit ratio to the athlete; critical sport-specific visual skills should be emphasized. The enhancement training programme for the tennis player may therefore have little in common with the enhancement training programme for the golfer.

When practitioners have limited experience with any particular sport, they should consult Table 2.1 or one of the several sports encyclopaedias available. A good source of sports visual task analysis information is the *Sports Vision Guidebook* available from the Sports Vision Section of the American Optometric Association (1993). Each chapter in the *Guidebook* discusses a specific sport and is based upon input from many experienced optometric practitioners for the primary purpose of providing task analytic information.

Visual performance skills

The evaluation of visual performance skills should be undertaken using a standardized norm-referenced testing battery such as the Pacific Sports Visual Performance Profile (PSVPP; Coffey and Reichow, 1990), and emphasis should be placed upon the specific visual skill areas that are critical in the athlete's sport. Because of the learned, developmental nature of most visual skills, athletes competing in different sports and at different competitive levels would be expected to develop different levels of visual ability; for example, it is anticipated that the developed visual skills of the professional golfer will differ from those of the young rugby player. Hence, any comparative analysis of an individual athlete's visual skills profile should be conducted with a reference group of athletes in the same sport or in sports with very similar visual task demands. Also, it has been shown that gender differences exist for many sport-related visual skills (Coffey and Reichow, 1990), so comparative analysis should be gender-specific.

Athletes

Several variables concerning the individual athlete should be carefully considered prior to proposing or providing an enhancement training programme. The level of competition and years of competitive experience are important variables. A different programme would be proposed for the professional tennis player than for the junior player with one year of experience. Enhancement training for the young athlete may involve activities designed to enrich visual development with emphasis upon the visual skills necessary for peak performance in a specific sport. For the experienced athlete who has attained a level of stable performance in terms of technique and motor skills, the visual enhancement training programme may be more narrowly focused to achieve consistent stable visual

function in the presence of higher levels of competitive stress, and to fine tune the visual system to increase sensitivity to subtle forms of visual information.

The motivation of the athlete must be considered, and the level of support provided by the parents, coach and team should be weighed up in the decision to provide the enhancement programme. Consultation with coaches should include a comparative analysis of their assessment of the athlete's overall sport performance and the optometrist's assessment of visual performance. It is often productive for the practitioner to make observations or predictions regarding the impact on overall performance of any diagnosed visual inefficiencies. These observations should then be compared to the coach's concerns regarding specific sport-related performance inconsistencies. Any parallels derived from these comparisons should be highlighted to the coach and athlete.

Athletes and their support groups should be well informed regarding the role of vision in sport. It is the responsibility of the practitioner to provide educational material such as brochures, article reprints, videotapes and demonstrations to increase the understanding of visual performance. A well-informed athlete is generally a more highly motivated, compliant and responsive athlete. The practitioner should strive at all times to explain evaluation and enhancement procedures in the context of the visual demands of the specific sport. Motivation in an enhancement training programme is better when the athlete can appreciate the sport-related significance of any procedures administered. For example, a short explanation to the baseball player of the value of depth perception in catching a fly ball, and a demonstration of reduced depth perception when monocular as compared to binocular, will give the binocularity enhancement training a level of meaning that is directly transferable to the competitive environment.

An athlete's competitive goals affect their overall motivation. The young downhill skier who is striving to attain a position on a National or Olympic team will generally bring a higher level of motivation to the enhancement training than will the recreational skier who wants to read the moguls better. On the other hand, it has been the experience of many sports vision practitioners that, because of varying motivation, professional athletes do not necessarily achieve the greatest success in enhancement training. It is often the younger, more coachable, goal-orientated athlete who attains the best results. These athletes are often seeking a competitive edge that will carry them to the next level of performance. For certain athletes with visual inefficiency, sports vision enhancement training may be the critical variable in the overall sports performance equation.

Visual enhancement: general principles

After completing the visual task analysis, visual performance evaluation and interview of the athlete and coach (and the athlete's parents, when appropriate), the practitioner is ready to determine whether or not a visual enhancement training programme will be recommended. If recommended, the athlete (and coach, parent, team personnel etc.) should be advised of the specific optometric goals of the programme, the relevance of those goals to sport performance, the estimated duration of the programme and follow-up, the expectations of the athlete regarding appointments and out-of-office training activities, the expectations of team support personnel and the costs. Practitioners vary somewhat in their preferred scheduling of training appointments, however it is typical that athletes are seen every one or two weeks for 60–90 minutes, and are expected to perform out-of-office training activities for 30–60 minutes per day. These activities serve to reinforce

training concepts presented during the office visits and are sometimes integrated into the athlete's ongoing training regimen. Such integration places optometric sports vision enhancement training beside weight training, cardiovascular training, skills training and other procedures included in the training repertoire of the successful athlete. Though most practitioners work with athletes in a one-on-one setting, some practitioners utilize sports vision trainers or conduct group training where the athletes have the opportunity not only to perform the training activities but also to teach others how to attain success in the enhancement programme, thereby strengthening the depth of understanding and integration. Transference of skills can be enhanced by developing training procedures and drills that can be practised in the actual competitive environment of the athlete (for example, in the arena, on the field, at the track).

The sports optometrist must relate, both by word and by action, enhancement training activities to the sports task demands faced by the athlete. Several general principles should be followed. The visual task demands of virtually all sports are in the distance, not at the nearpoint. Therefore, except in cases where a visual inefficiency has arisen due specifically to a nearpoint dysfunction, enhancement training activities should generally use target distances greater than 3 m. The enhancement training programme should usually proceed from skill isolation (enhancement of a specific skill or function) to skill integration (integration of the enhanced skill into the completion of complex sport-related tasks). Simple, foundational skills should be developed prior to complex skills involving many visual functions. Distractions and demands for multi-tasking or simultaneous cognitive processing should be incorporated only after the basic skills are sound and relatively automatic. In sports which involve movement and quick reactions, the training programme should eventually include procedures that are dynamic and emphasize fast responses. If balance or non-primary gaze demands are present in the athlete's sport these aspects should be eventually incorporated into the training environment. Developing the training programme with these points in mind improves transference and will help the athlete to appreciate the goals of the training, thus increasing motivation and improving the likelihood of a successful outcome.

Any enhancement training programme and, ideally, any compensating lens change, should be undertaken when the athlete is in the off-season, i.e. during that part of the year when the athlete is not involved in formal competition. Successful programmes of visual enhancement training usually cause a reorganization of visual function and visual perception. These changes can have temporary negative impacts upon the athlete's consistency of performance. Because of this, the sports vision practitioner strives to administer services during the off-season when the athlete can better tolerate performance inconsistency and can attend more fully to the training process.

A common error made by practitioners entering the field of sports vision care is to overstate the power of sports enhancement training. Although the discipline can provide the critical component of the sports performance equation for carefully selected athletes, it is not a panacea for all the vagaries of sports competition. Practitioners must strive to identify those athletes with potentially performance-limiting visual conditions that are amenable to optometric remediation and enhancement. Training goals must be carefully delineated and conveyed to the athlete in an understandable way. Above all, one must remember that vision is but *one* aspect, albeit an often neglected aspect, of the complex set of abilities necessary to attain peak performance in any sport. With careful evaluation, analysis and planning, the practitioner can achieve success. Success breeds success, while perceived failure can close many doors that are very difficult to reopen.

Visual skill areas addressed in enhancement training

Visual sensitivity

Visual sensitivity as used here refers to the individual's ability to resolve detail or contrast in the retinal image. The obvious first step in optimizing visual sensitivity is the provision of ophthalmic lenses (usually well-fitting contact lenses) to compensate for any refractive condition which compromises contrast sensitivity. This said, it is worthwhile noting that many accomplished amateur and professional athletes compete routinely and successfully with reduced visual acuity. The authors have had the clinical experience of providing compensatory lenses and demonstrating the positive effect of those lenses upon visual acuity and contrast sensitivity, only to have the athlete return months later to advise the authors that he discontinued lens wear for reasons he deemed more important than the improved visual sensitivity provided by the lenses. Although optometrists and ophthalmologists place great emphasis upon compensation of refractive conditions, one must carefully consider the sports task analysis to determine whether fine visual acuity is critical for the sport. To cite an extreme example, the sport of wrestling does not have great demands for precise visual acuity. A more thought-provoking example may be that of tennis. Due to the high speed of ball movement in that sport, and the associated difficulty in foveating the moving ball, some practitioners argue that fine visual acuity is not necessary for consistent peak performance. Little research is presently available to guide clinical practice, so the practitioner must depend upon professional judgement, background knowledge of sport task demands, and a comprehensive interview with the athlete. One must also consider the potential effects of compensatory lenses upon binocularity and spatial perception, particularly for the athlete who has successfully competed for a long period of time without lenses.

If visual sensitivity enhancement training is to be undertaken, the practitioner should use techniques that require precise discrimination of retinal information. Procedures involving lens and prism sensitivity may be useful. These procedures are performed monocularly while viewing a distance target and require the athlete to determine the spatial effects induced by the lens or prism. In the case of prism sensitivity, the athlete determines the direction of spatial shift caused by the insertion of prisms of progressively weaker power when an assistant inserts the prism with the base in random directions (up, down, left, right, diagonal). Lens sensitivity techniques require the athlete to discriminate between ophthalmic lenses of different powers. Emphasis is placed upon the determination of any spatial magnification or minification induced, changes in perceived target distance, and/or changes in perceived accommodative effort.

Sensitivity to subtle changes in retinal image size can be trained by means of comparative judgements of target size while viewing through iseikonic lenses, or through use of a modified Howard–Dolman apparatus. We have developed and utilize a simple Howard–Dolman apparatus which uses golf balls (or other types of sport balls) instead of pegs for targets. The golf balls provide a better representation of real-world target conditions that include monocular cues of texture and relative size. The athlete views the targets monocularly for progressively shorter periods of time (approaching, therefore, tachistoscopic presentation of stimuli, see Chapter 2) and makes a judgement of which ball appears closer.

Visual acuity training

Perhaps the best-researched method of visual sensitivity enhancement is used mostly outside optometry, although its early application can be traced to optometric sources (Woods, 1945; Ewalt, 1946; Rowe, 1947). Visual acuity training, using the method of fading with

feedback, has been repeatedly shown t[ ] up to two lines' improvement on the S[ ] acuity chart (Epstein et al., 1981). The[ ] nique involves the presentation of pr[ ] sively smaller stimuli using a mod___u method of limits (fading). The subject is asked to discriminate the targets and is given feed-back regarding the correctness of responses. Guessing is encouraged and the goal is to progressively reduce the threshold target size required for consistently accurate discrimina-tion by the athlete. It is often useful also to reduce the target exposure time as training progresses. The technique is frequently dis-missed by critics as 'nothing more than blur interpretation' or 'chart memorization' (Bail-liet et al., 1982), but it has been shown that the visual acuity training effect generalizes to untrained stimuli (Epstein et al., 1981; Gil and Collins, 1983; Collins et al., 1984; Ricci and Collins, 1988) and to contrast sensitivity (Gil et al., 1986), suggesting that the training effect may be occurring at a level above the retina or that the retinal sensitivity is in fact heightened due to the training. Because visual acuity enhancement training appears to transfer from a trained to an untrained eye, there is at least limited evidence to suggest that the effect occurs at a level above the retina (Epstein et al., 1981; Bailliet et al., 1982). In any case, many dynamic and reactive sports require the ability to interpret blur associated with fast-moving targets or objects, and improvement of that ability may yield more consistent overall performance.

Dynamic visual acuity

An area of much interest to the sports vision community that is frequently discussed in relationship to static visual acuity is dynamic visual acuity (DVA). DVA is usually defined as a measure of sensitivity to visual detail when there is relative movement between the target and the observer, although it is typically measured as visual acuity during ocular pur-suit of a moving target (Geer and Robertson, 1993). Many sports create visual task demands which involve DVA and it has been demonstrated that this skill is trainable and can be improved with practice in the laboratory setting (Long and Rourke, 1989; Long and Riggs, 1991). There is ongoing debate about the relationship between static visual acuity and DVA that is partly attributable to the fact that DVA testing involves not only contrast discrimination but also precise eye movement ability to foveate the moving target. Hence, compromises in visual sensitivity *or* in oculomotor function may have a negative impact on DVA. Most studies have found a relatively low degree of predictive relationship between static and dynamic acuities (Miller and Ludvigh, 1962; Bergenson and Suzansky, 1973; Hoffman *et al.*, 1981), except in cases where static visual acuity is poor, DVA is also poor (Morrison, 1980).

Athletes are generally very interested in and engaged by DVA testing. The primary impediment to further work in this area is the absence of a commercially available instrument to provide the DVA stimulus. Such a device should project the target stimuli at distances greater than 3 m and should be capable of providing both rotational and linear sweep stimuli at variable speeds and exposure durations. Most DVA research has been conducted using lateral sweep stimuli, and it is reasonable to recommend this procedure as a clinical testing standard. Enhancement training could be conducted by utilizing the rotational stimulus.

Accommodation and vergence facility

Facility of accommodation and vergence is important in any sport that requires shifts of visual attention to targets at different distances from the athlete. Facility refers to the speed and ease with which accommodation and vergence can be adjusted rapidly to provide clear, single, binocular vision when looking, for example, from the ball during the tennis serve to the opponent at the other end of the court, or from the gauges of a racing motorcycle to the track ahead. This skill is easily measured and is quite amenable to enhancement training. In our experience, accommodative–vergence facility as measured with the Haynes distance rock test (Haynes, 1979; Haynes and McWilliams, 1979) has been a good discriminator of visual function between athletes and non-athletes. The distance rock test is described in Chapter 2, p. 32. Faster facility is desirable for athletes in virtually all dynamic, reactive sports.

Accommodation and vergence facilities are easily accessible using procedures which have been developed within the discipline of vision therapy (Griffin, 1982; Birnbaum, 1993; Calorosso and Rouse, 1993). Lens rock (stimulating and relaxing accommodation by viewing a target, alternately, through minus and plus power lenses) and prism rock (stimulating and relaxing vergence by viewing a target, alternately, through base-out and base-in prisms) procedures are frequently used to enhance accommodative and vergence facility. It is good to remember that binocular lens rock and prism rock provide a measure of *relative* facility, i.e. the lenses and prisms place demands on the visual system which are not encountered in the real world. For example, when viewing a target binocularly through a base-in prism, and attempting to maintain clarity and unity of the target, the demand on the visual system is to posture vergence at a point in space that is beyond the target plane where accommodation must be maintained. This demand is likely to stimulate sensory suppression in many athletes, so these procedures should always be administered using anaglyphic (red–green) or vectographic (polarized) target materials to avoid the unintended embedding of a sensory suppression tendency. *Absolute* accommodative facility can be enhanced by using lenses alternately to stimulate and relax accommodation while the athlete views the target monocularly.

Accommodative–vergence facility can be trained in a way that is more similar to the demands of sport by utilizing distance rock procedures. These procedures involve the use of multiple targets that contain a challenging visual acuity demand placed at different distances from the athlete. The athlete's task is to shift attention between the charts and identify the visual stimuli at progressively faster speeds. A metronome can be used to pace the activity. Demands for non-primary gaze positions can be satisfied by varying target placement or head position during the procedure. Anaglyphic or vectographic targets can be used if control of sensory suppression is desired.

If the practitioner seeks to improve the flexibility between accommodation and vergence postures, techniques which provide opposite stimulation to accommodation and vergence can be employed. These procedures, referred to as BIM/BOP techniques, can be very challenging and should be used judiciously with a specific goal in mind. The BIM procedure involves negative vergence (BI, base-in demand) and positive accommodation (M, minus lens demand) while the BOP procedure involves positive vergence (BO, base-out demand) and negative accommodation (P, plus lens demand). BIM/BOP demands can be created by using lens and prism flippers combined correctly, or by using free space fusion targets which the athlete fuses first orthopically (BIM) then chiastopically (BOP). When anaglyphic or vectographic targets that create vergence demands are used, the BIM/BOP demands can be created by combining a red–green or polaroid flipper with a lens flipper. These procedures should always be used with targets that allow for control of sensory suppression and accommodative response to ensure that the demands of the training activity are being met by both the motor and sensory processes involved.

Vergence stability and control

Control and stability of the vergence postural system is important in sports that require the precise spatial localization of visual targets. Spatial localization information is derived from both retinal information and from information related to activity of the extra-ocular muscles. There is ample research to support the relationship between activity of the vergence system and spatial localization for relatively close target distances (Papp and Ebenholtz, 1977; Ebenholtz and Wolfson, 1979; Ebenholtz and Fisher, 1982; Shebilske et al., 1983), but the common perspective among classical vision scientists is that binocular information from the extra-ocular muscles is not important for spatial localization of targets that are more than 1 or 2 metres away from the observer. Despite this, it has been the experience of many sports vision practitioners that elite athletes tend to possess uncommonly acute visual systems, and that dependable, consistent spatial information provided by any visual process will be utilized to refine spatial judgement in the competitive environment. Supportive evidence for this phenomenon has recently been reported for players from the Professional Golf Association Tour. Compared to age-matched skilled amateur golfers, the professional golfers were found to have faster 6-metre speed of stereopsis for obvious stimuli, and a significantly higher likelihood of being able to discern very subtle stereopsis stimuli (Coffey et al., 1994).

Highly skilled, elite athletes routinely demonstrate supranormal visual abilities. Sports vision practitioners respect this fact and hesitate to generalize to the elite athlete population the classical limitations in visual function found in laboratory studies usually performed with college students as subjects. Practitioners are routinely amazed by the tested visual functions of skilled athletes. Indeed, one problem which must be addressed in sports vision is the development of testing instruments which can measure the acute and subtle visual skills found among athletes. These skills often exceed those of the general population for whom the tests were originally designed.

Binocular vision

Practitioners of vision therapy and orthoptics have long realized the value of developing large vergence reserves for efficient nearpoint function. It is common, for example, to provide training activities which enhance positive relative convergence for the patient who presents with symptoms related to high nearpoint exophoria. Following this logic, some sports optometrists advocate the development of large 6 m vergence ranges for athletes as a means of general enhancement of visual function in sport. Although such treatment may be beneficial to the athlete who has a large distance phoria or intermittent distance strabismus, there appears to be no basis for distance vergence range expansion as a means to improve visual function in sport. Six-metre vergence range data collected using the protocols of the PSVPP indicate that elite athletes tend to have significantly narrower 6 m vergence ranges than do age-matched non-athletes (Coffey and Reichow, 1990). It has been suggested that the narrower, tighter 6 m vergence range found among most elite athletes may be related in some way to greater stability or precision in spatial information provided by the vergence system. Such explanatory notions are perhaps logical, but remain speculative at this point in time.

It has been shown that skilled golfers who have unstable 4 m fixation disparities tend to have greater errors in putting alignment than do golfers with stable fixation disparities (Coffey *et al.*, 1990). The effect is more associated with *stability* of the fixation disparity rather than *magnitude* of the disparity, and is more pronounced among golfers who are esophoric. If, in fact, vergence posture fluctuation or instability influences spatial localization consistency, it may be desirable to improve the control and stability of the vergence system. The athlete should be provided with feedback regarding vergence posture using anaglyphic or vectographic fixation disparity (or associated phoria) targets. Variations in the vergence posture should be noted, then the athlete should be encouraged to develop a 'feel' for vergence misalignment and learn the subtle vergence control necessary to overcome fluctuations in vergence alignment. It is sometimes useful to employ prisms to magnify the variable alignment tendency and thereby make it more noticeable to the athlete. Speed in attaining vergence realignment after prism insertion and removal should be emphasized, and prism powers should usually not exceed three or four prism dioptres. The vergence stability is likely to change with increased stress levels, so loading procedures should be incorporated into the training. There is also a tendency for phoria and fixation disparity to shift in an eso-ward direction when the athlete uses non-primary positions of gaze (Coffey *et al.*, 1991). It is therefore important to work on control of vergence posture in all gaze positions that are important in the specific sport.

Vergence biofeedback can be powerful tool in developing conscious control of vergence function (Halperin and Yolton, 1986). The authors utilize an infrared eye movement monitor with a feedback tone to develop fine, precise control of vergence in free space. Not only is this procedure useful in the specific development of vergence control, it also requires a certain mental state to attain that control. Many athletes have commented that the attentional set necessary to be successful during vergence biofeedback training is very similar to the attentional focus they attempt to achieve during competition. This phenomenon has been particularly noted by athletes who compete in sports with a primarily internal locus of control such as golf, trap-shooting and gymnastics.

Visual spatial perception

The presence or absence of the SILO phenomenon is interpreted as an indication of the athlete's biases in processing visual spatial information. SILO is an acronym that refers to visual perceptual effects associated with viewing a target through prisms, lenses or during binocular procedures that stimulate vergence with no direct concomitant stimulation of accommodation. An individual with a positive SILO response will perceive a target to be smaller (S) and closer (inward, I) when viewing the target through base-out prisms compared to viewing without prisms, and will perceive the target to be larger (L) and farther away (outward, O) when viewing through base-in prisms. A positive SILO response is thought to indicate that the athlete is giving preference to information provided by the extra-ocular muscles in order to reach the perceptual outcome in the following way. When the base-out prism is placed before the eyes, the athlete must increase vergence output in order to maintain sensory fusion. Increased vergence output is normally associated with a closer target and increased retinal image size. Since retinal image size is unchanged, the perceptual conclusion that prioritizes the vergence change is that the target has moved closer and simultaneously become smaller (SI). Parallel logic can be applied to the LO perceptual effect associated with base-in prism. If the athlete does not give priority to spatial information provided by the vergence system, but rather prioritizes retinal image information, a SOLI response may result. The SOLI response to base-out prism is interpreted in the following way. The vergence system provides information that the target has moved closer, but there is no increase in retinal image size as would be expected for a real target. The perceptual conclusion is that the target has simultaneously become smaller (as in the case of SILO) but, because retinal image size information predominates the perceptual outcome, the athlete concludes that the target has moved away (outward, O), as would be the case with decreasing retinal image size for targets in real space. An alternative interpretation (Birnbaum, 1993) of SILO/SOLI phenomena relates the different perceptual outcomes to the predominance of current retinal information (SILO) or the predominance of logic and past experience (SOLI). SILO awareness and consistency may also be influenced by general quality of binocularity.

The SILO phenomenon is trainable, and it may be worthwhile to pursue such training for athletes who participate in sports where varying vergence demands and precise spatial localization of targets at different distances from the athlete are typical. Alternatively, it could be argued that SOLI perceptual responses are desirable in sports such as rifle shooting or archery which have predominantly static target distances and demands for careful evaluation of retinal image information. Training procedures can be developed using hand-held prisms or vectographic slides projected to a distance of 3–6 m. It is not uncommon to find athletes who give mixed SILO/SOLI responses at different times or with different targets, or athletes who are insensitive to either the size or distance dimensions of the perceptual phenomena.

Many sports have demands for precise localization of targets that occur at different distances from the athlete (i.e. on the Z-axis). Any sport which requires catching or hitting a thrown ball incorporates these demands, and the visual motor timing necessary to succeed in such sport tasks is dependent on the athlete's ability to judge where the ball is in space and its rate of approach. This far-to-near perception of motion is mediated by many visual processes, one of which is the level of activity present in the vergence system. The procedures discussed below for enhancement of Z-axis target localization presume the presence of good binocular depth perception and this ability should be fully developed before proceeding with the Z-axis localization sequence. Depth perception should be assessed using either vectographic projection materials (Coffey and Reichow, 1990) or the BVAT instrument available from Mentor Ophthalmic Instruments. The BVAT device was used by the authors at the 1992 Bausch & Lomb Olympic Vision Centres and has been incorporated into the current version of the PSVPP.

Procedures to enhance the calibration of Z-axis spatial localization often take the form of directly viewed or projected vectograms (such as the Quoits rings) which the athlete must localize in space by means of a long hand-held pointer. The precise localization of the (apparently) floating target is influenced by the vergence demand set of the vectogram, the viewing distance, the interpupillary distance and the presence of significant fixation disparity. When the practitioner is satisfied that the athlete has developed stable and accurate Z-axis spatial localization, the training procedures can be further developed in several ways. The stimulus materials can be tachistoscopically presented to enhance speed of Z-axis localization. Dual vectograms with differing vergence demands can briefly be presented and the athlete challenged to determine the relative spatial positions of the two targets. Contrast can be reduced by placing dark surfaces behind the vectographic images, thus incorporating a contrast discrimination component into the spatial localization task. Each of these variations on the Z-axis localization technique takes the enhancement training a few steps closer to the actual visual demands faced during competition and thus improves transference of the training to the sport environment.

Localization of targets on the X and Y axes is a visual task demanded by many sports such as trapshooting, football, basketball and racquet sports. There is little historical work regarding measurement or enhancement of this type of spatial localization. The authors have developed a procedure at Pacific University that has proved useful in this area. The athlete is seated and views a projection screen with a central fixation target. Targets are then presented tachistoscopically in the periphery of the screen. Immediately after target presentation, the athlete uses a small tripod-mounted laser to indicate the perceived position of the peripheral target. The procedure is useful in refining X–Y axis localization accuracy, and can easily be loaded by presentation of simultaneous central and peripheral targets or multiple peripheral targets.

We have experimented with several procedures designed to assess and enhance the accuracy of spatial imagery. It is often recommended that athletes practise imagery or visualization activities as an adjunct to active physical skills training. Such training activities are considered to have the best efficacy if the imagery is vivid, multisensory and accurately calibrated in terms of temporal and spatial factors (Harris and Harris, 1984). If imagery activities do, in some sense, replace (or supplement) active practice, it seems important that the spatial aspects of the mental imagery be accurately calibrated in terms of real space. A procedure that may provide insight to these issues requires the athlete to make real space judgements based upon a visual image stored in short-term memory. The athlete is first asked to toss beanbags to an array of targets placed on the ground in an arc at varying distances. An assessment is made of any habitual error tendencies. The targets are then moved slightly, the athlete views the array and generates an image of the new target locations. The athlete then closes the eyes and is asked to toss the beanbags to each target in a random order given by the practitioner. After all the beanbags have been tossed, the athlete and practitioner review the tosses for any rightward, leftward, long or short error tendencies which may be present in the imaged spatial array that were not present when tossing the beanbags initially with the eyes open. This procedure is confounded by the many motor variables involved, but has been well received by athletes as a means of improving the vividness and precision of spatial imagery.

Visual processing speed

Tachistoscopic procedures have been used for over forty years by vision therapists and other professionals interested in improving the perceptual speed or span of visual recognition (Olsen, 1956; Dumler, 1958). These procedures have been adopted by many sports vision practitioners and may have utility in the context of reducing the amount of time the athlete must look at a target or situation in order to derive meaning from the visual information available. This ability has obvious application in dynamic, reactive sport situations. Most of the classical tachistoscopic procedures have used, as stimuli, number or letter sequences presented in the centre of the visual field. Such targets tend to engage the verbal aspects of information processing which may be relevant to tasks such as reading, but which probably have much less relevance to the task demands of sport. As such, it is perhaps more appropriate to use targets other than letters or numbers when using tachistoscopic procedures for the purpose of optometric sports enhancement training. Perhaps the best targets for this training would be provided by virtual reality technology (Rheingold, 1991) and would portray actual sport situations and require visual decision making. Unfortunately, useful and affordable vitual reality devices are not yet available. Nor are 35 mm projection slides that could be used with conventional tachistoscopes. Targets which require visual search for a specific target amidst an array of novel geometric forms may have some utility, as, perhaps, would targets which require some type of spatial judgement related to the task demands of the particular sport.

Visual reaction and response speed

Speed of reaction and response to visual information is a critical component of performance in dynamic, reactive sports. These factors are important also in many non-dynamic sports where a motor response must be precisely timed to coincide with a particular imagery state or attentional focus. Visual reaction speed is defined as the elapsed time between the onset of a visual stimulus and the

initiation of a motor response to that stimulus. Response speed is defined as the elapsed time between the onset of visual stimulus and the completion of a motor response to that stimulus (Coffey and Reichow, 1990). The authors utilize the Reaction Plus instrument as the standard for evaluation of eye–hand and eye–foot visual reaction and response speeds, and also as the instrument of choice for determining efficacy of procedures designed to improve these abilities. Though reaction and response speeds can likely be positively influenced by many different enhancement procedures, most sports optometrists use some type of eye–hand coordinator to enhance these skills.

Eye-hand coordination

Several manufacturers have developed eye–hand coordination training instruments. The Wayne Engineering Saccadic Fixator (described in Chapter 2) was the first instrument to be marketed and has been redesigned at least twice to add new features. This device is probably the most widely used eye–hand coordinator available. A newer device, the AcuVision 1000 (International AcuVision Systems Inc.) incorporates state-of-the-art technology and can be connected to a computer for storage and analysis of athletes' testing and training results. The AcuVision has been redesigned since its initial entry into the market, and the current model is lightweight and easily portable. Other devices such as the EyeSpan (the instrument used in the development of the early PSVPP normative data) and the DynaVision, while offering desirable features for enhancement training, are either no longer available or have unreliable distribution and service networks.

Probably both the Saccadic Fixator and the AcuVision have a place in sports vision practice. The AcuVision 1000 differs from the Saccadic Fixator in that it presents a larger target area for stimulus presentation (Figure 8.1), records an analysis of the athlete's per-

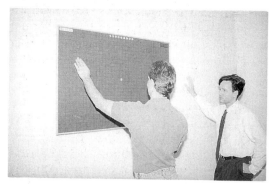

Figure 8.1   AcuVision 1000 (International Acu-Vision Systems Inc.)

formance in different quadrants of the target field, enables variable stimulus light intensities and utilizes pressure-sensitive film switches which require precise spatial responses to the target stimuli. The Saccadic Fixator enables the connection of accessory response devices which may be useful for other aspects of evaluation or training. It utilizes mechanical switches which require less precision to depress than those of the AcuVision. The difference in switching between the two instruments probably makes the Saccadic Fixator more appropriate for response *speed* training while the AcuVision is more appropriate for response *precision* training.

In studies at Pacific University, it has been found that relatively brief training periods (15 days at 10 minutes per day) using basic eye–hand coordination training procedures will yield a significant improvement in eye–hand response speed, and will also yield significant gains in eye–hand reaction speed for some individuals (Reichow and Coffey, 1986). These studies utilized training activities which emphasized speed of response. When the training emphasis is placed upon precision of the response (for example requiring the athlete to respond to target lights using only the tip of one finger versus using the entire surface of the hand), the positive effect upon response speed is reduced. When utilizing eye–hand coordination training, the sports vision practitioner must carefully consider the

visual task demands of the athlete's sport to determine whether speed or precision training (or both) should be emphasized in the athlete's programme. Speed training, for example, might be emphasized for the hockey player or football receiver, while precision training might be emphasized for the fencer, trapshooter or gymnast.

When improvements in visual reaction and response speeds are a goal of an enhancement training programme, we often recommend that the athlete participate in other sport activities which require fast eye–hand responses. Racquet sports such as table tennis, racquetball and squash are useful as supplemental training activities. We have also found it useful to consult with coaches and physical trainers who specialize in speed training. Such interaction can open new doors for training approaches, and provides mutual education for optometrists and sports training personnel.

Peripheral vision

Many sports require fast responses to peripheral visual information, particularly team sports in which the players must maintain awareness of the ball or goal in central vision while simultaneously tracking team mates and opponents in peripheral vision. The eye–hand coordinator devices may be useful in improving integration of central and peripheral visual processing, especially if the practitioner uses training procedures that require central processing (such as calling letters from a chart or playing catch with beanbags) simultaneously with peripheral processing (such as depressing the target buttons on the eye–hand coordinator).

Another device available from Wayne Engineering, the Peripheral Awareness Tester/Trainer (PATT) (Figure 8.2), is a rather odd-looking instrument which is useful not only for testing peripheral eye–hand response speed, but also for training integration of central and peripheral visual processing. In

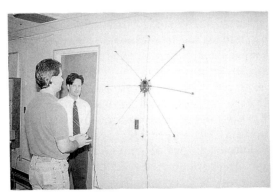

Figure 8.2 The Peripheral Awareness Tester (Wayne Engineering)

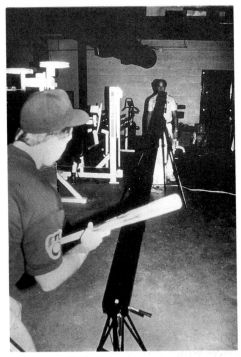

Figure 8.3 The Bassin Anticipation Timer (Wayne Engineering). (From Berman, 1993, by permission of Appleton and Lange Inc.)

the training mode, the device presents a blinking central fixation light and random stimulus lights in the periphery. The athlete must time the motor response (via a hand-held joystick) to the peripheral stimulus to coincide with the moment when the blinking central stimulus is on. The instrument is self-pacing, so that the blink rate of the central stimulus is increased when the athlete is successful in training and decreased when errors occur. The difficulty of the training task can be modified by adding loading activities or by changing illumination levels.

Visual motor reaction and response speeds are critical components of visual anticipation timing. Anticipation timing is a larger concept that encompasses not only the reaction and response speeds as such, but also the timing of the visual motor actions when a visual target can be seen moving prior to the response. The Bassin Anticipation Timer (Figure 8.3) is the standard instrument for assessing anticipation timing, and it is also used in different ways for enhancement training. It consists of several interlocking rails with a row of red lights which sequentially illuminate at different rates of speed. The sequential illumination of the lights simulates a moving target. By positioning the athlete in different areas, the simulated moving stimulus can appear to move toward or away from the athlete, or from right to left or left to right. In any case,

the athlete's task is to make a motor response at the precise moment that the last light on the rail illuminates. The control panel then displays the temporal relationship (amount of time early or late) between the motor response and the onset of the final stimulus light. The authors recommend using a set of rails at least 6 m in length and using a protocol which encourages the athlete to become internally calibrated regarding visual-motor timing characteristics. After each response, the athlete should be asked whether they think the response was early or late, and training should be structured to refine the precision of the response and also the internal awareness of any response errors. Speed of stimulus movement can be adjusted over a wide range, and the rails can be adjusted to mimic the types of target movement typically encountered in different sports.

Biofeedback

Biofeedback is used for the purposes of monitoring many physiological processes which are predominantly controlled by the autonomic nervous system. Processes which are routinely monitored for the purpose of biofeedback include heart rate, skin temperature, respiration and muscle tension. Optometric biofeedback procedures have been utilized for remediation of many categories of visual dysfunction (Halperin and Yolton, 1986), and have been previously recommended in this chapter for the purpose of developing conscious control of vergence function. Roncagli (1993) has endeavoured to integrate biofeedback procedures into the practice of sports optometry for two primary purposes: to facilitate the development of automaticity of visual functions deemed critical in sport performance, and to provide athletes with feedback regarding physiological stress responses while they practise visually dependent sport skills.

Information presented at the beginning of this chapter discussed how visual inefficiency may cause an excessive draw upon our moment-to-moment limited pool of attentional energy. Excessive attentional demands may elicit a generalized stress response that will compromise sport performance. Visual abilities that have been developed to a skilled level require less attention and become more automatic or reflexive. For overall performance to remain unaffected by visual factors, all visual skills that are critical in a given sport should be developed to a level of automaticity. Automaticity implies stress-free function even in demanding competitive situations. Biofeedback procedures may be helpful in attaining automaticity of visual skills that have been enhanced in a training programme. After athletes have developed good control of particular visual abilities and can maintain these abilities with progressively greater loading, they can be provided with an appropriate form of biofeedback that will generate an auditory or other signal when the stress response rises above a permissible level. The biofeedback is incorporated into the final stages of the enhancement training until the athlete can maintain accurate visual function in the presence of external stressors without experiencing a negative physiological stress response. As an example of this principle, consider the soccer player with an intermittent exotropia of the divergence excess type. With training, the athlete will develop the ability to overcome the intermittent strabismus and to maintain fusion during competition. Initially, it may require a significant commitment of conscious attention to make the convergence movement necessary to overcome the exo strabismus without a concomitant over-accommodation causing blur. With further training, the compensation for the exo tendency becomes increasingly automatic until the athlete is able to perform multiple soccer-related tasks without losing binocular sensory fusion and accurate spatial perception. The biofeedback is added at this point to facilitate the development of full automaticity of the binocular skills without eliciting a negative stress response.

Roncagli (1993) has taken this enhancement procedure one step further by fitting athletes with small portable biofeedback devices which can be used during practice for competition. The strategy is to create a situation that closely mimics actual competition, then to present the athlete with competitive situations that incorporate the visual functions that have been the target of the enhancement training programme. The goal of athletes is to respond appropriately to the competitive tasks while maintaining a state of nervous system arousal that does not exceed their range of optimal function.

Stress, and the physiological changes which comprise the stress response, are inherent in competitive sport. Elite athletes have developed ways to control their stress response in order to stay in the zone of optimum physiological arousal that allows the best overall sensory motor function. Since many aspects of visual function are susceptible to stress responses, it seems reasonable that biofeedback procedures may well have a place in the repertoire of the successful sports vision practitioner.

Summary

This chapter presents an introduction and overview of visual performance enhancement training in sports optometry. Several general and specific enhancement procedures are discussed. These procedures represent a modest sampling of the varied approaches that have been created and developed by sports optometry practitioners. Many additional techniques exist that expand the concepts presented here. The authors hope that this small contribution to the growing literature related to sports vision will encourage other practitioners to share their ideas, approaches and findings so that we may all become more successful in assisting athletes to reach their competitive potentials. While some practitioners argue against any degree of standardization within the discipline, the very lack of standardization makes it much more difficult to disseminate accurate and useful knowledge to practitioners and athletes alike. Without a shared, standardized core of knowledge, sports vision specialists are less able to communicate with each other. This inability to communicate impedes progress in the discipline and presents the public with a very uneven impression of sports optometry practice. As our knowledge base grows, so too does our responsibility to share that knowledge with fellow practitioners and with the sporting public.

Acknowledgements

Some of the principles and concepts presented in this chapter were derived from experimental work supported by Pacific University, Bausch & Lomb, and Vistakon Inc. The authors gratefully acknowledge their support in the ongoing development of the discipline of sports optometry.

References

Bailliet, R., Clay, A. and Blood, K. (1982) The training of visual acuity in myopia. *Journal of the American Optometric Association*, **53**, 719–24

Bergenson, P.E. and Suzansky, J.W. (1973) An investigation of dynamic and static visual acuity. *Perception*, **12**, 343–56

Berman, A.M. (1993) Clinical evaluation of the athlete. *Optometry Clinics*, **3**(1), 1–26

Birnbaum, M.H. (1993) *Optometric Management of Nearpoint Vision Disorders*, Butterworth-Heinemann, Stoneham, Mass.

Broadbent, D.E. (1982) Task combination and selective intake of information. *Acta Psychologica*, **50**, 253–90

Caloroso, E.E. and Rouse, M.W. (1993) *Clinical Management of Strabismus*, Butterworth-Heinemann, Stoneham, Mass.

Christenson, G.N. and Winkelstein, A.M. (1988) Visual skills of athletes versus nonathletes: development of a sports vision testing battery. *Journal of the American Optometric Association*, **59**, 666–75

Coffey, B. and Reichow, A.W. (1987) Guidelines for screening and testing the athlete's visual system, part III. Optometric Extension Program Foundation. *Curriculum II*, **59**(7), 355–68

Coffey, B. and Reichow, A.W. (1990) Optometric evaluation of the elite athlete: the Pacific Sports Visual Performance Profile. *Problems in Optometry*, **1**(2), 32–58

Coffey, B. and Reichow, A.W. (1993) Athletes vs. nonathletes: static visual acuity, contrast sensitivity, and dynamic visual acuity. *Journal of the American Optometry Association*, submitted for publication.

Coffey, B., Mathison, T., Viker, M. *et al.* (1990) Visual alignment considerations in golf putting consistency. In *Science and Golf* (ed. A.J. Cochran) E & FN Spon, London

Coffey, B., Reichow, A.W., Colburn, P.B. and Clark, D.L. (1991) Influence of ocular gaze and head position on 4m heterophoria and fixation disparity. *Optometry and Vision Science*, **68**, 893–8

Coffey, B., Reichow, A.W., Johnson, T. and Yamane, S. (1994) Visual performance differences among professional, amateur, and senior amateur golfers. In *Science and Golf II* (eds A.J. Cochran and M.R. Farrally) E&FN Spon, London

Collins, F.L., Pbert, L.A. and Gil, K.M. (1984) The effects of behavioral training for improving visual acuity in emmetropic and myopic volunteers. *Behavioral Medicine Abstracts*, **5**, 142–4

Downing, C.J. and Pinker, S. (1985) The spatial structure of visual attention. In *Attention and Performance XI* (eds M.I. Posner and O.S.M. Marin) Lawrence Erlbaum Associates, Hillsdale, NJ, pp 171–87

Dumler M.J. (1958) A study of factors related to gains in the reading rate of college students trained with the tachistoscope and accelerator. *Journal of Educational Research*, **52**, 27–30

Ebenholtz, S.M. and Fisher, S.K. (1982) Distance adaptation depends upon the plasticity in the oculomotor control system. *Perception and Psychophysics*, **31**, 551–60

Ebenholtz, S.M. and Wolfson, D.M. (1979) Perceptual after-effects of sustained convergence. *Perception and Psychophysics*, **17**, 485–91

Epstein, L.H., Greenwald, D.J., Hennon, D. and Heldorn B. (1981) Monocular fading and feedback training. *Behavior Modification*, **5**, 171–86

Ewalt, H.W. (1946) The Baltimore myopia control project. *Journal of the American Optometric Association*, **17**, 167–85

Finke, R. (1986) Mental imagery and the visual system. *Scientific American*, **254**(3), 88–95

Geer, I. and Robertson, K.M. (1993) Measurement of central and peripheral dynamic visual acuity thresholds during ocular pursuit of a moving target. *Optometry and Vision Science*, **70**, 552–60

Gil, K.M. and Collins, F.L. (1983) Behavioral training for myopia: generalization of effects. *Behavioral Research and Therapy*, **21**, 269–73

Gil, K.M., Collins, F.L. and Odom, J.V. (1986) The effects of behavioral vision training on multiple aspects of visual functioning in myopic adults. *Journal of Behavioral Medicine*, **9**, 373–87

Griffin, J.R. (1982) *Binocular Anomalies: Procedures for Vision Therapy*, 2nd edn, Professional Press Books, New York

Halperin, E. and Yolton, R.L. (1986) Ophthalmic applications of biofeedback. *American Journal of Optometry and Physiological Optics*, **63**, 985–98

Harris, D.V. and Harris, B.L. (1984) *The Athlete's Guide to Sports Psychology: Mental Skills for Physical People*, Leisure Press, New York

Haynes, H.M. (1979) The distance rock test – a preliminary report. *Journal of the American Optometric Association*, **50**, 707–13

Haynes, H.M. and McWilliams, L.G. (1979) Effects of training on near–far response time as measured by the distance rock test. *Journal of the American Optometric Association*, **50**, 715–18

Heil, J. (1984) Imagery for sport: theory, research, and practice. In *Cognitive Sport Psychology* (eds W.F. Straub and J.M. Williams), Sport Science Associates, Lansing, NY, pp. 245–52

Hoffman, L.G., Rouse, M. and Ryan, J.B. (1981) Dynamic visual acuity: a review. *Journal of the American Optometric Association*, **52**, 883–7

Long, G.M. and Riggs, C.A. (1991) Training effects on dynamic visual acuity with free-head viewing. *Perception*, **20**, 363–71

Long, G.M. and Rourke, D.A. (1989) Training effects on the resolution of moving targets – dynamic visual acuity. *Human Factors*, **31**, 443–51

McLeod, B. (1985) Field dependence as a factor in sports with preponderance of open or closed skills. *Perceptual and Motor Skills*, **60**, 369–70

Miller, J.W. and Ludvigh, E. (1962) The effect of relative motion on visual acuity. *Survey of Ophthalmology*, **7**, 83–116

Morrison, T.R. (1980) A review of dynamic visual acuity. *National Aerospace Medicine Research Laboratory Monograph 28*, Pensacola, Fla

Navon, D. (1985) Attention division or attention sharing? In *Attention and Performance XI* (eds M.I. Posner and O.S.M. Marin), Lawrence Erlbaum, Hillsdale, NJ, pp 133–46

Olsen, E.A. (1956) Relationship between psychological capacities and success in college athletes. *Research Quarterly of the American Association for Health and Physical Education*, **27**, 79–89

Papp, K.R. and Ebenholtz, S.M. (1977) Concomitant direction and distance after-effects of sustained convergence: a muscle potentiation explanation for eye-specific adaptation. *Perception and Psychophysics*, **21**, 307–14

Posner, M.I. (1980) *Chronometric Explorations of Mind*, Lawrence Erlbaum, Hillsdale, NJ

Poulton, E.C. (1957) On prediction in skilled movements. *Psychological Bulletin*, **54**, 467–78

Raiport, G. (1988) *Red Gold*, Jeremy Tarcher, Los Angeles, CA

Reichow, A.W. and Coffey, B. (1986) Enhancement of visual abilities associated with sports vision training. Abstract, in *American Journal of Optometry and Physiological Optics*, **63**(10), 80P

Reichow, A.W. and Coffey, B., Walker, C.M. and Velenousky, D.A. (1985) Visual evaluation of the elite athlete: optometric visual performance profiling. Abstract in *American Journal of Optometry and Physiological Optics*, **62**(10), 81P

Rheingold H. (1991) *Virtual Reality*, Touchstone Simon & Schuster, New York

Ricci, J.A. and Collins, F.L. (1988) Visual acuity improvement following fading and feedback training – III: effects on acuity for stimuli in the natural environment. *Behavioral Research and Therapy*, **26**, 475–80

Roncagli, V. (1993) Uses of biofeedback in sports optometry. Paper presented to the Annual Meeting of the American Optometric Association Sports Vision Section, Anaheim, Ca. Tape-recorded transcript available from American Optometric Association Sports Vision Section, St Louis, Mo.

Rowe, A.J. (1947) Orthoptic training to improve the visual acuity of a myope. *Journal of the American Optometric*

Association, **24**, 494

Shebilske, W.L., Karmiohl, C.M. and Profit, D.R. (1983) Induced esophoric shifts in eye convergence and illusory distance in reduced and structured viewing conditions. *Journal of Experimental Psychology: Human Perception and Performance*, **9**, 270–7

Sports Vision Section, American Optometric Association (1984, 1985, 1988, 1993) *Sports Vision Guidebook*, St Louis, Mo.

Suinn, R.M. (1984) Imagery and sports. In *Cognitive Sport Psychology* (eds W.F. Straub and J.M. Williams), Sport Science Associates, Lansing, NY, pp. 253–71

Woods, A.C. (1945) Report from the Wilmer Institute on the results obtained in the treatment of myopia by visual training. *Transactions of the American Academy of Ophthalmology and Otolaryngology*, **49**, 37–65

Setting up a sports vision practice

Alan Berman

Philosophy of sports vision

The basic premise of sports vision depends on the concept that the eyes feed information to the brain which in turn interprets the information to set the arms, hands, legs, feet and the body's balance system in motion. This happens within a fraction of a second, over and over again, for the duration of play. However, if the eye's message is inaccurate, incomplete or not at the correct time – performance may suffer.

The range of services provided by people who call themselves sports vision specialists may vary from fitting a contact lens, or supplying protective eye wear to providing a detailed diagnostic battery of sports vision tests or assisting with enhancement or training to help any weak areas. It does not matter which level of care is provided, the important thing is that the athlete is helped to maximize his or her potential and perhaps improve their competitive edge.

There are some unique responsibilities for those becoming involved in this specialty. First, one should learn the rules and regulations of the game and know the specifics and nuances of each sport. One should also read up about sports, attend every local game, as far as possible, listen to radio and television broadcasts or, preferably, actively participate in sports oneself. This will give the most understanding of any particular sport and vision's role in it. Secondly, it helps to keep informed about local teams, and know the standings and the names of the players. Finally, a vision consultant to a team is responsible for being on hand to replace lost contact lenses or provide on-site first aid for ocular trauma. Therefore, as most games are not normally played during office hours, the sports vision specialist must be ready to provide round-the-clock coverage.

The market

Many people ask whether there is a market for sports vision: however, to understand the potential fully one should look at the demographics of sports participation. The world is sports crazy! Millions of people participate in sports activities, whether it be in a team or as an individual. Moreover, many sports activities have demonstrated significant growth, and in some cases numbers of participants have almost doubled in recent times. All activities have sizeable bases of millions of participants providing potential market opportunities. A market survey undertaken on behalf of the Institute of Sports Vision concluded that in many activities over 50% of those involved in any sport had been so for at least four years (Payne, 1991, p. 31). Many of the most frequent participants in a sport also participate in many other sports during the year and at least one-third of the participants are also involved in at least five other sports (Payne, 1991, p. 37). From a marketing perspective, this makes it very easy to reach the active sport participant. Collectively, as a group, participants in many sporting activities have very attractive demographics, and advertisers spend enormous sums of money to attract them. While demographics vary from one sport to another, generally speaking, participants are relatively young, affluent and professional (Loran, 1992) and reside in metropolitan market environments, which make them relatively easy to reach with a message. More specifically, many of these participants are already of an age where glasses are usually or imminently needed, have an income high enough to afford spending on improving their performance and some may have health insurance which covers the costs associated with examinations and training. Sports enthusiasts spend a significant amount of money annually on equipment to participate in activities and to improve their performance. In the United States, enthusiasts spent almost $30 billion in 1989 on various products associated with their sports (Payne, 1991, p. 42). In the equipment market, large sums were spent in golf, hunting, fishing and camping. In total, it was estimated that over $300 million was spent specifically on optical goods alone related to these activities (Payne, 1991, p. 42).

History

Prior to the sports vision examination, a thorough visual history is necessary. In addition to general health questions, a sports-specific questionnaire such as that shown in Figure 9.1 should be given to the athlete. This should include questions regarding the form of visual correction used on the field; visual symptoms such as blurred or double vision experienced while playing; consistency of performance under various lighting conditions; concentration ability and goals from an athletic and visual standpoint. This gives the practitioner an understanding of how the athlete perceives his or her problem, how it affects the athletic performance and how motivated the athlete is to correct it. This questionnaire aims to extract information which will, in turn, lead to a positive effect on the athlete's performance both on the field and in everyday life. Sports vision specialists should create their own sports case history questionnaire or these can be obtained from some of the various contact lens manufacturers.

Examination and instrumentation

Surprisingly little space is needed to provide sports vision services in a practice. A small room can be used for sports vision diagnostic testing. Training requires more equipment, but this can usually be stored relatively easily. If a larger room is available, then a careful plan is required as to where all the equipment should go. Room for walking rails, balance boards and wall space for certain instruments should be considered. The room should be set up so that the athlete can move freely from one test to another according to the battery of tests provided. When sports vision testing is carried out on-site, however, one must adapt to the space allotted. Testing in strange places, such as the visiting team locker or shower room, is remarkably frequent. Things should be planned so that there is a smooth flow from one test to the next, with adequate lighting and clear markings where the athlete should stand for each test (Figures 9.2, 9.3).

Initially, a comprehensive eye examination should be undertaken, including refraction and testing of binocular function. Any pathol-

CASE HISTORY QUESTIONNAIRE

This evaluation is designed specifically for athletes. The purpose is to evaluate the efficiency of those visual skills necessary for peak sports performance. Our goal is to assist you in reaching your potential. Please consider all questions carefully and answer as thoroughly and accurately as possible.

☐ Yes ☐ No   1. Have you ever had a complete visual examination by an eye care practitioner?
    a. If yes, when was your first examination? _____
    b. If yes, when was your most recent examination? _____

☐ Yes ☐ No   2. Have you ever been involved in a visual training programme? _____
    a. If yes, when and for what reason(s)? _____
    b. If yes, do you feel it was successful? _____
    Explain _____

☐ Yes ☐ No   3. Do you wear glasses?
    a. If yes, how old are they? _____
    Are they satisfactory at present? Yes No
    When used? Near distance Far distance Both
    During sports? Yes No
    b. If you do not wear glasses, have you ever had glasses in the past? Yes No
    If yes, when and why did you stop wearing them? _____

☐ Yes ☐ No   4. Do you presently wear contact lenses? If yes, what type?
    soft rigid gas permeable
    a. If yes, do you wear them during your sport? Yes No
    Do you wear them all day? Yes No
    When did you last have them checked by your eye doctor? _____
    List any problems with your present lenses _____
    b. If you do not wear contact lenses, have you ever had contact lenses in the past? Yes No If yes, when and why did you stop wearing them? _____

☐ Yes ☐ No   5. Do you ever see blur?
    a. If yes, where? Near distance Far distance How often? _____
    b. During sports? Yes No How often? _____
    If yes, please describe _____

☐ Yes ☐ No   6. Do you ever see double?
    a. If yes, where? Near distance Far distance How often? _____
    b. During sports? Yes No How often? _____
    If yes, please describe _____

☐ Yes ☐ No   7. Do you ever feel you have difficulty 'keeping your eye' on a moving object? If yes, please cite examples and describe _____

☐ Yes ☐ No   8. Do you notice variations in your performance during a game or event?
☐ Yes ☐ No   9. Do you notice variations in your performance over a period of time such as in a tournament?
    10. Performance is most consistent _____ (during) sports performance.
    a. early b. later c. equal throughout
☐ Yes ☐ No 11. Is performance consistent during critical competition situations?
☐ Yes ☐ No 12. Is your performance the same for night competition as for day competition?
☐ Yes ☐ No 13. Do you experience loss of concentration during sports performance?
    Explain _____
☐ Yes ☐ No 14. Cite examples related to questions 8–13. _____

☐ Yes ☐ No 15. Are you experiencing any visual difficulties? If yes, please describe _____

    16. a. Please rate your feeling regarding the importance of vision in your sport (1 = not important, 9 = extremely important) 1 2 3 4 5 6 7 8 9
    b. How do you feel vision is important in your particular sport? _____

☐ Yes ☐ No 17. Do you use visualization/imagery techniques? If yes, please describe _____

☐ Yes ☐ No 18. Have you ever suffered head injury: or have you ever had injury, surgery, infection, or disease involving your eyes? _____

    19. Further information (list any other visual performance concerns that you may have) _____

Figure 9.1 Sports vision case history questionnaire. (After B. Coffey and A.W. Reichow, 1990; adapted from the Pacific Sports Vision Performance Profile)

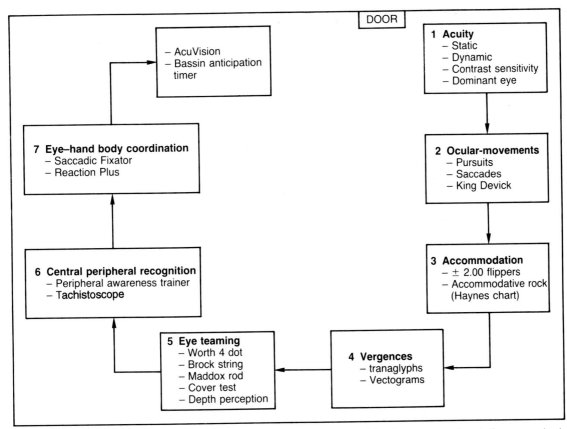

Figure 9.2 Flow diagram of equipment arranged so that the subject can move freely from one test to another

ogy should be noted, which should include the taking of retinal photographs as they are important regarding combat sports, such as boxing. Visual fields should also be documented as it is important to note any blind areas which the player may be unaware of. The second half of the examination consists of tests given in free space to evaluate such factors as peripheral skills, eye–hand–foot coordination, reflexes, dynamic visual acuity, depth perception, contrast sensitivity, eye dominance and other visual reflexes. After the evaluation, complete sports vision training programmes can be developed to improve and correct specific deficiencies.

There are many instruments that can be used in a sports vision work-up which do not necessarily have to be sophisticated or expensive. Indeed, a handful of simple tests, using very inexpensive equipment, can reveal significant information regarding how an athlete's eyes are affecting his or her performance (Table 9.1). If further insight into the role of different visual skills on the playing field is required, then specialized sports vision equipment can be purchased (Table 9.2). The battery of diagnostic tests should relate to the specifics of the sport itself (Table 9.3) and the practitioner should pick and choose which tests to perform on each individual athlete. Athletes are highly dynamic and therefore the instruments should be as closely related to the sport as possible; existing instruments should be adapted to meet the needs of each sport. The most effective testing should be performed in free space in the athlete's particular

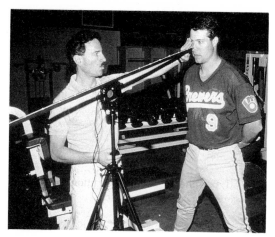

Figure 9.3 An athlete is shown being tested with the Visflex which is an electronic version of the Brock string (Wayne Engineering). Other equipment is seen in the background

position, such as the crouch of the hockey goalie or the basketball player looking up at the rim, and also in the nine cardinal positions of gaze. The optimum training involves all of the above, but with added stress to enhance the performance or make it harder – prisms, plus or minus lenses, on a balance board or with noise in the background. Most importantly, however, it is necessary to know the sport and its visual demands (see Table 2.1). One excellent source of this information is the *Sports Vision Guidebook* (Carlson, 1991), published by the American Optometric Association, which considers each sport as follows: an overview of the sport; visual skills important to the sport; terminology of the game; testing procedures specific to those visual skills; vision training techniques to remedy or enhance those skills; the most common ocular injuries; emergency first aid; protective eye wear for that sport; a bibliography for the sports vision consultant with reference to that sport. Additionally, as mentioned in the introduction to this chapter, the practitioner should observe or preferably play the sport.

When undertaking a sports vision evaluation, an explanation should be given regarding the test being done and how it relates to

the particular sport so that it makes sense to both the athlete and coach. Ensure that the tests are applied as closely as possible to the sport situation, such as measuring a phoria in upgaze for volleyball or in downgaze for hockey. Do not give in-instrument and near-point training unless the athlete performs at that distance, which very few do.

A new practice management tool is now available to help those in the eye care business. This is a computer software program which runs on an IBM compatible system. A demonstration disc is available from the company, Bright Eye-Deas, Inc. (see Appendix 2). It is called OPIS (Optometric Patient Information System) and it allows the eye care professional with creative means to instantly produce detailed eye care reports summarizing a particular patient's examination findings and eye care recommendations. It is a menu driven system which allows the user to customize a report by simply keying in to those items on the menu that pertain to the patient's ocular and visual conditions. In addition to the reports (which can be used to

Table 9.1 Basic sports vision equipment

Accommodative rock charts (i.e. Hayne's chart)
Aperture rule
Balance beam
Bar readers
Brock string
Depth perception test
Dominant eye card (hole in card or tube)
Flippers
Loose lenses
Maddox rod card
Marsden ball
Pegboard rotator
Projected King-Devick saccade test
Prisms
Strobe light
Tachistoscope
Vectograms
Worth 4 dot

Source: Institute for Sports Vision

Table 9.2   Advanced sports vision equipment

AcuVision saccadic board (AcuVision Systems, Inc.)

Bassin anticipation timer (Lafayette Instrument Co.)

Computer orthoptics (R.C. Instruments)

Contrast sensitivity chart (Stereo Optical, Vector Vision)

Dynamic visual acuity tester (J.W. Engineering)

Peripheral awareness trainer (Wayne Engineering)

Quick Feet (Sports Robots, Inc.)

Reaction Plus timer – hand/foot speed (W.R. Medical Electronics)

Saccadic Fixator (Wayne Engineering)

Saccadic Fixator options (balance board, accommodative board, visual stick-ups, speed track)

Visflex Automated Brock string (Wayne Engineering)

Source: Institute for Sports Vision
See also Appendix 2.

Table 9.3   Sports vision tests

Acuity: static, dynamic, contrast sensitivity

Oculo-movements: saccades, pursuits, projected King-Devick

Accommodation: ±2.00 flippers, distance accommodative rock (Hayne's chart)

Vergences (base-in/base-out): vectograms, (tranaglyphs)

Eye teaming: depth perception, Worth 4 dot, Maddox rod, cover test, Brock string

Central/peripheral visual recognition: peripheral awareness trainer, tachistoscope

Eye–hand–body coordination: AcuVision 1000, Bassin anticipation timer, Quick Feet, Reaction Plus

Miscellaneous: colour vision; night vision; strobe (visual concentration); dominant eye/hand/foot; retinal photography; automated visual fields (perimetry)

give to the patient or as a referral letter to another health professional), OPIS has other sections relating to specialty areas such as contact lenses, vision therapy, low vision, eye wear dispensing and sports vision. The sports vision section is a good overview for the general practitioner who wants to incorporate sports vision into his practice. The menu includes some of the following items: a description of how the patient's eye condition may affect his or her particular sport; visual skills important to sport in general; a description of each sports vision testing procedure and how it relates to each sport; specific office policies regarding training sessions, payment schedules and other practice management guidelines.

Staffing the practice

Some practices already employ a general vision therapist, whose role is to train vision skills (see Chapter 11). However, a prerequisite for any sports vision therapist is a genuine interest in sport. Candidates for sports vision therapists should preferably have flexible hours and might include other staff members, patients that have received vision therapy themselves, teachers and coaches. The therapist must be available when the patients need them, which may include weekends and evenings. Sufficient time must be given to train the vision therapist who must have a thorough understanding of the visual skills important to sports and how they relate to sports performance. They must be competent with each piece of equipment, practising on the optometrist and other staff members at first, before working with the athlete/'patient'. The flow from optometrist to therapist can work in the following manner – at the end of the general examination and sports vision work-up, therapy is discussed with the patient. If the patient expresses an interest in continuing, then an introduction to the therapist is arranged. At that time insurance forms together with the procedural and diagnostic codes are given to the sportsperson to send to the insurance companies to alert them to the participation in the programme. Prior to the patient starting therapy, the practitioner should sit down with the therapist to discuss the patient's strengths, weaknesses, goals and therapy plan and only after the therapist understands what is trying to be accomplished should the patient be contacted to set up training.

At sports vision screenings or projects the therapist can be primarily responsible for designing the test flow, can set up the equipment and be one of the testing personnel. The therapist can be a valuable public relations person for the practice and should be available to lecture to athletic groups, trainers and school or community groups. It is most important that the therapist has good communication skills and can convey information to sportspeople in simple terms on how eye conditions can affect sports performance.

Establishing a practice

In order to get started and achieve a better understanding of sports vision, the practitioner should probably affiliate with a sports vision organization. The International Academy of Sports Vision was established in 1984 and is the only group where optometrists, ophthalmologists, opticians, coaches and trainers are affiliated together and meet to exchange views and ideas. The American Optometric Association Sports Vision Section provides many of the above services and also provides the *Sports Vision Guidebook* as a member benefit. Being a member of both organizations has its advantages. Outside the United States, practitioners have access to the European Academy of Sports Vision, the Dutch/Belgian Council on Sports Vision, the

Sports Vision Sections of both the Australian and Canadian Optometric Association, and the Sports Vision Association in the United Kingdom. The addresses of some sports vision associations are given in Appendix I.

When you are establishing a sports vision practice, it is important to make yourself and your services known in the community you wish to serve. For this, the right people must be contacted: for example at high school level this would be the coaches and the athletic directors; at collegiate level, coaches, athletic directors and trainers; while with professional players and teams, it is important to cover all contingencies by contacting the owners, managers and trainers. The latter are really the key once a practitioner has gained approval to work with the team, as it is the trainer who is responsible for the athlete's health. The next step is to carry out a sports vision screening session.

Sports vision testing

Holding a local sports vision screening is recommended as a good way of letting people know what a sports vision practice can offer. This may be done in one of two ways. First, it can be done at the office, where stations need to be set up and staff should probably assist in the testing. In this situation, to minimize confusion and maintain a smooth flow at all times to avoid any backlog at a particular test area, generally three athletes at a time can be run through the different stations. The advantages of having this at the office are: all the equipment at is at the practitioner's fingertips, allowing a more in-depth analysis and any extra test that might be needed beyond what was planned for; it gets the athlete to know the office location for any future eye services that might be needed and for referrals; it shows the athlete that the practice offers other things besides sports vision (i.e. contact lenses, low vision aids etc.). Alternatively, sports vision screening can be done on-site, such as at the school, gym, playing field or locker room. This approach may be more convenient for the team to fit into its time-table, shows that the practitioner takes them seriously and also is flexible and willing to accommodate them within the practice's busy schedule. The advantage of being on location is that other people in the area such as parents, secretaries, ground staff etc. can see what is being done and may take an interest in the service. In this situation, the practitioner can be more flexible in the order of testing players. What generally happens is that a group of athletes comes by for the evaluation in between their practice sessions or drills. There may be much time spent waiting around for the players to come, but once they do, the practitioner must be ready to go and get the players through on time, so that they can quickly return to their practice. The disadvantage of on-site testing, however, is that not all of the equipment can be taken along, so there might be slightly less 'in-depth testing'. Care should be taken with the priority of equipment chosen for transport to the test area.

On a local level, it really helps to have either the coach or trainer visit the practice to see what is on offer, or alternatively the practitioner can take a video tape and some demonstrations to them. Sometimes the hardest part of testing a team is convincing the coach or trainer about the importance of what sports vision has to offer, as they tend to want to know everything about their sport and may be apprehensive because they do not know how sports vision fits in. Generally both the coach and trainer should be run through the work-up first to allow for more detailed explanation on how each testing area relates to the specifics of that sport. Again, it is important to ensure the tests do relate to the specifics of the sport itself and the visual demands of the sport. For example, an archer should not be trained in peripheral awareness; in this sport concentration and visualization should be emphasized.

Developing links

Let us now imagine that you, as a sports vision specialist, have convinced a local team of the value of your services, and have been hired to work with the players. How should you proceed? First of all, it is very important to work around the coach's schedule. Do not interfere with practice schedules; players should be tested between drills. At a later stage tests may become a regular part of the pre-season activities.

Ensure that the sports vision practitioner is not seen as a threat to the coach and do not pretend to have all of the answers. If providing sports vision therapy or enhancement, do not present a whole battery of things to the trainer or coach for them to do, but concentrate on one or two specifics first and then add more later on. If you find that a player has a visual problem that can be helped by training, it is best to work with that player during the off season so as not to interfere with concentration. Athletes are very superstitious and may unjustly blame you for their poor performance if vision therapy is carried out during the season. It is probable that the player has already compensated in some way for the vision problem, so again it is best to wait to work with the individual after the season has ended. Also be careful how the visual problems are presented to players. It should not be made to sound like a major problem, as this may shake their confidence and may put a serious doubt in their minds about their ability. Preferably point out that they are good athletes now, but by carrying out sports vision training or enhancement, they can perhaps be even better.

Any player with a visual weakness should definitely be reported to the trainer in person. If contact lenses or glasses are needed, speak to the trainer about insertion/removal, solutions, spare lenses, safety frames, etc. A follow-up letter should also be sent to the owner, club management or whoever employed you. Conversely, the players with exceptional visual skills should likewise be established and reported, as this is also important information.

The bottom line in establishing a sports vision practice is that once you get the coach's, trainer's and definitely the players' confidence, then and only then will you be able to provide a worthwhile service.

Marketing

In the practice

How do you let your practice patients know that you are providing sports vision services? Sport is one thing that so many people have in common, either as a spectator or a participant. To begin with, you should talk about sports during the routine optometric examination if the patient is interested. In the office, a sports atmosphere can be created in the following ways.

1. Have pre-written sports vision pamphlets in the waiting room. They are available from the American Optometric Association, the Optometric Extension Program, and various contact lens companies (see Appendix 1).
2. Create your own brochure. This can give more detail on what visual skills are related to sports and what you can offer as a sports vision specialist. It gives a little more credibility to your commitment to this specialty area.
3. Have general sports photos or pictures around the office to create a sports theme.
4. Display photos of some projects that you have done with some known individuals.
5. Have a protective eye wear display in the dispensary.
6. Have articles about sports vision in the waiting area, especially ones that you have authored.
7. If you have a newsletter, write a short article on sports vision.
8. In your waiting room, have a bulletin board of news clippings of your patients who excel in sports.
9. Create a sports vision logo that identifies your office as a sports vision centre. Include it on your business card, stationery and signs outside your building.
10. Liaise with the contact lens and optical manufacturers who market their products with regard to sports (see Appendix 2) and who can assist the practitioner with marketing ideas, office posters and general help in establishing a sports vision practice.

In the community

It is necessary not only to promote sports vision in the practice but also in the community. Initially, you should lecture to various organizations such as community civic groups, little league or high school coaches' conferences, hospitals, community lecture series, police (who require the same ocular skills as athletes, but are reliant on them in a life and death situation), parent–teacher organizations at local schools and health clubs. Health clubs are a perfect area to market your sports vision services. Many clubs have a health lecture series, utilizing various health professionals in the local community. Clubs and medical health centres often have health programmes giving their members a total body analysis (i.e. fat percentage, cardiovascular output, aerobic capabilities etc.) using exercise physiologists, physical therapists and nutritionists. This is a good avenue for the sports vision specialist to pursue. Speak to the fitness director at the local health club about being included in providing services to their members. When giving a presentation to an organization, use audio-visual aids. Slide presentations and video tapes are available from the International Academy of Sports Vision, American Optometric Association, the Sports Vision Association in the UK and various manufacturers. When lecturing to a lay audience include personal slides and provide a demonstration that is fun and different and include the audience in some of the tests.

The problem with any form of advertising is that detailed information is necessary to explain sports vision adequately. Radio is difficult because of the short time period which is available to get the information across to the listener, and while television can be very descriptive, the cost factor is very limiting. In general newspaper or magazine feature articles are more valuable than advertising as they give more credibility to the information. Health and science editors both in newspapers and on radio are always looking for newsworthy items.

Active participation could include sponsoring, coaching or playing with a local team or league which might promote your name and logo in the public eye and newspaper ratings. Arrange a fitness/health display at a health forum or symposium, if possible, or show a video tape of someone undergoing testing. Show slides, hand out brochures and even have some hands-on equipment to demonstrate. Put on a seminar for local coaches, trainers, physical education instructors etc. The topics can be contact lenses, visual skills important to sports or first aid for common eye injuries. Have an 'open house' function in your sports vision facility and invite the general public as well as coaches, trainers and athletes.

Economics of sports vision

Sports vision can be profitable given a reasonable fee structure, which may be undertaken in one or more of the following methods.

1. Donate time to a team to get established with them and show that you care about the players.
2. At the local level, charge a reasonable minimum fee per player for a sports vision screening. It gives your services more value and players will pay a little more attention to you when they have paid.
3. Charge a total sum that covers the whole team. Many local colleges and high schools prefer this, due to their limited budget.
4. On a professional level you can charge in one of two ways:
   (a) Retainer: such a fee may amount to many thousands of dollars. The disadvantage of this is that you might have to be available at any time and be required to leave your practice at a moment's notice, which can be inconvenient and interfere with your private practice.
   (b) Standard professional fee per player plus expenses: this may go into hundreds of dollars per player depending on the depth of the evaluation. The provision of appliances such as contact lenses or protective goggles is invoiced separately.

For the private patient, a complete visual examination can be undertaken initially followed by a sports vision diagnostic battery test. This may take a number of hours, so you must schedule the time appropriately and charge accordingly. Office sports vision therapy should be charged at the regular vision therapy rate and can be based on an individual or group setting. Often insurance coverage is available when there is a related visual skill problem associated with the need for therapy. Sports vision can be financially rewarding, especially when a therapist is incorporated in the practice so that it does not take away from the practitioner's general examination time.

Levels of sports vision practice

There are various levels of sports vision practice. Each requires a different amount of investment, both in terms of money and the amount of time the practitioner dedicates solely to sports vision. **Level 1** does not require additional expenditure. Ask all patients in what sports they participate and use a sports questionnaire (see Figure 9.1), remembering to consider unusual or non-competitive sports such as snowboarding, aerobics or hiking. Emphasize the role of contact lenses in sports where they may be useful in improving the game for far less than is often spent on other sports equipment. Dedicate a section of the office to sports vision using counter cards, sports photos or posters and ensure that employees are educated, informed and involved in promoting sports vision to patients. **Level 2** could involve holding an open house with a free trial pair of contact lenses for sports. A protective eye wear company could demonstrate frames at the same time. Advertising public relations materials developed by various companies can be used to augment the sports vision effort. A sports vision screening could be arranged for a local team, where it will be found that approximately 20% of the athletes will fail, leading to further involvement for the practitioner. At **level 3** the practitioner becomes a sports vision specialist, a consultant to a local professional team or a visual performance enhancement consultant to a competitive amateur or professional athlete. At this level investment in terms of time and equipment becomes maximal.

The future

While sports medicine was traditionally retrospective, the trend with exercise physiologists, physical therapists, sports psychologists and now sports vision is increasingly towards prevention and enhancement. More and more professional teams are realizing the importance of vision in their sport and are incorporating sports vision into their programmes. In North America some teams now have optometrists or ophthalmologists on their staff. This is a trend that can only increase.

Sports vision is now gaining credibility with research and data to support the findings and claims. Optometry schools are currently providing more sports vision in their curricula. Sports vision is fun, offering a chance to travel, meet interesting people, players and colleagues and provide a service that is appreciated by everyone: coaches, managers, but most importantly the players. This exciting new specialty offers its practitioners a great deal of satisfaction.

References

Carlson, N.J. (1991) *Sports Vision Guidebook*, American Optometric Association, St Louis, Mo

Coffey, B. and Reichow, A.W. (1990) Optometric evaluation of the elite athlete. *Problems of Optometry*, **2**, 32–59

Loran, D.F.C. (1992) Eye injuries in squash. *The Optician*, **203**, 18–26

Payne, E. (1991) *Market/Business Overview for the Institute for Sports Vision*, Institute for Sports Vision, Ridgefield, CT

Further reading

Christensen, G.N. and Winkelstein, A.M. (1988) Visual skills of athletes versus non-athletes: development of a sports testing battery. *Journal of the American Optometric Association*, **59**, 947–50

Classé, J. (1993) Clinical evaluation of the elite athlete. *Optometry Clinics*, **3**, 1–26

Falkowitz, C. and Mendel, H. (1977) The role of visual skills in batting averages. *Optometric Weekly*, **68**, 577–80

Gregg, J.R. (1987) *Vision and Sports*, Butterworths, Stoneham, Mass

Martin, W.F. (1987) *An Insight into Sports: Featuring Trapshooting and Golf*, 3rd edn, Sports Vision Inc., Seattle

Melcher, M.H. (1988) Wisconsin Sports vision project, *NASV Highlights*, **4** (2), 17–18, 21

Spinell, M.R. (1989) A design and consideration of contact lenses for athletes. *National Academy of Sports Vision Newsletter*, **5**, 4–14

Sherman, A. (1983) A method of evaluating eye–hand coordination and visual reaction time in athletes. *Journal of the American Optometric Association*, **54**, 801–2

Sherman, A. (1990) Sports vision testing and enhancement: implications for winter sports. In *Winter Sports Medicine* (eds M. Casey, C. Foster and E. Hixson), F.A. Davis, Philadelphia

Stine, C.D., Arterburn, M.R. and Stern, N.S. (1982) Vision and sports: a review of the literature. *Journal of the American Optometric Association*, **53**, 627–33

Forensic sports vision
Steve P. Taylor

Introduction

For the majority of the population, sporting activities are merely pastimes and therefore are not treated with the consideration that they may otherwise be given. Even professional sportsmen and women may not be fully aware of the ramifications and implications of their work. This chapter sets out to explore the areas of product liability, personal liability and third party liability in relation to sports vision and to examine how different parts of the world view these problems.

Product liability

Whenever consumers use a product they have a right to expect that it will meet their described needs. This holds as true for spectacles as it does for any other consumer goods. While there may be variations in the detail of consumer law, the fundamental elements are the same. When reviewing product liability with regard to optical correction it is possible to subdivide the elements into:

- Standard spectacles
- Protective or impact-resistant spectacles
- Specialist spectacles, e.g. sports eye protectors
- Contact lenses
- Other appliances

Product liability law states that if a consumer is using a product for its intended purpose and without substantial alteration, and the consumer is injured by a defect in that product then the designer, manufacturer or seller of the product is liable for the assumed injuries. This applies regardless of the care that went into the design, manufacture or sale of the product.

If a case were brought under product liability, the court reviewing the case would need to consider details such as:

- The manner in which the product was marketed.
- The instructions or warnings accompanying the product.
- The conditions under which the product might reasonably be used.
- When the product was supplied.

The normal situation of 'innocent until proven guilty' does not strictly apply in cases of damage under product liability law. While it needs to be shown that a defect in the product caused the damage, once this is established liability may only be avoided if it can be proved that:

- The product was not supplied (e.g. was stolen or counterfeit).
- The state of scientific and technical knowledge at the time of supply was such that a producer of products of the same description as that being

investigated would have been unable to discover the defect.

- The defect resulted inevitably from complying with the law.
- The supplier did not sell the product but supplied it as a gift or donation.
- If the product was made from components manufactured by different producers, the component producer will not be liable where it is shown that the design of the completed product is deficient or where incorrect component specifications have been given by the producer of the finished product.

Inevitably, a greater number of product liability cases have been brought in the United States of America than elsewhere because of the large population, the high profile of the legal system and the substantial settlements made in the past.

If supplying a specialist product, e.g. goggles designed specifically for sports, then it is important that care is taken to ensure they are effective. Additionally, if special instructions are required to accompany the goggles, for example with regard to limitations in protection, then these must be explained to the customer – it is not acceptable to expect the customer to have read through instructions to discover the limitations for themselves. In the case of *Whitacre* v. *Halo Optical Products, Inc. and Optical Dispensary* (1987) the court found in favour of the plaintiff (Classé *et al.*, 1988). Whitacre, a 41-year-old male racquetball player, purchased a pair of lensless Rec Specs goggles but was not informed by the dispenser that to obtain protection they would need to be glazed with plano polycarbonate lenses. Furthermore this requirement was not pointed out in the accompanying literature. The case was brought when Whitacre was injured by a ball which had softened and become elongated sufficiently to pass through the unglazed frame damaging the eye.

A similar situation arises with the provision of contact lenses. If a squash player who normally uses prescription polycarbonate lenses is fitted with contact lenses the need for a plano polycarbonate pair of spectacles to provide the same protection when using contact lenses should be discussed. Contact lenses do not protect the eyes and wearers require the same degree of eye protection as non-wearers.

Standards of product

When dealing with athletes it is essential to offer advice on the suitability of products dispensed. If, for example, a patient indicates that they play cricket or baseball it would be foolhardy for the practitioner to supply standard glass lenses and not to discuss the benefits of polycarbonate material. The responsibility on the practitioner is to provide the most suitable correction for the individual's needs but in the case of athletes and sportspeople there are no accepted international standards laid down. In this case, therefore, it is necessary to review the national standards that exist for sports vision and the more general standards relating to eye protection which may be applicable (American National Standards Institute, 1987a, 1987b, 1989; British Standards Institution, 1987; Taylor, 1994). The general standards may be categorized as:

1. General purpose, which covers normal wear lenses which will offer little or no protection to high velocity particles or low velocity high mass particles.
2. Protective eye wear, which covers impact resistant lenses and which meets specific standards as regards the drop ball test or equivalent, minimum centre thickness and complete appliance assessment.

While there is no specific standard for sports vision in the USA, performance standards to be expected from selected sports eye ware have been offered by the American Society for Testing and Materials (1986). These are not legal standards but their existence means that a court of law could take them into account when making judgment on whether a practitioner provided the most suitable appliance for the particular athlete's situation. The 'standard' covers four categories of protection:

Type 1   In this category the lens and frame are moulded as a single unit and the sides are fitted separately to complete the appliance.

Type 2   Lenses are produced independently of the frame either as plano or prescription and then fitted to the frame to complete the appliance.

Type 3   These are the lensless protectors in which the viewing aperture is restricted in size to prevent the object in play from reaching the eye.

Type 4   Covers the full face shield to give facial rather than just ocular protection.

Further details of standards for eye protectors for specific sports can be found in Chapter 5.

The Standards Association of Australia (1992) has published a standard covering eye protection in racquet sports. Based on a draft put out for comment, this project arose in response to the results of a survey on sports-related eye injuries and the design of sports eye protectors. The standard covers quality and tolerances of lenses and visor and integral moulded units, minimum dimensions of the protector, restrictions to the visual field, luminous transmission for tinted and non-tinted materials in addition to impact resistance requirements. The standard also reviewed eye protectors without lenses and identified that slit widths greater than 13 mm were not protective against a squash ball but that slit sizes smaller than this would be too narrow to provide an adequate field of view.

Canada also has recommendations for sports eye protectors (Canadian Standards Association, 1982). Since the introduction and implementation of these recommendations/standards it has been noted that no significant eye injury has been recorded for a person playing racquet sports while wearing an eye protector meeting the relevant recommendation/standard.

At the time of writing, there is no current British standard available for sports eye pro-

tection although the British Standards Institution are currently investigating a standard for racquet sports eye protectors (British Standards Institution, 1993).

It has been suggested that the industrial eye protection standards such as BS 2092 in the UK and ANSI Z87.1 in the USA could be used. There is evidence to show that these are not entirely suitable for the particular conditions that are present in the sporting environment. The frames used for industrial protection have been found to be too weak in the sporting arena (Bishop et al., 1982; Feigelman et al., 1983), with breakages to the frame material and damage at the hinge. With the exception of polycarbonate material, lenses suitable for industrial use are not suitable for sports and furthermore the size and shape of many industrial frames do not give adequate protection to objects travelling from frontal directions (Gregg, 1987).

The increasing awareness of sports injury has concentrated attention on the matter and hopefully an internationally acceptable standard can be produced for eye protection in racquet sports in the near future. It will then require clubs and sports bodies to enforce the use of such protectors if the full impact of such a standard is to be seen on the eye injuries resulting from participation in racquet sports.

Negligence

For practitioners, the issue of negligence is likely to prove the most serious case in which they could become involved. Negligence may be defined as 'conduct which falls below a standard established by the law for the protection of others against an unreasonable risk of harm' (Classé, 1989). To succeed in an action for negligence the plaintiff is required to prove the following:

● There exists a duty of care owed personally by the defendant to the plaintiff.

That duty of care has been broken.
Harm has been suffered as a result of the breach of duty.

As far as an eye care professional is concerned, the requirement is for the plaintiff to demonstrate that harm was suffered as a result of the practitioner not conforming to the standard of care expected of like practitioners acting under the same or similar circumstances. This means that a practitioner who indicates a greater expertise in sports vision would be expected to demonstrate higher standards of care in sports vision matters than a practitioner not indicating special skills.

Returning to the three elements which are required to be proven for a case of negligence to succeed, let us examine them in more detail.

Duty of care

Following the case of *Le Lievre* v. *Gould* in the UK in 1893, it has been said that a man may be as negligent as he pleases towards the whole world, if he owes no duty to them. The important question therefore is does such a duty of care arise in real life?

A broad definition of the duty of care was provided as follows by Lord Atkin (Redmond, 1970) following the case of *Donoghue* v. *Stevenson* in 1932:

1. You must take reasonable care to avoid acts or omissions which you can reasonably foresee would be likely to injure your neighbour.
2. Who then is my neighbour? The answer seems to be persons who are so closely and directly affected by my act that I ought reasonably to have them in contemplation as being so affected when I am directing my mind to the acts or omissions which are called into question.

When the court hears a case of negligence they must therefore compare the actions involved with the likely actions of a reasonable person with the same qualifications or special ability acting under the same or similar circumstances. Comparison will only

be made with like for like, i.e. the actions of an optometrist would be compared with those of another optometrist but not with those of an ophthalmologist in similar circumstances.

Frequently in cases of negligence, to prove a duty of care it is necessary to hear expert testimony to establish the expected peer view standard of care. The professional bodies set their own minimum standards of conduct which form the basis for establishing this peer view.

Broken duty of care

Once the practitioner–patient relationship has been established, the former is obligated to provide a service with all due care. This due care extends through identification of the individual patient's problem, selection and implementation of the means of dealing with the problem and ensuring adequate follow-up. To demonstrate that, at any point, the duty of care has been breached it is again necessary to determine a peer group view of the minimum requirements below which liability would be considered. While this may seem straightforward, the determination of a minimum acceptable level is not always easy, as professional viewpoints can differ markedly.

Harm has been suffered as a result of the breach of duty

The final piece in the jigsaw to complete the picture regarding negligence is for the plaintiff to show that harm has been suffered as a result of the breach of duty. The term 'harm' according to Classé (1989) includes 'all forms of injury that the mind can conjure up whether temporary or permanent, petty or disabling, hidden or evident.'

Liability for negligence is not, however, strict and there is no liability to guard against damages which a reasonable man could not foresee by the exercise of reasonable prudence. In a sporting context, for example, where a cricket ball was propelled by a quite exceptional hit beyond the cricket ground resulting in injury to a woman standing in the road beyond the fencing of the ground, this was not considered as negligent (*Stone* v. *Bolton*, 1951).

Ignorance of the law

In general it is considered that mistakes of either law or fact are no defence in court. Within this context the maxim '*ignorantia legis non excusat*' – ignorance of the law is no excuse – would apply.

Claims against practitioners by sportspeople

Classé (1993) has suggested that areas where claims have been brought by sportspeople against practitioners include:

- Failure to prescribe the material of choice (polycarbonate).
- Failure to warn of the diminished impact resistance of alternative materials.
- Failure to inspect and verify the ophthalmic materials dispensed.
- Failure properly to manage an ocular injury or its sequelae.

When the court considers each of these situations, the basic question it will ask, as has already been suggested, is what would a reasonable practitioner have done under similar circumstances?

Failure to prescribe the material of choice

An example of this would be where a spectacle wearer indicated that they played cricket or baseball and the practitioner failed to prescribe polycarbonate of sufficient thickness as the material of choice. The possibility of a hard ball hitting the lens is raised in these sports and therefore polycarbonate should be provided.

A similar approach should be taken when prescribing for a squash, badminton, tennis or racquetball player, but here it is also important to consider the possibility of the racquet striking the lens as well as the ball.

In any instance where there is a possibility of an object striking the lens, polycarbonate should be the material of choice and any prescription provided should be marked accordingly (Young, 1989). It is essential that even when a patient decides to select a different material the advice in favour of polycarbonate is recorded and the patient's decision documented.

Failure to warn of the diminished impact resistance of alternative materials

This is an extension of the first category and would occur if, in the example given, glass or standard plastic (CR39) lenses had been prescribed, without informing the patient of the higher impact resistance of polycarbonate lenses. Any subsequent accident resulting in injury would prompt the court to look at why polycarbonate was not discussed. If it were considered that it was necessary for the patient's activities as they had been described and that a 'reasonable practitioner' would have offered polycarbonate the practitioner could be found at fault.

The need to warn of impact resistance limitation was demonstrated by the case of *Grady* v. *American Optical Corp. et al.* (1985). While carrying out his work in a steel plant, a worker was hit by an acetylene torch and his safety spectacles broken sending glass splinters into his eye. The spectacles were made to the applicable ANSI Z87.1 standards for impact resistance but the company was sued on the basis of not warning that the lenses could shatter and cause eye injury. A substantial judgment in favour of the worker was made following a jury trial.

Failure to inspect and verify the ophthalmic materials dispensed

Having determined that a polycarbonate lens is required and prescribed accordingly there is a duty on the dispenser to ensure that the lenses received are as prescribed. In the case of a qualified optician or optometrist carrying out the dispensing, they would be held responsible for correctly ordering and verifying. In the case of an unqualified person verifying the dispensing, however, the liability would fall to the optometrist or ophthalmologist involved for not ensuring adequate follow-up to the prescription. The exception would be where the patient took the prescription away and had spectacles made by an unregistered supplier over whom the clinician had no control.

Frame suitability is also important and selection of a suitable frame to hold the lenses would fall within the area of care. Using a frame that is patently not suitable to protect in the given circumstances could render the dispenser liable. Classé (1987) cites the case of the manager of a raquetball club who purchased a pair of lensless safety goggles sold as providing protection when playing racquetball, squash or handball. Unfortunately while playing racquetball the man was struck in the eye by a ball which penetrated the lensless opening and a traumatic cataract resulted. When the manufacturer was sued, evidence was presented that the Canadian Sports Standards Commission had conducted tests on the goggles to show that a high velocity racquetball could penetrate the lens opening and strike the eye. The case was settled in favour of the plaintiff.

Management of sports-related ocular trauma

Depending on the severity of any ocular trauma caused through a sports accident the patient may attend their trainer, team physician, optometrist, general practitioner, hospital casualty unit or ophthalmologist. In all cases it is important that the patient is examined adequately and given the appropriate treatment and advice. If there is any doubt about the ocular damage the patient should be referred to an ophthalmologist for specialist assessment which, if there is any suggestion of an intra-ocular foreign body, should include an X-ray. As with all clinical examination, a careful history should be recorded and attention paid to the visual acuity, the pupil reactions, motility, visual fields and examination of the eye, details of which should be fully recorded. Patients should be warned of the possible sequelae of injury such as infection, retinal detachment or glaucoma and adequate follow-up must be provided. In the case of the optometrist being the first to examine the patient a letter should be sent to the patient's general practitioner indicating the findings and the proposed follow-up arrangements.

According to Classé (personal communication, 1994) blunt trauma to the eye can cause:

1. Immediate secondary injury such as the rebleeding of a hyphaema, shortly after the initial injury.
2. Complications arising some months after the initial injury, such as retinal detachments.
3. Long-term disease, such as unilateral glaucoma.

The example cited (Bettman, 1980) is of a woman struck in the face with a fist who was found by an ophthalmologist to have a hyphaema and depressed fracture of the orbit. After 2 months of treatment her problems resolved and she was discharged from care. Eight months later she experienced a retinal detachment but because she had not been warned of possible symptoms the woman failed to seek treatment until it was too late and the ophthalmologist was successfully sued for failure to warn.

One special case relates to eye injuries in boxers, and the American Academy of Ophthalmology has issued details of 'reforms for the prevention of eye injuries in boxing'. It is known that although there is high incidence of ocular injuries in boxers many of the conditions are treatable if detected early. The British Boxing Board of Control also laid down regulations concerning medical assessment of suitability to box and to continue to box; these are general but currently under review.

In all cases of sports-related ocular trauma, it is obviously imperative that patients are warned of the symptoms to watch for and that practitioners keep full records and maintain adequate follow-up after the injury.

Volenti non fit injuria

Translated as 'no injury can be done to a willing person', this defence in a civil action for damages is obviously applicable to the sporting arena. Essentially, a person who has voluntarily consented to the commission of an injury by taking part in an activity in which such injury is a known possibility cannot sue if such an injury occurs. A boxer, for example, voluntarily runs the risk of being punched in the face by his opponent and cannot therefore complain if this occurs within the rules of boxing and damage results. A further example would be where a soccer player kicks the ball towards goal and in the process the ball strikes another player in the face breaking his nose – there would be no grounds for action as the participants voluntarily undertake to run the lawful risks and hazards which form part of the game.

There are situations, however, in which there would be grounds for legal action. If, for example, in a game of rugby, while in a scrum one player deliberately and intentionally gouges the eye of another player, this would be actionable. Gouging is against the laws of the game and may therefore be considered as falling outside the limits of what a participant in the game could reasonably have expected to happen when acting as a willing participant.

It is possible also for the officials to be caught up in this situation. The role of an official is to ensure that the game is played according to the rules and in so doing offer protection to the participants. If an official consistently fails to enforce the rules and as a result of this injury occurs, the injured party may be able to sue the official. This may extend even beyond those directly involved and if, for example, a football match was arranged to take place at a time when, according to medical advice, the temperature and humidity would make play dangerous, and a player was subsequently harmed due to the conditions, the organizers may find themselves open to action. This would particularly be the case if the player involved was not aware of the medical advice given. Similarly if a coach or trainer was to play an individual knowing that the individual suffered from an injury which would put them at increased risk of further damage, and did not warn the player of this, then there is a possibility that the trainer could be sued.

It is considered that any sportsman taking part in a dangerous activity while giving consent does so in the expectation that no external factors apply. If, as in *Gillmore* v. *LCC* (1938), a person participating in a sporting activity is injured due to defective flooring of which he had been unaware, *volenti non fit injuria* would not apply and the owners of the venue could be sued.

The principle of *volenti non fit injuria* applies beyond those involved in the sport to spectators who voluntarily undertake the lawful risks in attending sports meetings and who may have no cause for action if they are injured while attending an event. An example of this is the case of *Hall* v. *Brooklands Auto Racing Club* (1935). In this case Hall paid for admission to the race course to watch motor car racing. Unfortunately following a collision during one of the races a car went over the barrier and killed two spectators. Despite regular racing at the track this was the first time that a car had cleared the barrier. The court decided that the precautions taken by

Brooklands were adequate and that the danger to spectators was inherent in this sport and that therefore Hall must be taken to have assented to the risk of such an accident.

The fact that spectator safety is given a high priority by organizers has been displayed by the recent changes to requirements in football stadia in the UK following a tragedy at the Hillsborough stadium (Taylor, 1990). It was decided that areas of terracing which allowed movement and surging of crowds were a danger and stadia have had to meet new strict safety regulations on seating for spectators.

Inevitable accident

This defence occurs where the happening cannot be avoided by the taking of ordinary precautions. The appellant would need to show that this accident could have been foreseen and action taken to prevent it from taking place. An example of this is the case of *Stanley* v. *Powell* (1891). Powell, while involved with a shooting party, fired a shotgun but unfortunately one of the pellets hit a tree and ricocheted into the eye of Stanley who was acting as a beater with the shoot. After consideration the court held that Stanley had failed to prove the case that Powell had been negligent resulting in damage.

Club and sport rules

As a responsibility is placed on those organizing activities and operating venues to ensure safety most clubs or organizations will issue rules and regulations. Where such rules are issued and a condition of membership or use of facilities is compliance with these then failure to comply could remove the right to compensation if injury was to occur. If, for example, protective eye wear must be worn when playing squash at a club and a player suffers an injury through a raquet supplied by the club breaking and hitting the eye while failing to wear protection then any claim for compensation is likely to be dismissed or substantially reduced on the grounds that compliance with the rules would have prevented the injury.

Record keeping

Case records are the fundamental cornerstone for a defence in the courts (Taylor and Austen, 1992), although good records which show mismanagement can also be its downfall! It is essential that information is recorded at each visit and that all records include:

- Date of examination
- Reason for attendance
- Details of previous history
- Lifestyle details
- Examination findings, including specialist tests performed
- Recommendations and action taken
- Special instructions given
- Details of recall period and follow-up arrangements

It is important that at subsequent visits, however short these may be, the details are recorded. This may appear over cautious, but it is those brief visits that tend to have least attention paid to them in the records which are frequently associated with difficulties, where good records provide solid defence should a claim be lodged.

When presented as evidence the records need to be neat, legible and complete. Where records are poorly written or are filled with jottings and therefore indecipherable the court is less likely to put store by the practitioner's testament as a whole, assuming that it is of the same nature. It is essential that a record of nothing seen or detected is made – leaving a blank would be interpreted as indicating that nothing was done.

When dealing with specialist areas such as sports vision it is worth bearing in mind that you can prevent problems by your approach to the patient and by ensuring that you carefully record all actions and, if necessary, get the patient to sign the record. A patient cannot sign away their statutory rights but can sign to indicate that information has been passed on. What then should you do to help protect against problems?

- Never say that a lens is unbreakable – all lenses are breakable under certain conditions. Never say a lens is shatterproof or describe a protective lens as a safety lens.
- If any manufacturer's warnings accompany products, e.g. sports goggles not suitable for specific sports, ensure that the purchaser is told and note on the records that the purchaser has been informed. If goggles are only suitable when glazed with polycarbonate lenses then do not, even at the patient's request, glaze them with anything else.
- When you check and verify an optical aid returned from the laboratory, in addition to the optical correction check that the lenses are free from defects and that they fit well into the frame. Once checked note on the record that the appliance has been checked and sign alongside the date.
- If a lens is specified as meeting standards ensure that it genuinely does conform to the requirements of the standard and if necessary ask the manufacturer for a written statement supporting this.
- Offer the most suitable material to patients for their own specific needs and explain the advantages and disadvantages of the alternatives available. Note the selected material on the record and indicate if the patient selects an alternative and ask the patient to sign that they have selected knowing the pros and cons.

While the above is not an exhaustive list and compliance is no guarantee against liability, if the information is recorded, the strength of the defence would be substantially enhanced. It is important to record the date with entries and retrospective entries to records should be avoided.

Third party liability

It is important when taking part in any sport that every attempt is made to protect those not involved directly, e.g. spectators or those involved in a separate unrelated but proximal game. It is also important to protect property. For the most part this is straightforward, however in some sports, for example golf, there is a possibility of injury to persons or damage to property not related to the participants. In such cases it is possible to take out insurance to cover claims made. Many insurance companies have developed specialist policies to protect the amateur and the professional athlete. The cost of taking out such a policy is normally modest for the protection provided.

Summary

The increase in leisure time, when health consciousness has also been raised, has seen a rapid increase in the numbers becoming involved in sport. A high profile legal system, particularly in the United States of America, has resulted in a greater number of product liability cases being brought which have a real bearing on if not direct involvement with sport. The need to provide adequate international standards for products and clubs involved in sport is demonstrated. Additionally, details such as good record keeping are outlined, which health care practitioners of all disciplines should follow to ensure they satisfy patient needs and minimize the risk of legal action.

List of cases

Donoghue v. *Stevenson* [1932] A.C. 562; 147 L.T. 281
Grady v. *American Optical Corp.* et al. (1985) 702 S.W. 2d 911 (Mo. App.)
Hall v. *Brooklands Auto Racing Club* [1933] 1 K.B. 205
Le Lievre v. *Gould* [1893] 1 Q.B. 491
Stanley v. *Powell* [1891] 1 Q.B. 86; 60 L.J.Q.B. 52
Stone v. *Bolton* [1951] A.C. 850
Whitacre v. *Halo Optical Products, Inc. and Optical Dispensary* (1987) 501 So. 2d 994 (La. App.)

References

American National Standards Institute (1987a) Z80.3 (1986) *Recommendations for Non-prescription Sunglasses and Fashion Eyeware*, ANSI, New York

American National Standards Institute (1987b) Z80.1 *Recommendations for Impact Resistance of Prescription Ophthalmic Lenses*, ANSI, New York

American National Standards Institute (1989) Z87.1 *Practice for Occupational and Educational Eye and Face Protection*, ANSI, New York

American Society for Testing and Materials (1988) F803–88 (Standard Specification for Eye Protectors for use by Players of Racquet Sports) ASTM, Philadelphia

Bettman, J.W. (1980) A review of 412 claims in ophthalmology. *International Ophthalmology Clinics*, **20**, 131–42

Bishop, P.J. Kozey, J. and Caldwell, G. (1982) Performance of eye protectors for squash and racquetball. *Physician and Sports Medicine*, **10**(3), 63–9

British Standards Institution (1987) BS 2092 *Eye Protectors for Industrial and Non-industrial Use*, BSI, London

British Standards Institution (1993) *Draft Specification for Eye Protectors for Squash and Other Racket Sports*, Document 93/307794, BSI, London

Canadian Standards Association (1982) CSA P400-M1 *Racquet Sports Eye Protectors*, CSA, Ontario

Classé, J.G. (1987) Legal aspects of prescribing for athletes and sportsmen. *Journal of the American Optometric Association*, **58**, 674–9

Classé, J.G. (1989) *Legal Aspects of Optometry*, Butterworths, Stoneham, Mass.

Classé, J.G. (1993) Legal aspects of prescribing for athletes and sportsmen. *Sports Vision*, **9**(2), 28–34

Classé, J.G., Gold, A.R. and Harris, M.G. (1988) A review of five recent cases of significance for optometrists. *Journal of the American Optometric Association*, **59**, 964–8

Feigelman, M.J., Sugar, T., Jednock, N. *et al.*, (1983) Assessment of ocular protection for racquetball. *Journal of the American Medical Association*, **250**(24), 3305–9

Gregg, J.R. (1987) *Vision and Sports*, Butterworths, Stoneham, Mass.

Redmond, P.W.D. (1970) *General Principles of English Law*, 3rd edn, M & E Handbooks, London

Standards Association of Australia (1992) AS/NZS 4066 *Eye Protection in Racquet Sports*, Standards Association of Australia, Sydney

Taylor, Right Honourable Lord Justice (1990) *The Hillsborough Stadium Disaster*, CM 962, HMSO, London

Taylor, S.P. (1994) Playing safe at work. *The Optician*, **5449**, 29–31

Taylor, S.P. and Austen, D.P. (1992) *Law and Management in Optometric Practice*, 2nd edn, Butterworth-Heinemann, Oxford

Young, J.M. (1989) Liability in ophthalmic lenses. *Optical World*, April, pp. 16–25

The future of sports vision

Alan W. Reichow and Brian R. Ariel

The final chapter presents views on the future of the sports vision discipline within North America and elsewhere. It is based upon the demonstrated growth of the specialty over the past two decades, and the present involvement of the sports, academic, corporate and eye care practitioner communities. A brief overview of the history behind sports-related vision care services is necessary to provide the foundation for projections presented later. Current trends can be demonstrated by looking at the activities of various sports vision associations, corporations and academic institutions while surveys of the optometric community and college and professional athletic programmes demonstrate growth in utilization of sports vision services. Future projection of the continued expansion of sports vision can then be made, based upon the history, current level of involvement and demonstrated need for services. The chapter is in two parts. First Alan Reichow explores the North American perspective, then Brian Ariel looks at the future of sports vision elsewhere in the world.

1. THE NORTH AMERICAN PERSPECTIVE

The scope of sports vision

In order to discuss the past, present and future of sports vision in North Amercia it is necessary first to define its scope. Based upon clinical experience and the orientation, quality and extent of professional training, this is fairly challenging as each practitioner, coach and athlete possesses a different viewpoint. To many, sports vision is limited to '20/20', '6/6', '1.0' (clarity of sight in each eye) meaning remediation of any refractive error through the application of contact lenses or spectacles. To others, it is primarily a matter of injuries and ocular protection. Whilst to some, reme-dial vision therapy and enhancement vision training are major aspects. With the scope of vision care varying so much, even in the eyes of practitioners within the same profession, it is not surprising to find so many uninformed and misinformed coaches, trainers and athletes (Zieman et al., 1993).

Based upon clinical experience and contribution from practitioners, the following definition was published in 1986:

> Sports vision encompasses *performance-oriented* comprehensive vision care programs involving the education, evaluation, correction, protection and enhancement of the athlete. Each of the above areas should be

addressed in a performance-oriented manner. This means that the practitioner should consider all of his or her services from a performance standpoint. Improved visual performance resulting in enhanced athletic performance must be the ultimate goal of sports vision regimens. (Reichow and Stern, 1986a).

Sports and recreational activities constitute a major commitment of time by the general public. Unfortunately, the term 'sports vision', or 'sports optometry' has a general connotation of high profile sports, such as soccer, basketball and ice-hockey. In practical terms, the majority of sports vision patients present as general clinic patients on a daily basis. A large percentage of patients enjoy a sport or recreational activity outside of the workplace or school, such as cycling, tennis and golf. Often these patients are unaware of the potential benefits of comprehensive vision care services, and therefore enter the practice without this in mind. Similarly, despite the common practice of incorporating a specific question regarding hobbies and interests on the case history questionnaire, relatively few practitioners pursue questioning beyond this level. Additionally, the practitioner is often unaware of the benefits their services may provide to the patient's recreational interests. Often, a beneficial opportunity is missed by both clinician and patient.

Organized sports vision associations

American Optometric Association Sports Vision Section

Practitioners have been practising sports vision as long as eye care has been provided. Sports vision, a sub-category of environmental vision, is applied whenever the practitioner provides consultation, diagnostic, protective, remedial or enhancement services to the sports- or recreational-minded patient. Formalization of the sports vision discipline within North America began with the establishment of the Sports Vision Section within the 30 000 member American Optometric Association in June, 1978. That same year the section began a vision care service for athletes of the United States Olympic Committee. That programme, varying in scope over the years, has continued to this day.

The Sports Vision Section has grown to a membership of 730 with an annual growth rate of approximately 15%. The purpose of the American Optometric Association's Sports Vision Section is to:

- Promote, advance and enhance sports vision care
- Promote visual fitness
- Enhance the vision/eye care of the public
- Provide and promote education and research
- Serve as an information source
- Provide a forum for those members of the American Optometric Association with a common interest in sports vision

The section provides educational symposia, a semi-annual publication entitled *News and Views*, patient brochures, educational audio and video tapes, membership directory and research funding. The desire for international cooperation is being pursued and lecturers from Canada, Australia and Europe have made presentations during past symposia. Other projects include development of a current sports vision bibliography which includes articles dating back to 1924. This bibliography is maintained with annual updates.

The *Sports Vision Guidebook* is a long-term project for the purpose of educating eye care practitioners regarding vision care in sports and recreational activities with which they may be unfamiliar, or inadequately prepared to provide vision care for. Each sport chapter addresses not only the visual requirements and suggestions for enhancing visual skills pertinent to that particular sport, but also gives a historical overview of the sport, terminology dictionary, vision screening/testing procedures, related problems and solutions, ocular injuries and first-aid, and a bibliography. The *Guidebook* briefly familiarizes the practitioner with each sport so as to allow the athlete to receive more appropriate services. Future plans are to complete a chapter for every known sport and recreational activity, with continued emphasis on completing all Olympic sports as soon as possible.

In addition to the services provided for the United States Olympic Committee, the section is also involved with other sports organizations, including the International Special Olympics, the second largest sports organization in the world with approximately one million participants representing more than 160 countries. Vision care programmes, which included optometrists from throughout North America, have determined that an unmet need for comprehensive eye care exists within the International Special Olympics population (Stern and Reichow, 1986; Reichow *et al.*, 1994). Areas of greatest concern include the large number of competitors never having received vision care (nearly one-third of the athletes participate with uncompensated or residual refractive error) and the increased risk of ocular trauma resulting from the lack of eye protection. At present there are no vision care requirements for participation in Special Olympics. Efforts are under way to develop mandatory requirements for the future. To facilitate such a large undertaking, international cooperation will be necessary.

Sports Vision Section of the Canadian Association of Optometrists

The Sports Vision Section of the Canadian Association of Optometrists was established in 1987, and currently has fifty members. The stated purpose of this section mirrors that of the American Optometric Association's Sports Vision Section. The section, in its early development stages, is planning to grow, with a membership campaign being developed.

International Academy of Sports Vision

The International Academy of Sports Vision (formerly the National Academy of Sports Vision) was founded in 1984. It is dedicated to the promotion and advancement of research development and education in the field of sports vision. Membership consists of ophthalmologists, optometrists, opticians, researchers, athletic trainers, coaches and other athletic specialists. The organization has developed affiliations with the National Athletic Trainers Association (NATA), the National Association of Collegiate Directors of Athletics (NACDA), the United States Sports Academy (USSA), the National Strength and Conditioning Association (NSCA) and the National Youth Sports Coaches Association (NYSCA).

The academy provides educational symposia, a quarterly research publication, a newsletter, audio and visual library, and a referral service. The academy, through its various programmes, will continue to encourage sports vision awareness to ensure comprehensive vision care for athletes of all ages and abilities.

Eye injury prevention

Without question the single most important role of the eye care practitioner is protecting the vision already present. Senseless eye injuries have for long plagued the sports world in North America (Clark and Lord, 1976; Pashby, 1979; Vinger, 1980). These injuries continue at an alarming rate despite such efforts as Prevent Blindness America (formerly the National Society to Prevent Blindness) to educate both the general public and eye care practitioners regarding the incidence, needless suffering and health care costs related to these injuries. Prevent Blindness America was created to act as a clearinghouse for information pertaining to cause, incidence and prevention of visual loss. They estimate that approximately 90% of all sports-related eye injuries are preventable given application of *appropriate* protective athletic eye wear (Stephens, 1994).

The American Society for Testing and Materials, recognizing the need, developed rigorous criteria for sports protective eye wear which are even more demanding than the requirements for industrial protective eye wear (ASTM, 1988). They recommend the use of polycarbonate plastic lenses mounted in a sturdy frame with foam nose pads and posterior flanges to hold the lenses in place. In 1977 the Canadian Standard Association established standards for eye protectors in ice-hockey (CSA, 1982). The standard, which is performance-orientated, involved small aperture wide masks for all players. These steps have significantly reduced eye injuries in ice-hockey (Vinger, 1981).

Despite increasing measures to protect the eyes in sports and recreation, eye injuries continue to occur at an alarming rate. As many as 10–20% of all serious eye injuries in the United States may be related to sports and other recreational activities (Stephens, 1994). Prevent Blindness America estimates that approximately 50 000 sports and recreational eye injuries were treated in hospital emergency rooms in 1992. This figure is perhaps two to three times greater when ocular injuries treated elsewhere are considered. Basketball, closely followed by the baseball/softball sports, are the top causes of these injuries. More than half of these occur to people between the ages of 5 and 24.

Various North American sports organizations have rules, regulations or recommendations regarding eye protection. Among these are ice-hockey, squash and racquetball. However, as identified previously, the high risk sports of basketball and baseball have no eye protection requirements at present. Future efforts by optometrists, ophthalmologists and

opticians must address this epidemic of easily preventable athletic eye injuries.

In addition to the lack of regulations, limited awareness of injury and prevention by the general public, and various compliance issues, there has been a problem with inadequate athletic eye wear. Prior to the mid 1980s availability of sports eye wear was relatively limited in terms of the number of manufacturers, eye wear size availability, adequacy of protection and cosmetic appeal. Recognizing the potential for growth in this market, many more sports eye wear manufacturers now exist. The improved quality, selection and size availability now provide the practitioner with the tools necessary to promote and protect the athlete. It is the responsibility of every practitioner to investigate and consult the patient regarding any ocular risk they may face.

Academic programmes

The first formal sports vision course in the professional curriculum of eye care practitioners began in 1980 at Pacific University College of Optometry, Forest Grove, Oregon. The programme, which consists of 4 lecture hours on sports optometry in a core course (entitled Environmental Vision) and 32 contact hours in the elective course (entitled Sports and Recreational Vision), has also provided clinical continuing education and research services for the past 15 years.

Since then, positive growth in course content and/or curriculum has been made in optometric education programmes to address the increasing interest in sports vision. In 1986, ten of the seventeen optometric institutions in North America included lectures on sports vision (Reichow and Stern, 1986b). Four of these programmes also offered additional training through sports vision elective courses. By 1992, all optometric professional programmes surveyed by Classé provided sports vision coverage in their curriculum (see Table 11.1).

Table 11.1   Optometry sports vision curriculum survey for 1992

School	Curriculum	Total hours	Lecturer
Berkeley	Lectures: bincoular vision, ophthalmic optics	4	Burton Worrell Jim Sheedy
Ferris State	Lectures: primary care courses, vision screenings	12	James Miller
Houston	Lectures: environmental vision	6	Ralph Herring
Illinois College	Lectures: binocular vision, ophthalmic optics	3	Steve Beckerman
	Elective course: sports vision	8	
Indiana	Lectures: environmental optics, binocular vision, contact lenses	10	Steve Hitzman
Missouri	Lectures: vision performance, binocular vision	3	Michael Wolf Kevin Fete
	Elective course: sports vision[a]	8	
New England	Lectures: environmental vision, binocular vision, ophthalmic optics	10	Jack Richman Stan Hatch
Northeastern	Lectures: environmental vision, binocular vision, ophthalmic optics	8	Bill Monaco Hank Van Veen W.C. Maples
Ohio State	Lectures: binocular vision, senior seminar, vision screening	6	Jeff Doty Paulette Schmidt
Pacific	Lectures: environmental vision	4	Al Reichow
	Elective course: sports vision	32	
Pennsylvania	Elective course: sports vision	12	Michael Spinell Michael Gallaway
Southern College	Lectures: vision therapy, ophthalmic optics	10	Glenn Steele
Southern California	Lectures: 4th year seminar	4	Graham Erickson Alan Winkelstein
New York	Lectures: binocular vision, ophthalmic optics	4	Carl Gruning Jeff Cooper
Alabama	Required course: sports vision	10	John Classé

[a] Not currently being offered due to cuts in academic programme.
   Source: Courtesy of J.G. Classé

Knowledge, utilization and practitioner role expansion potential

To date, only a limited number of projects have attempted to assess the utilization of vision care services in the sports world. In 1974, eighty-four ophthalmologists in the United States were surveyed relative to a variety of factors considered in the prescription of contact lenses for athletes (Goss *et al.*, 1974). The authors reported the increased use of flexible lenses as the 'main general trend'. In 1980 and 1983 unpublished surveys conducted at Pacific University College of Optometry sampled random optometrists, various college and university athletic programmes and the major professional sports teams throughout North America (Barton *et al.*, 1981; Helmick, 1983). They were designed to measure utilization and specific attitudes of optometrists and sports programme personnel about sports vision. Five years later the survey was expanded and repeated to assess the growth in both the optometric and athletic communities (Zieman *et al.*, 1993).

The same 100 optometrists were surveyed in each of the three postal surveys (see Table 11.2). More than 85% of the optometrists in each of the three surveys felt there was potential for growth of sports vision services. Growth was noted in the percentage of practitioners considering the specific visual demands of the athlete when prescribing, and in those providing vision training in their practices for athletes. Most practitioners preferred contact lenses over spectacles for refractive correction, and demonstrated concern for eye injury prevention.

Professional and collegiate sports teams were also surveyed (see Tables 11.3 and 11.4). Of particular interest was the dramatic increase in the number of vision care specialists affiliated with these teams, including those compensated. Despite this increase, the number of teams incorporating a vision screening programme, no matter how limited, remained surprisingly low as compared to the percentage of teams with an affiliated vision care specialist. An increasing number of team athletic trainers advocated the use of contact lenses over spectacles, and maintained spare contact lenses in a trainer's kit. Teams utilizing vision training services remained fairly constant.

At the time this book went to press, a follow-up survey was being conducted to once again assess any growth in the knowledge and utilization of vision care services for athletes throughout North America.

Standardization and certification

With growth in any discipline, the demands for quality education, research and instrumentation increase – needs which should come as no great surprise. Unfortunately, for all the effort, time and financial commitment to date, much of the development in this discipline has been far less efficient and productive than it may have been, primarily due to lack of standardization and certification. Skill level, knowledge base and approach to clinical care vary considerably among practitioners. These differences are not necessarily reflective of experiential backgrounds, as even those highly recognized in the field provide vision care services with relatively little common protocol. Difference is beneficial to growth and expansion, but a minimal level of professional conformity is essential. The art of practising sports vision is to modify, adapt and expand certain standardized techniques and approaches for the needs of the specific patient.

At present, a coach, athlete, trainer or fellow practitioner may look at a sports vision association directory with the perception that each practitioner is equally qualified in all aspects of vision care for the athlete. If this indeed were the case it would ensure a more unified effort, allowing better communication between practitioners, stronger scientific foundation through numbers and more effi-

Table 11.2   Optometric sports vision longitudinal data

100 optometrists surveyed	1987–8	1983	1980
Percentage response	49	51	64
Optometrists consulting to athletic teams at the high school, collegiate, and/or professional level	14% (7/49)	16% (8/51)	9% (6/64)
Optometrists paid vs volunteering services	5/7 paid 2/7 volunteer	1/8 paid 4/8 volunteer 3 not specific	2/6 paid 4/6 volunteer
Optometrists indicating a potential for growth in the area of sports vision	90% (44/49)	90% (46/51)	85% (54/64)
Optometrists considering the specific visual demands of the athlete separately when prescribing lenses	80% (39/49)	65% (33/51)	75% (46/61)
Optometrists preferring contact lenses over spectacles for athletes	94% (45/48)	84% (43/51)	93% (59/64)
Optometrists preferring soft contact lenses, rigid lenses or no preference	85% soft 5% rigid 10% no pref.	NA	NA
Optometrists advocating the use of extended wear contact lenses.	21% (9/42)	NA	NA
Optometrists including vision training in their practice for athletes	46% (22/48)	39% (20/51)	25% (16/64)
Vision training techniques utilized	2 not specified	7 not specified	
Vision enhancement	9/20 (45%)	4/13 (31%)	
Remedial training	3/20 (15%)	2/13 (31%)	
Combination of both techniques	8/20 (40%)	7/13 (54%)	
Optometrists advocating the use of athletic eyewear for the athletes.	90% (43/48)	NA	NA
Optometrists including athletic eyewear in their dispensary	87% (40/46)	NA	NA

NA: Denotes information was not available for specific survey subset.

Source: Courtesy of the American Optometric Association

cient growth. What we find is that practitioners are not equally skilled, knowledgeable or in agreement.

To gain maximal acceptance within the sports world and related health care fields, expanded standardization supported and fol-lowed by each of us is necessary. When one reviews literature or attends lectures on vision assessment, remediation or enhancement, the variability reveals itself. For instance, with regard to visual skills assessment, each 'authority' has a different set of tests and

Table 11.3 College/university sports vision longitudinal data

Colleges and universities surveyed	1987–88	1983	1980
Total response rate	61% (49/80)	26% (21/80)	36% (27/75)
Vision care specialists affiliated with college athletic programmes	65% (32/49)	26% (7/27)	24% (5/21)
Vision consultants paid vs volunteering their services	50% paid (16/32)	14% paid (1/7)	20% paid (1/5)
Degree of vision consultant (optometrist, ophthalmologist, or both)[a]	78% OD 34% MD (21/32, OD) (17/32, MD) 4 teams used both	71% OD (5/7, OD)	100% OD 20% MD (14/5, OD) 1 team used both
Teams using a vision screening programme	59% (29/49)	57% (12/21)	NA
Mean of athletes failing vision screenings	15%	4.5%	NA
Range of responses for failing screenings	0–33%	0–30%	0–15%
Recommendation of contact lenses over spectacles for athletes	83% (40/48)	67% (14/21)	NA
Percentage of players requiring visual correction utilizing contact lenses	53%	42%	NA
Ratio breakdown of soft lens wearers to the total of all rigid and soft lens wearers			
100–76% soft	32	21	11
75–51% soft	6	2	3
50–26% soft	1	0	1
25–0% soft	0	0	0
Athletes' most frequent problems with contact lenses	Irritation and loss	Irritation and loss	Irritation and loss
Teams keeping extra contact lenses available in case of loss or damage	60% (28/47)	43% (9/21)	36% (8/22)
Teams with someone available to remove a contact lens from an injured athlete	90% (43/48)	76% (16/21)	86%
Athletic teams utilizing visual training	23% (11/49)	24% (5/21)	Approx. 5%
Vision training techniques utilized	6 not specified		
Vision enhancement	2/5 (40%)	3/5 (60%)	NA
Remedial training	1/5 (20%)	0/5 (0%)	
Combination of both techniques	2/5 (40%)	2/5 (40%)	
Team and/or player improvements associated with vision training	70% (7/10)	80% (4/5)	NA

[a] May not equal 100% due to shared use of optometrists and ophthalmologists by some teams.
NA: Denotes information was not available for study subset.
Source: Courtesy of American Optometric Association

Table 11.4   Professional sports vision longitudinal data

Professional athletic programmes surveyed	1987–8	1983	1980
Response rate	56% (53/94)	32% (35/108)	38% (27/72)
Vision care specialists affiliated with professional athletic programmes	93% (49/53)	40% (14/35)	33% (9/27)
Vision consultants paid vs volunteering their services	95% paid (38/40)	86% paid (12/14)	78% paid (7/9)
Degree of vision consultant (optometrist, ophthalmologist, or both)[a]	38% OD 81% MD (9/48, OD) (30/48, MD) (9/48, both)	50% OD (7/14, OD) (7/14, MD)	33% OD (3/9, OD) (6/9, MD)
Teams using a vision screening programme	68% (34/50)	70% (19/27)	NA
Mean of athletes failing vision screenings	6% failure	3% failure	1–4% failure
Range of responses for failing screenings	(0–30%)	(0–20%)	
Recommendation of contact lenses over spectacles for athletes	96% (44/46)	62% (18/29)	Approx. 75%
Percentage of players requiring visual correction utilizing contact lenses	72%	62%	75%
Ratio breakdown of soft lens wearers to the total of all rigid and soft lens wearers			
100–76% soft	38	11	12
75–51% soft	6	9	4
50–26% soft	0	2	0
25–0% soft	0	3	5
Athletes most frequent problems with contact lenses	Irritation and loss	Irritation and loss	Irritation and loss
Teams keeping extra contact lenses available in case of loss or damage	96% (50/52)	80% (28/35)	75%
Teams with someone available to remove a contact lens from an injured athlete	98% (51/52)	91% (32/35)	100%
Athletic teams utilizing visual training	35% (17/49)	29% (10/35)	Football–25% Baseball–65%
Vision training techniques utilized	3 not specified	4 not specified	
Vision enhancement	7/14 (50%)	2/6 (33%)	NA
Remedial training	7/14 (50%)	2/6 (33%)	
Combination of both techniques	6/14 (43%)	2/6 (33%)	
Team and/or player improvements associated with vision training	73% (8/11)	40% (4/10)	NA

[a] May not equal 100% due to shared use of optometrists and ophthalmologists by some teams.
NA: Denotes information was not available for study subset.
Source: Courtesy of American Optometric Association

norms, which quite often cannot be replicated. There is even a lack of consistent agreement and implementation among the most active providers with regards to such basic concerns as the minimum level of refractive error requiring lens correction, or even which sports indicate the need for proper eye protection.

The development of the Pacific Sports Visual Performance Profile (PSVPP), in response to the request of the United States Olympic Committee and the Sport Vision Section of the American Optometric Association, was a major step towards standardization (Coffey and Reichow, 1990). The PSVPP has been evolutionary in nature, due in part to feedback from practitioners. Based on practitioner education and utilization of the profiling system, a strong database has been created and serves to validate much of the work.

Standardization does not end with testing; a certain level is also desirable for diagnosis, remediation and enhancement. Future growth in sports vision must certainly address these needs. Meanwhile, in order for this discipline to evolve more efficiently, certification of practitioner skill and knowledge would seem in order. Currently, certification does not exist within North America. The Optometric Extension Program, an international organization, has recognized the need for standardization and certification, and is developing a new specialty track curriculum, one which will include a course sequence on sports vision.

Research

An adequate discussion of North American research related to vision and athletic performance is certainly beyond the scope of this chapter. As a perspective though, both the quality and quantity of research addressing this field has steadily risen. This is quite apparent in the scientific literature as well as in the proceedings of scientific meetings (Sherman, 1980; Stine *et al.*, 1982; Hitzeman and Beckerman, 1993).

In 1988, the Sports Vision Section of the American Optometric Association formed a research committee with the mission to promote research efforts. Similarly, the International Academy of Sports Vision began to publish quarterly issues of the *International Journal of Sports Vision*, a refereed journal devoted to the dissemination of research. These efforts are necessary for the proper and timely expansion of the discipline.

In review of the literature, it becomes apparent that the majority have addressed visual performance differences between athletes and non-athletes, with some emphasis on sport-to-sport comparisons. Future work must expand to assess performance characteristics, validity, reliability and transference issues relating to such factors as athletic eye wear, instrumentation, corrective lens intervention, remedial therapy and enhancement vision training.

Technological advances

The market creates the demand for services and materials. Despite the apparent growth in the demand for sports vision services, noteworthy improvements in instrumentation have been relatively limited. With technological advances such as video games and, more recently, virtual reality, the future is promising for significant improvement in commercially available diagnostic, remedial and enhancement equipment.

Conclusion

This section has presented a view of the future of sports vision in North America from the basis of a review of the past and present involvement of the sports, academic, corporate and eye care communities. It is the author's hope that this will stimulate careful thought, concern and creativity in providing comprehensive performance-oriented vision care services to the athletic community.

2. THE NON-AMERICAN PERSPECTIVE

The specific optimizing of safe and efficient vision in sports – or sports vision – has only recently been accepted outside North America as a specialty in its own right (Brown, 1993; *Sports Vision Association*, 1993). If the development of international sports vision follows the North American model it seems likely that a significant minority of eye care practitioners will become increasingly involved in the screening and training of athletes' vision. The concept of both individual athletes and teams appointing their own sports vision consultants in a similar manner to trainers, coaches, psychologists and physicians should follow. Furthermore, the involvement of eye care professionals in concert with sports authorities could constitute an accepted multi-disciplinary approach to sports vision. To facilitate sports vision development, a number of organizations have now been established outside North America in Australia, Belgium, Canada, Holland, Italy and the UK (see Appendix 1). It is anticipated that all these sports vision associations, together with teaching and research institutes, the professional bodies and associations, will all play a significant role in the future development of sports vision. As depicted in Figure 11.1, the future of sports vision will lie in three interconnected directions.

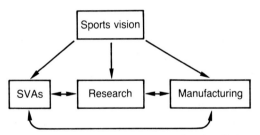

Figure 11.1 The three interconnected directions for sports vision

Sports vision associations

It is anticipated that sports vision associations (SVAs) will play a key role in the development of sports vision, since, among other concerns, will be their involvement with research and development. Their stated aims are 'to maximize visual ability, promote eye protection and to investigate the use of sports vision for the enhancement of visual performance in the sport concerned' (Sports Vision Association, 1993); in short, to optimize visual ability with,

if necessary, the best optical correction and protection. The sports vision practitioner will function as a specially qualified expert to the sporting fraternity and will be in a unique position to give advice, especially if the practitioner is a sports participant.

At the time of writing, sportspeople including cricketers, tennis players and cyclists are increasingly wearing sports spectacles such as eye protectors, tinted and reflective lenses or yellow filters. Rather than the media providing an explanation as to why such a course of action had been taken, these sports people were derided on TV and in the newspapers. The press officers of the SVAs will be in a position to enlighten them, by giving the media a reasoned explanation of such action. Figure 11.2 illustrates the way the development of sports vision will progress.

Increasing public awareness through schools, colleges and the sporting community is seen as an important function of SVAs in addition to educating sports vision practitioners through symposia, lectures, articles, demonstrations and research projects. If a practitioner feels unable to fulfil the vision needs of the sportsperson, that practitioner will be able to refer to the sportsperson to a sports vision specialist. A directory of practitioners will be produced, listing the specialty of each eye care practitioner and will be distributed to sports organizations and to fellow eye care practitioners in order to help the sportsman and woman in their quest for

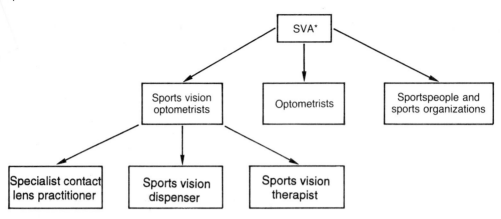

Figure 11.2 The way in which sports vision may develop

improved sporting performance. Advice could be given in the following areas: determining the visual problems affecting sports performance; correcting abnormalities with optical aids or vision enhancement training or, in extreme cases, surgery, and protecting sportspeople from ocular hazards. These areas could lie within the province of a single sports vision specialist who could, after offering suitable advice, refer the sportsperson to a number of other sports vision specialists, including the following.

Sports contact lens practitioner

Contact lenses may be needed for optical correction and/or protection. Although there are very many contact lens practitioners, only a few have the specialist knowledge in fitting lenses to those involved in the more arcane sports, for example scuba diving, sand-surfing or fell-running. Such specialists would be aware of the problems associated with the visible ocular hazards of water, sand and dirt respectively (see Figure 11.3).

Sports vision dispenser

Such a person would dispense specialist sports spectacles or visual aids, for example snooker spectacles, monocular aids for ballistic sport or golf bifocals. They would also

supply eye protectors (with or without a prescription), to protect the eyes from trauma or from environmental hazards such as ultraviolet light ('blue light').

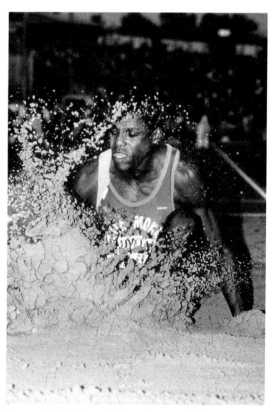

Figure 11.3 The obvious hazard of sand when long jumping into the wind with corneal contact lenses. (After Mark Brennan, with permission.)

Sports vision therapist (SVT)

A sports vision therapist works with equipment designed continually to evaluate and train the sportsperson when wearing the most suitable refractive correction. The sports vision therapist identifies defects and works on them through exercises tailored to each individual. The requisite exercises are instituted after a sports vision questionnaire, which is designed to highlight the sportsperson's weaknesses, and after a full ophthalmic examination (see Table 9.1).

Every sport has its own vision profile; from sprinting, with its relatively low visual input, to motor-racing, with its enormously high visual input. The public acknowledges the racing driver's visual skills which need little clarification, but think of sprinting as simply running 'hell for leather' from gun to tape. However, athletes are, almost by definition, very competitive and are always seeking some advantage over rivals. By following a sports vision training programme they may well obtain that vital edge over opponents. The sprinter with a sports vision therapist could need to work on the following sports vision programmes.

Auditory reaction time – in order to react as quickly as possible to the starter's gun.

Visual reaction time – in order to react positively and very quickly to any sudden acceleration by an opponent (this so-called reflex action is, in fact, an anticipation facet).

Central–peripheral awareness – which encourages the sprinter to keep the head continually facing forward to the finishing line and not to look askance to see his position in the race. Turning the head he would actually slow progress, and although this may only be a matter of hundredths of a second, it could make the difference between a gold and a silver medal (Figure 11.4).

Spatial location – to locate the finishing tape precisely, since diving for it too soon or too late could, once again, make the difference between winning and losing.

In team sports the profile may vary slightly or greatly according to the position of the player

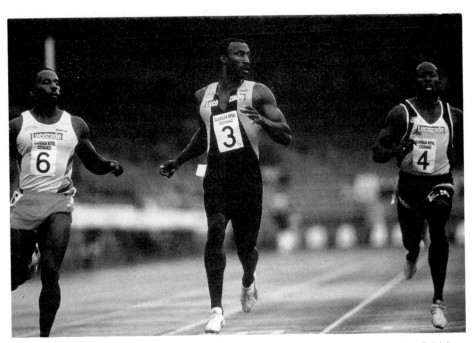

Figure 11.4 Sprinter looking askance at one of his rivals when close to the finishing line and subsequently losing the race. (After Mark Brennan, with permission.)

on the team. For example, in cricket or baseball, a close fielder will need different visual abilities from an outfielder. The former will need a high level of dynamic visual acuity, a fast reaction time, good eye–hand–foot coordination and good saccadic movements, whereas the outfielder's principal needs are good spatial location and pursuit movements. All these visual abilities can be worked on by a sports vision trainer.

Once sportspeople and their coaches accept the concept of visual evaluation, proper optical correction and sports vision training within their regular training programme, then sports vision will grow. If they claim that their sporting improvements are due, at least in part, to seeking sports vision advice, so much the better.

Taking sports vision equipment out of the consulting-room and on to the playing area of the sport is essential, to bring in all the likely variables of wind, light, heat etc., which are normally encountered. Assessing the athlete on sports vision training equipment when the athlete is stressed, tired, overheated etc. is ideal, perhaps during some respite from play (Wood, 1981).

It is anticipated that in the near future the SVAs will accumulate large databases storing information regarding the elite and the recreational sportsperson to which researchers, sports vision practitioners and manufacturers may refer.

Research

It is generally accepted that the functional properties of the neurones in the visual pathway and cortex are fixed by adulthood and that no amount of visual training will change them (ten Napel 1993). However, the concept of learning to use the existing pathways more effectively lies at the heart of sports vision enhancement, i.e. training the visual system. At present the literature contains mostly anecdotal evidence as to the efficacy of sports vision training. Sceptics argue that there is no scientific proof of its value and that it merely acts as a placebo or a confidence boosting exercise (Cockerill, 1981; ten Napel, 1993).

The future, therefore, could see numerous research projects being undertaken. There are many variables (diet, peaking, visualizing, conditioning etc.) that make it difficult to prove beyond doubt either that improved results on sports vision equipment in the laboratory or consulting room are transferable to the sporting arena or that improvements in sporting performance are due, even in part, to sports vision training. However, research will tell us how some visual skills are affected when the body is tired and/or stressed and that different lighting conditions affect different aspects of vision. It may be the selection of the appropriate tint, not just for protection but for comfort as well, which will give the sportsperson a better visual performance. Sports vision is in an early stage of development and needs to be supplemented by scientific research. The following list suggests some possible research projects:

1. Determining if filters actually improve vision performance, including contrast sensitivity. If a significant improvement can be demonstrated further research could be directed to determine the most suitable filter for specific sports and ambient conditions.
2. Assessing the effect, if any, of contact lenses on contrast sensitivity.
3. Evaluating how best to overcome the problem of a sporting emmetropic presbyope who cannot see the 'split-times' on his watch when training or racing.
4. Measuring the characteristics such as transmission and impact resistance of commercially available, and often expensive, sports spectacles.
5. Determining the most suitable colour for the ball, shuttlecock etc. in the prevailing light, and the most suitable colour clothing for the players in order to obtain the best colour contrast.
6. Assessing the effect of sports spectacles on vision and sports performance.
7. Determining whether peripheral awareness can really be improved with appropriate training techniques.

8. Improving indoor and outdoor lighting for optimal and comfortable sports performance.
9. Probably most important is the establishing of scientifically controlled and designed experiments to validate or otherwise the efficacy of sports visual enhancement training.
10. Establishing international standards for sports eye protectors.
11. Ascertaining the effects of fatigue on vision, colour discrimination and sports performance.
12. Establishing whether visual concentration can be sustained through longer periods of sports vision training.
13. Determining methods to reduce or eliminate the problem of disability glare encountered under varying circumstances in different sports, e.g. the tennis lob or pole-vault bar in direct line of the sun.
14. Reducing ocular trauma in sport by evaluating the preventable causes of eye injuries and the role of protection.
15. Assessing binocular status with an aim to improve function with an orthoptic prescription/utilization of monocular cues.

The answers to these and many other problems encountered in sport will hopefully be found, but undoubtedly new problems will emerge with the introduction of new rules, different colours of playing surface and the increasing speed of most games.

Manufacturing

The future may see increased cooperation between manufacturer, sports vision associations, research and sportspersons. Looking into a crystal ball through rose-tinted polycarbonate lenses, manufacturers of protective frames or goggle eye wear will need to improve their products for the requirements of sportspeople. The new generation aids will have to have non-misting, non-scratchable, impact-resistant, hydrophobic, dirt-repellent lenses which are fitted into unbreakable, well-ventilated, hydrophilic, lightweight and comfortable frames (American Society for Testing and Materials, 1988; Canadian Standards Association, 1982; Prestage, 1990). Photo-electric lenses, with their ability to react instantly

to changing light conditions, will improve and may well supersede photochromic lenses, not only in spectacles but also in contact lenses. New sports vision equipment will almost certainly be developed which will simulate sporting situations with much more verisimilitude, possibly in a similar form to video games on television supplemented by intense, video orientated home exercises. Tests of dynamic stereo vision will probably be devised using the concept of virtual reality. The quality of such appliances should ideally be controlled by approved standards organizations.

Conclusion

At present, sports vision is one of the less developed areas of optometry and sports medicine outside of North America. Once ophthalmology, optometry, orthoptics, visual physiology, sports science, standards organizations, vision sciences, coaching and manufacturing pool their combined knowledge in the development of this specialty, it will become a fast developing part of vision care practice. The eye care practitioner should find it a viable, worthy, interesting and satisfying part of his work. The day will then soon dawn when people will no longer have to ask, 'What exactly *is* sports vision?'

References

American Society for Testing and Materials (1988) F 803–88 *Standard Specification for Eye Protectors for use by Players of Racquet Sports*, ASTM, Philadelphia.

Barton, D., Cahill, K. and Link, L. (1981) Knowledge, present utilization and potential for expansion of the optometric role in sports vision. Unpublished doctoral thesis project, Pacific University College of Optometry, Forest Grove, Oregon

Brown, M. (1993) Chasing sport's top prizes, *The Times*, 9 June, p. 32

Canadian Standards Association (1982) CSA 400-M1 *Racquet Sports Eye Protectors*, Canadian Standards Association, Ontario

Clark, M. and Lord, M. (1976) And now, tennis eye. *Newsweek*, July, p. 73

Cockerill, I. (1981) Peripheral vision and hockey. In *Vision and Sport* (eds I. Cockerill and W. McGillivary), Stanley Thornes, Cheltenham, p. 54

Coffey, B. and Reichow, A.W. (1987) Guidelines for screening and testing the athlete's visual system, part III. Optometric Extension Program Foundation. *Curriculum II*, **59**(7), 355–68

Coffey, B. and Reichow, A.W. (1990) Optometric evaluation of the elite athlete: the Pacific Sports Visual Performance Profile. *Problems in Optometry*, **1**(2), 32–58

Goss, D.A., Cary, W. and Holyk, D.M. (1974) Contact lenses for the athlete. *Optometric Weekly*, **67**, 1071–3

Helmick, K. (1983) Optometric trends in sports vision; knowledge, utilization, and practitioner role expansion potential. Unpublished doctoral thesis project, Pacific University College of Optometry, Forest Grove, Oregon

Hitzeman, S.A. and Beckerman, S.A. (1993) What the literature says about sports vision. In *Optometry Clinics*, 3(1) (ed. J.G. Classé), Appleton and Lange, Norwalk, Conn., pp. 145–69

Pashby, T.J. (1979) Eye injuries in Canadian hockey: phase III. Older players now at risk. *Canadian Medical Association Journal*, **121**, 663

Prestage, M. (1990) Eye protection in racquet sports, the need for a European Standard. In Eye *Protection in Racquet Sports*, Joint Symposium organized by the Royal National Institute for the Blind and The City University, London

Reichow, A. (1993) An overview of sports vision. In *Transactions of the First Symposium of the Sports Vision Association*, The City University, London

Reichow, A.W. and Stern, N.S. (1986a) Athlete and optometrist: performance-oriented. Optometric Extension Program Foundation. *Curriculum II*, **59**(1), 35–42

Reichow, A.W. and Stern, N.S. (1986b) Optometric trends in sports vision. Optometric Extension Program Foundation. *Curriculum II*, **59**(7), 355–68

Reichow, A.W., Berman, P.E., Bleything, W.B. *et al.* (1994) A descriptive study of the Special Olympic Athletes' vision care needs. *Journal of the American Optometric Association*, submitted for publication

Sherman, A. (1980) Overview of research information regarding vision and sports. *Journal of the American Optometric Association*, **7**, 661

Sports Vision '93 (1993) *Conference and Exhibition Journal*, International Academy of Sports Vision, Harrisburg, PA

Sports Vision Association (1993). Constitution.

Stephens, G.L. (1994) Sports eyewear takes off. *Optometric Economics*, March, pp. 10–14

Stern, N.S. and Reichow, A.W. (1986) Special Olympics vision care program. Paper presented to the Annual Meeting of the American Public Health Association, Las Vegas, Nevada

Stine, C.D., Arterburn, M.R. and Stern, N.S. (1982) Vision and sports: a review of the literature. *Journal of the American Optometric Association*, **53**(8), 627–33

ten Napel, J. (1993) Can visual training improve athletic performance? In *Transactions of the First Symposium of the Sports Vision Association*, The City University, London

Vinger, P.F. (1981) Sports eye injuries; a preventable disease. *Ophthalmology*, February, pp. 108–13

Vinger, P.F. (1994) The eye and sports medicine. In *Clinical Ophthalmology* (ed. W. Tasman and E.A. Jaeger), J.B. Lippincott, Philadelphia, **5**(45), 1–103

Wood. G. (1981) Effects of exercise – small induced fatigue on visual reaction times. In *Vision and Sport* (eds I. Cockerill and W. McGillivary) Stanley Thornes, Cheltenham, p. 81

Zieman, B.G., Reichow, A.W. and Coffey B. (1993) Optometric trends in sports vision: knowledge, utilization, and practitioner role expansion potential. *Journal of the American Optometric Association*, **64**(7), 490–501

Appendix 1
Sports vision organizations

American Optometric Association,
Sports Vision Section,
243 North Lindbergh Boulevard,
St Louis, MO 63141
314 991–4100

Australian Optometric Association,
Sports Vision Section,
Dublin Terrace,
204 Drummond Street,
Carlton,
Victoria, 3053
03 663 6833

British Blind Sport,
Heygates Lodge,
Elkington,
Yelvertoft,
Northants, NN6 7NH
01858 575584

Canadian Optometric Association,
Sports Vision Section,
1785 Alta Vista Drive,
Suite 301,
Ottowa,
Ontario, K1G 3Y6
613 738 4412

College of Optometrists in Vision
Development,
PO Box 285,
Chula Vista, CA 92012
619 425 9191

The Dutch/Belgian Council on Sports Vision,
Postbus 129,
2100 AC Heemstede,
Nederlands
23 339179

The European Academy of Sports Vision,
48015 via Parini 9,
Cervia,
Italy
546 972301

International Academy of Sports Vision,
200 South Progress Avenue,
Harrisburg, PA 17109
717 652 8080

International Blind Sports Association,
Secretariat,
42 rue Louis Lumière,
7502 Paris,
France
403 14500

Optometric Extension Program Foundation,
2912 S. Daimler Street,
Santa Ana, CA 92705
714 250 8070

Prevent Blindness America,
500 East Remington Road,
Schalmburg, IL 60173
708 843 2020

The Sports Vision Association,
Bridge House,
233–234 Blackfriars Road,
London, SE1 8NW
0171 261 9661

Appendix 2
Manufacturers of sports vision equipment

AcuVision Systems Inc.,
4425 Bayard Street,
Suite 230,
San Diego, CA 92109
800 944 2141

Bernell Corporation,
750 Lincolnway East,
PO Box 4637
South Bend, IN 46601
46634 4637

Bright Eye-Deas Inc.,
PO Box AE – Route 134,
South Dennis, MA 02660
508 760 3937

J.W. Engineering,
8 Dike Drive,
Wesley Hill, NY 10952
914 354 8025

BiofeedTrac Inc.,
26 Schermerhorn Street,
Brooklyn, NY 11201
800 852 2SEE

Humphrey Instruments Inc.,
2992 Alvarado Boulevard,
San Leandro,
CA 94577
800 227 1508
Fax 510 351 0792

Layfayette Instrumentation Co.,
PO Box 5729,
Sagamore Parkway,
Layfayette, IN 47903
800 428 7545

Liberty Sport,
380 Verona Avenue,
Newark, NJ 07104
800 444 5010

North American Coating Laboratories,
Division of Wilson Optical Laboratories,
190 Alpha Park,
Cleveland, OH 44143
800 326 NACL

Polycarbonate Lens Council,
22330 Hawthorne Boulevard, Suite 201,
Torrance, CA 90505–2536
800 477 5652
Fax 310 378 3165

Mentor O and O Inc.,
3000 Longwater Drive,
Norwell, MA 02061
800 992 7557

Stereo Optical,
3539 North Kenton Avenue,
Chicago, IL 60641
800 344 9500

Wayne Engineering,
1825 Willow Rd,
Northfield, IL 60093
708 441 6940

WR Medical Electronics Company,
123 North Second Street,
Stillwater, MN 55082
612 430 1200

Appendix 3
Olympic Vision Centre, Lillehammer, 1994:
findings of the Bausch & Lomb survey*

During the 1994 Olympic Games in Lilleham-mer, Norway, Bausch & Lomb tested the visual skills of 342 athletes (92 females and 250 males) representing 46 countries and 12 sports groups. Athletes tested ranged in age from 16 to 41 (average age 25). The following provides data collected from visual perform-ance history questionnaires and specific tests, as reported by Vittorio Roncagli, PhD, FAAO, co-founder of the European Academy of Sports Vision and chief consultant to the Olympic Vision Centre (OVC).

Previous eye examination

- More than 50% of the athletes have never received a complete visual examination. This finding is consistent with OVC data collected during the 1992 Olympic Games.
- None of the athletes tested in Lillehammer from Bulgaria, Greece, Hungary and Romania had previously ever received a complete vision examination.
- 58.3% of those who rated the importance of vision a '3' (with '5' being the most important) had never had a complete visual examination.

* After Bausch & Lomb (1994) with permission.

Injuries

- 18.42% of athletes examined said they had had an eye or head injury or trauma, or infection or surgery.
- The highest percentage of self-determined trau-mas was recorded for athletes of:
  Freestyle (30% of athletes examined for this sport).
  Ice-hockey (28% of athletes examined for this sport).

Contact lenses

- 15.5% said they wear contact lenses.
- 90.5% of lens wearers are using soft lenses.
- 94.3% of contact lens wearers use them for sports.
- 69.8% of lens wearers use them every day.

Glasses

- 19.59% said they wear spectacles.
- Only 3.2% said they use glasses for sports.

Vision training

- Only 4.6% said they followed a vision training programme.

Vision difficulties

- 18.1% of the athletes examined said they were currently experiencing visual difficulties.
- The highest percentage of visual difficulties were recorded for athletes of:
  Nordic Combined (44% of athletes examined for this sport).
  Alpine Ski (35% of athletes examined for this sport).

Static visual acuity

- 4.6% of athletes had binocular visual acuity below 20/20.
- 12.5% had visual acuity below 20/20 in one eye.

Visualization

- 36.8% of athletes examined said they use visualization/imagery techniques.
- The highest percentage of athletes using visualization were recorded for athletes of:
  Short Track (67% of athletes examined for this sport).
  Freestyle (63% of athletes examined for this sport).

Importance of vision during sports

- On a scale from 1 to 5 (with 5 being extremely important), 62.5% responded with '5'.
- The average rating for this question was 4.39.

- The highest rate was recorded for athletes of:
  Ice-hockey (4.73)
  Alpine Ski (4.71)
  Biathlon (4.69).
- 90.5% of those using contact lenses rated the importance of vision with '4' or more.

Near stereopsis (18')

- Only 44.4% of athletes were able to discriminate all the stereoscopic targets at near.

Distance stereopsis

- 5.2% of athletes had no measurable stereopsis at 6 m.
- Only 36.8% of athletes were able to discriminate all the stereoscopic targets at 6 m.

Fixation disparity

- 2.9% of athletes had suppression of one eye during fixation disparity and stereopsis tests.
- 19.2% of athletes showed unstable fixation disparity.

Note: Since this behavior affects stereopsis, we may speculate that these athletes need specific vision care (either adjusted vision correction and/or vision training).

Accommodation/vergence flexibility

- 2 athletes (0.5%) were able to reach the amazing performance of 30 cycles in 30 seconds on the 20/80 target test. This test measures how quickly one can shift focus from near to far and back again.
- 4 athletes (1.1%) were not able to reach at least 10 cycles in 30 seconds.

Contrast sensitivity

- Only 4 athletes (1.1%) could discriminate all 8 targets (100% of targets).
- 5.8% of athletes significantly failed the test, not being able to discriminate an average of at least 4 targets (50% of targets).

Peripheral awareness time

- 24.8% of athletes tested had a significantly low average peripheral awareness time (time slower than 0.40 seconds), as compared to other elite athlete scores.
- 20.4% of athletes tested had a time better than 0.30 seconds.
- 4 athletes showed excellent performance (time better than 0.25 seconds).

Eye-hand reaction/response speed

- 15.4% of athletes tested performed very well (time below 0.20 s).
- On average, better performances were recorded for athletes in Ski Jump and Short Track.

Eye-foot reaction/response speed

- 6.7% of athletes tested performed very well (time below 0.21 s).
- Better performances were recorded for athletes in Alpine Ski and Ski Jump.

Glossary*

Abrasion (corneal)
Removal of an area of the epithelial surface of the cornea.

Aspherical or non-spherical design (D.F.C. Loran)
A surface designed without transitions which continuously alters its radius of curvature.

Accommodation (C.J. MacEwen)
Adjustment of the dioptric power of the eye in order to clearly see objects in the distance and those close to the eye.

Alphabetical syndrome or A&V patterns (C.J. MacEwen)
Horizontal squint in which the deviation increases or decreases in upgaze or downgaze, e.g. a convergent squint with a V pattern increases in downgaze and decreases in upgaze.

Amblyopia (after Millodot)
A condition characterized by a reduction in corrected vision without any apparent organic lesion of the eye or visual pathways.

Anaglyphs
Sterograms consisting of two superimposed laterally displaced drawings or photographs of the same scenes but taken from two directions and in complementary colours (usually red and green).

Analgesics (C.J. MacEwen)
Pain killers.

Aniseikonia (after Millodot)
A difference in the size or shape of the ocular images as perceived by each eye.

Anisometropia
Condition in which the refractive state of a pair of eyes differs and therefore one eye requires a different lens correction from the other.

Astigmatic keratomy (D.F.C. Loran)
Corneal surgery to eliminate or reduce corneal astigmatism.

Astigmatism
A condition of refraction in which the image of a point object is not a single point.

---

* Unless specified to the contrary, the definitions quoted are reproduced with permission from Millodot (1993). Other definitions are by contributors to this book, or have been compiled from reference works cited in the Bibliography.

Avulsion (Lid) (C.J. MacEwen)
Tearing of the lid away from its insertion.

Binocular
Pertaining to both eyes.

Biofeedback (after B. Coffey and
A. Reichow)
The self regulation of physiological processes
due to positive or negative feedback process.

Carcinoma (C.J. MacEwen)
Malignant growth of epithelial cells.

Cataract (C.J. MacEwen)
Opacity of the lens of the eye.

Chiastopic fusion (Cline *et al.*, 1992)
Fusion obtained by converging voluntarily in
order to fixate directly two fusable targets,
laterally separated in space such that the right
eye fixates the left target and the left eye the
right target (syn. crossed disparity).

Chromophores (C.J. MacEwen)
Chemicals or structures within cells that are
coloured (and therefore may absorb and
reflect different wavelengths of light).

Concomitant squint (C.J. MacEwen)
A squint in which the deviation does not vary
with direction of gaze or fixing eye.

Conjunctiva
A thin, transparent mucous membrane lining
the posterior surface of the eyelids and the
anterior eyeball where it merges with the
cornea at the limbus.

Contrast
Subjective assessment of the difference in
appearance of two parts of a field of view seen
simultaneously or successively.

Contrast sensitivity
The ability to detect luminance contrast; in
psychological terms, the reciprocal of the
minimum perceptible contrast.

Contusion (C.J. MacEwen)
A bruise.

Convergence
Movement of the eyes turning inwards or
toward each other.

Cornea
The transparent anterior portion of the fibrous
coat of the globe of the eye. The cornea is the
first and most important refracting surface of
the eye.

Cycloplegic
Paralysis of the ciliary muscle resulting in less
accommodation.

Depth perception (J.J. Gardner, and
A. Sherman)
The perception of relative or absolute differ-
ence in distances of objects from the observer.
(See Stereoscopic acuity)

Diabetic retinopathy (C.J. MacEwen)
Condition of the retina due to underlying
diabetes.

Dialysis iris (D.F.C. Loran)
Separation of the iris from the ciliary body.

Dialysis retina (D.F.C. Loran)
Separation of the retina from the retinal
pigment epithelium at the ora serrata, due to
vitreo-retinal traction.

Diplopia
A condition in which a single object is seen as
two rather than as one.

Divergence
Movement of the eyes turning away from
each other.

Divergence excess
A large exophoria or tropia at distance associated with a much smaller exophoria or
tropia at near.

Dynamic visual acuity (Geer and Robertson, 1993)
A measure of sensitivity to visual detail when there is relative movement between the target and the observer.

Emmetropia
The refractive state of the eye in which, with the accommodation relaxed, the conjugate focus of the retina is at infinity. In this condition, vision is normally clear without spectacles.

Emmetropization
A process that is presumed to operate to produce a greater frequency of emmetropic eyes than would otherwise occur on the basis of chance.

Erythrocytes (C.J. MacEwen)
Red blood cells.

Esophoria
A latent squint in which the eye turns inwards.

Esotropia
A manifest squint in which the eye turns inwards.

Exophoria
A latent squint in which the eye turns outwards.

Exotropia
A manifest squint in which the eye turns outwards (see Strabismus).

Eye movements (Leigh and Zee, 1991)
Nystagmus (quick phases) To direct the fovea towards the oncoming visual scene during self rotation.
Optokinetic To hold images of the seen world steadily on the retina during sustained head rotation.
Saccades To bring the object of interest onto the fovea.
Smooth pursuit To hold the image of a moving target on the fovea.

Vestibular To hold the image of the seen world steady on the retina during brief head rotation.
Vergence (version) To move the eyes in opposite directions so that the image of a single object is placed on both foveae.

Facility of accommodation and vergence (B. Coffey and A. Reichow)
The speed and ease with which accommodation and vergence can be adjusted rapidly to provide clear, single, binocular vision.

Fixation disparity (after Millodot)
Binocular vision in which the two retinal images do not fall on corresponding points at the fixation point. This may cause under- or over-convergence of the eyes.

Glare
A visual condition in which the observer either feels discomfort and/or exhibits a lower performance in visual tasks and is produced by a relatively bright source of light within the visual field.

Glare (direct)
The glare produced by a source of light situated at or near the object of fixation.

Grating
A series of black and white bars orientated vertically or horizontally.

Hypermetropia
Refractive condition of the eye in which distant objects are focused behind the retina when accommodation is relaxed. (Syn. far sight, long sight, hyperopia.)

Hyphaema
Haemorrhage or bleeding into the anterior chamber of the eye.

Illuminance/Illumination
The quotient of the luminous flux incident on an element of a surface divided by the area of that element of surface.

Incomitance

Condition in which a manifest or latent squint differs according to which eye is fixating or in which direction the eyes are looking.

Infrared (IR)

Radiant energy of wavelengths between the extreme red wavelength of the visible spectrum and a wavelength of a few millimeters (abbreviated IR)

IR–A

The wave bands comprising radiation between 760 and 1400 nm.

IR–B

The wave bands comprising radiation between 1400 and 3000 nm.

IR–C

The wave bands comprising radiation between 3000 and 10 000 nm.

Intensity, luminous

The quotient of the luminous flux leaving the source, propagated in an element of solid angle containing the given direction, diverted by the element of solid angle.

Iseikonic lens

A lens designed to correct aniseikonia.

Kerataconus

A developmental anomaly in which the centre of the cornea becomes thinner and bulges forward in a cone-shaped fashion.

Keratopathy (C.J. MacEwen)

Non-inflammatory disease of the cornea.

Keratitis (C.J. MacEwen)

Inflammation of the cornea.

Laceration (C.J. MacEwen)

A wound caused by cutting or tearing.

Light, visible

Electromagnetic vibration capable of stimulating the receptors of the retina and producing a visual sensation which is comprised within the wavelength 400–760 nm.

Lumen

The flux emitted within a unit solid angle of one steradian by a point source with a luminous intensity of 1 candela.

Luminous efficacy

The conversion of electrical energy into light energy, expressed as lumens per watt.

Luminous flux

Flow of light which produces a visual sensation, measured in lumens.

Metabolism (C.J. MacEwen)

Transfer of energy in a living organism.

Miosis (C.J. MacEwen)

Constriction of the pupil.

Motor fusion

One of the components of vergence in which the eyes move until the object of regard falls on corresponding retinal areas.

Myopia

Refractive condition of the eye in which images of distant objects are focused in front of the retina when the accommodation is relaxed. (Syn. short sight, near sight.)

Non-ionizing radiation (W.N. Charman)

Electromagnetic radiation of wavelengths between 100 nm and 1 mm which is incapable of ionizing the surrounding media.

Oedema (C.J. MacEwen)

Excessive fluid within the intercellular spaces.

Orthopic fusion (Cline et al., 1992)

Fusion obtained by voluntarily converging to fixate directly two fusible targets laterally separated in space, such that the right eye directly fixates the right target and the left eye the left target.

Parallel processing (D.F.C. Loran)
A mechanism in which data is simultaneously transmitted through more than one pathway.

Perception
The mental process of recognizing an object through one or more of the senses.

Peripheral awareness (D.F.C. Loran)
The ability to maintain awareness of objects in the periphery while maintaining central fixation.

Photorefractive keratectomy (PRK)/Laser refractive keratoplasty (Loran, D.F.C.)
A surgical procedure which aims to reduce or eliminate refractive errors by using the excimer laser to alter the shape and power of the cornea.

Photochromic lens (D.F.C. Loran)
One which alters in colour as a result of changes in incident heat or light intensity.

Photopic (vision)
Vision at high levels of luminance (above 10 cal/m^2) and resulting from the functioning of the cornea.

Pinguecula
Proliferation of conjunctiva on the nasal side of the cornea.

Polarized light
Light which is composed of transverse wave motion in only one direction is said to be polarized and may be obtained by passing light through a polarizer (e.g. Tourmaline crystals or a polarizing material such as polaroid).

Polarizer
An optical element such as Tourmaline crystals which polarizes light.

Presbyopia
A refractive condition which is a normal ageing process in which the accommodative ability of the eye becomes insufficient for satisfactory near vision without the use of corrective convex or plus lenses.

Proptosis (exophthalmos)
Abnormal protrusion of the eyeball from the orbit.

Pterygium (C.J. MacEwen)
Wing-shaped membrane extending from the conjunctiva to the cornea in the interpalpebral fissure.

Pulfrich phenomenon
If an object swings in the frontal plane and an observer places in front of one eye a light-absorbing filter (any value between 5% and 40%) that object will appear to move along an ellipse (syn. Pulfrich effect; Pulfrich stereophenomenon)

Purkinje shift
Reduction in the luminosity of a red light relative to a blue light when the luminances are reduced in the same proportion without changing the respective spectral distribution.

Radial keratomy (RK)
A surgical procedure on the cornea aimed at curing or reducing myopia by making radial incisions in the peripheral cornea to flatten it centrally and thereby reduce its power.

Radiation
Emission or transfer of energy in the form of electromagnetic waves or particles.

Reaction (AcuVision, 1992)
Response to an action.

Refraction
The process of measuring the refractive error of the eyes.

Relative amplitude of accommodation
The total amount of accommodation which the eye can exert while the convergence of the eyes is fixed. It can be either positive using

concave lenses until the image blurs or negative using convex lenses until the image blurs.

Response speed (B. Coffey and A. Reichow)
The elapsed time between the onset of a visual stimulus and the completion of a motor response to that stimulus.

Retina
The light-receptive innermost nervous layer of the eye.

Retinal disparity (C.J. MacEwen)
If images from a single object do not fall on to corresponding retinal points, retinal disparity is present. This may result in either diplopia, or the perception of a single image which has depth, depending on the distance between the disparate points.

Sclera
The tough, white, opaque, fibrous, outer layer of the eyeball which is continuous with the cornea.

Scotoma (C.J. MacEwen)
An area of reduced vision or blindness surrounded by an area of normal vision.

Scotopic vision
Vision at low levels of luminance which results from the stimulation of rods.

Sensory fusion
A neural process by which the images on each retina are integrated into a single percept.

Sight
The special sense by which the colour, form, position, shape etc. of objects is perceived when light from these objects impinges upon the retina. (See *vision*.)

Spatial frequency (J.R. Cronly-Dillon, personal communication)
The number of cycles per degree of the visual angle of a grating.

Spectrum
Spatial display of a complex radiation produced by separation of its monochromatic (single colour) components.

Sports visual task analysis (after B. Coffey and A. Reichow)
The examination of a sport to determine which visual skills and environmental factors are most critical to meet the visual demands of that sport.

Stereopsis
Direct awareness of depth due to retinal disparity.

Stereoscopic acuity
The ability to detect the smallest difference in depth between two objects expressed as the angle of steropsis in seconds of arc.

Strabismus
The condition in which the lines of sight of the two eyes are not directed towards the same fixation point when the subject is actively fixating an object. (Syn. heterotropia, squint, tropia).

Strabismus, convergent
Strabismus in which the deviating eye turns inwards. (Syn. esotropia.)

Strabismus, divergent
Strabismus in which the deviating eye turns outwards. (Syn. exotropia.)

Suppression
The process by which the brain inhibits the retinal image (or part of) of one eye, when both eyes are simultaneously stimulated.

Static visual acuity (Riggs, 1961)
The ability to resolve details of a stationary object in the field of view.

Syneresis (D.F.C. Loran)
Liquefaction of the vitreous body.

Tachistoscope
An instrument which presents visual stimuli for a brief and variable portion of time (usually less than 0.10 seconds).

Ultraviolet (UV)
Radiant energy of wavelengths smaller or shorter than those at the visible end of the spectrum and longer than 1 nm.

UV–A
The wave band comprising radiation between 320 and 400 nm.

UV–B
The wave band comprising radiation between 280 and 320 nm.

UV–C
The wave band comprising radiation between 100 and 280 nm.

Vectogram
A polarized stereogram consisting of two polarized images at right-angles to each other. When viewed through polarized filters, it presents one image to one eye and one to the other.

Vergence posture (after B. Coffey)
The alignment tendency of the vergence system when viewing a target at a given distance. It is usually indexed by measuring the heterophoria in prism dioptres.

Vision
The appreciation of difference in the external world such as form, colour, position, resulting from the stimulation of the retina by light.

Vision (J.J. Gardner and A. Sherman)
The interpretation of that which is seen, the ability to gain meaning from what the eyes see.

Vision, binocular
Condition in which both eyes contribute towards producing a percept which may or may not be fused into a single image.

Vision, intermediate
Vision of objects situated beyond 40 cm from the eye but closer than say 1.5 m.

Vision, near
Vision of objects situated 25–50 cm either from the eye or, more commonly, the spectacle plane.

Vision, distance
Vision of objects situated at infinity or, more usually, 5 or 6 m.

Visual acuity
See *Dynamic visual acuity; Static visual acuity.*

Visual reaction time (or speed) (B. Coffey, and A. Reichow)
The elapsed time between the onset of a visual stimulus and the initiation of a motor response to that stimulus.

Visual sensitivity (B. Coffey, and A. Reichow)
An individual's ability to resolve detail or contrast of the retinal image.

Visual task analysis (after B. Coffey and A. Reichow)
The examination of a task to determine which visual skills and environmental variables are most critical to meet the skills of that task.

Visualization
The ability to form a mental visual image of an object not present to the eyes.

Bibliography

AcuVision (1992) *CAS/AcuVision Training Manual*, International AcuVision Systems Inc., San Diego

Cline, D., Hoffsetter, H.W. and Griffiths, J.R. (1992) *Dictionary of Visual Science*, 5th edn, Chiltern Book Co., Radnor

Geer, I. and Robertson, K.M. (1993) Measurement of central and peripheral dynamic acuity thresholds during ocular pursuits of a moving target. *Optometry and Vision Science*, **70**, 552–60

Leigh, R.J. and Zee, D.S. (1991) *The Neurology of Eye Movements*, F.A. Davis & Co., Philadelphia

Ludvigh, E. and Miller, J.M. (1958) Study of dynamic acuity during ocular pursuits of moving test objects. I. Introduction. *Journal of the Optical Society of America*, **48**, 799–802

Millodot, M. (1993) *Dictionary of Optometry*, 3rd edn, Butterworth Heineman, Oxford

Riggs, L.A. (1961) Visual acuity. In *Vision of Visual Perception* (ed. C.G. Graham), Wiley, New York

Index